Push your Career Publish your Thesis

Science should be accessible to everybody. Share the knowledge, the ideas, and the passion about your research. Give your part of the infinite amount of scientific research possibilities a finite frame.

Publish your examination paper, diploma thesis, bachelor thesis, master thesis, dissertation, or habilitation treatises in form of a book.

A finite frame by infinite science.

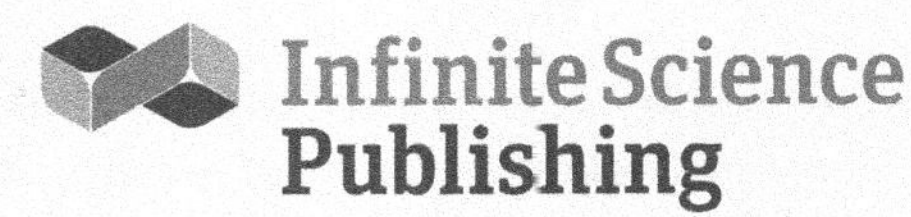

An Imprint of
Infinite Science GmbH
MFC 1 | Technikzentrum Lübeck
BioMedTec Wissenschaftscampus
Maria-Goeppert-Straße 1
23562 Lübeck
book@infinite-science.de
www.infinite-science.de

Ein Imprint der Infinite Science GmbH,
MFC 1 | BioMedTec Wissenschaftscampus
Maria-Goeppert-Straße 1
23562 Lübeck

Umschlaggestaltung, Illustration: Uli Schmidts, metonym
Lektorat: Universität zu Lübeck

Verlag: Infinite Science GmbH, Lübeck, www.infinite-science.de
Druck: Books on Demand GmbH, Norderstedt

ISBN Paperback: 978-3-945954-00-3

Bibliografische Information der Deutschen Nationalbibliothek:
Die Deutsche Nationalbibliothek verzeichnet diese Publikation in der Deutschen Nationalbibliografie; detaillierte bibliografische Daten sind im Internet über http://dnb.d-nb.de abrufbar.

Student Conference Medical Engineering Science

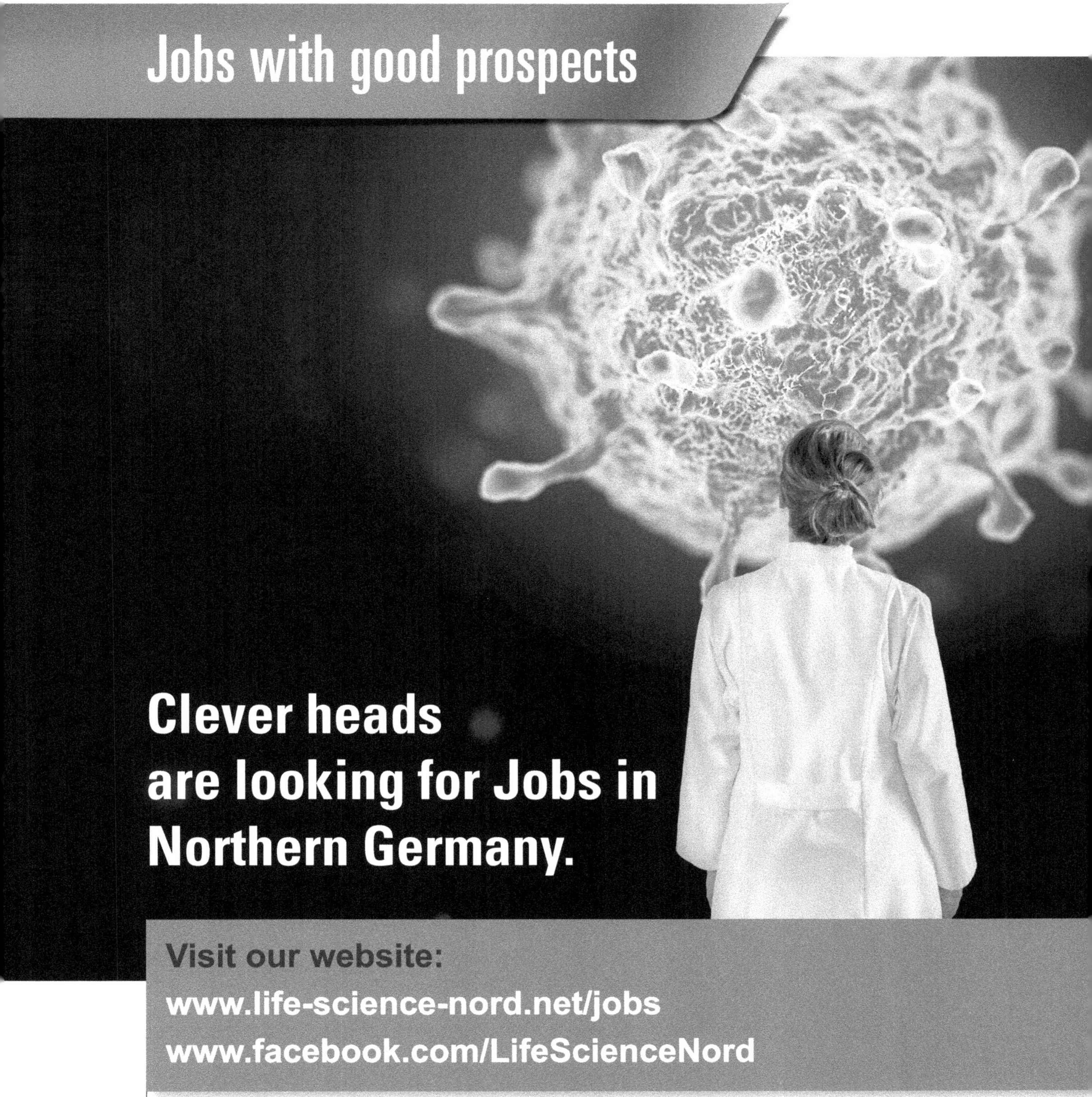

Student Conference
Medical Engineering Science

Proceedings 2015

Conference Chair

Thorsten M. Buzug (Chair), Institute of Medical Engineering, Universität zu Lübeck
Hartmut Gehring (Co-Chair), Department of Anesthesiology, UKSH
Stephan Klein (Co-Chair), Center for Biomedical Technology, Lübeck University of Applied Sciences

Local Coordination

Kanina Botterweck, Medisert, BioMedTec Science Campus
Martina Galler, Medisert, BioMedTec Science Campus
Christian Kaethner, Institute of Medical Engineering, Universität zu Lübeck
Christina Debbeler, Institute of Medical Engineering, Universität zu Lübeck
Gisela Thaler, Institute of Medical Engineering, Universität zu Lübeck

Scientific Program Committee

Reginald Birngruber, Institute of Biomedical Optics, Universität zu Lübeck
Ralf Brinkmann, Institute of Biomedical Optics, Universität zu Lübeck
Thorsten M. Buzug, Institute of Medical Engineering, Universität zu Lübeck
Thomas Gutsmann, Biophysics Group, Research Center Borstel
Heinz Handels, Institute of Medical Informatics, Universität zu Lübeck
Mattias Heinrich, Institute of Medical Informatics, Universität zu Lübeck
Horst Hellbrück, Center for Electrical Engineering and Computer Science, Lübeck University of Applied Sciences
Christian Hübner, Institute of Physics, Universität zu Lübeck
Gereon Hüttmann, Institute of Biomedical Optics, Universität zu Lübeck
Martin Koch, Institute of Medical Engineering, Universität zu Lübeck
Martin Leucker, Institute for Software Engineering and Programming Languages, Universität zu Lübeck
Kerstin Lüdtke-Buzug, Institute of Medical Engineering, Universität zu Lübeck
Erik Maehle, Institute of Computer Engineering, Universität zu Lübeck
Thomas Martinetz, Institute for Neuro- and Bioinformatics, Universität zu Lübeck
Alfred Mertins, Institute for Signal Processing, Universität zu Lübeck
Jan Modersitzki, Institute of Mathematics and Image Computing, Universität zu Lübeck
Hauke Paulsen, Institute of Physics, Universität zu Lübeck
Ramtin Rahmzadeh, Institute of Biomedical Optics, Universität zu Lübeck
Fred Reinholz, Institute of Biomedical Optics, Universität zu Lübeck
Philipp Rostalski, Institute of Medical Electronics, Universität zu Lübeck
Michael Scharfschwerdt, Department of Cardiac and Thoracic Vascular Surgery, UKSH
Christian Schmidt, Isotope laboratory of the Natural Sciences Section, Universität zu Lübeck
Achim Schweikard, Institute for Robotics and Cognitive Systems, Universität zu Lübeck
Alfred Vogel, Institute of Biomedical Optics, Universität zu Lübeck
Stephan Wehrig, Faculty of Building Trade and Construction, Lübeck University of Applied Sciences

Preface and Acknowledgements

After the great success of the three previous meetings from 2012 to 2014, the 4th Student Conference on Medical Engineering Science 2015 shows continuing growth both in quality and quantity of scientific contributions. The experienced organization team of the BioMedTec Science Campus Lübeck in cooperation with Life Science North Management GmbH, the North German Life Science Cluster Agency, has spared no effort to provide an excellent conference, where master and diploma students of the campus present their recent research results to a broad public of academics and industry. The contributions show how physics, engineering and computer sciences can advance medicine, health and health care. Moreover, this conference offers a good opportunity for both students and companies to get in touch at the industrial exhibition and to get to know each other from a different point of view.

Students from the Life Sciences programs at the BioMedTec Science Campus present their results from projects carried out at the laboratories and institutes of Lübeck's Universities, in international research facilities or research-oriented industrial companies. The conference focus has been placed on topics from medical engineering. This interdisciplinary field has been established at the Lübeck University of Applied Sciences for decades and Medical Engineering Science (Medizinische Ingenieurwissenschaft – MIW) is an important bachelor and master program at the Universität zu Lübeck as well. Both universities jointly offer the international master degree course Biomedical Engineering (BME). This is complemented with further life science oriented programs of the University (Computer Sciences, Medical Computer Sciences, Mathematics in Medicine and Life Sciences, Molecular Life Science, Medicine) which contribute to the success of the Medical Engineering Science and Biomedical Engineering programs.

The 4th Student Conference on Medical Engineering Science 2015 has been complemented by concepts and designs of students of architecture of Lübeck University of Applied Sciences, which perfectly illustrates the dynamic development of the BioMedTec Science Campus – towards a broader variety of topics and an increasing identification with the campus itself.

I want to thank all the people who worked with enthusiasm and dedication to make the conference a successful event. I have to thank the companies who support the meeting. Moreover, my thanks go to the technology transfer platform Medisert of the BioMedTec Science Campus. The professional management of Kanina Botterweck and her Medisert team has contributed substantially to the success of this conference. Personally and on behalf of all colleagues of the BioMedTec Science Campus,

I especially want to thank Christian Kaethner and Christina Debbeler from the Institute of Medical Engineering. They have been the first contact point for all questions of students and the program committee members. Their in-depth overview of all details of this event is the key to the success of the 4th Student Conference at the BioMedTec Science Campus.

Lübeck, March 11–13, 2015

Prof. Dr. Thorsten M. Buzug
Vice President of the Universität zu Lübeck
Chair of the 4rd Student Conference
on Medical Engineering Science 2015

Contents

Biomedical Engineering

Safety and Quality I

Safety and Quality II

Medical Imaging

Signal Processing I

Signal Processing II

Image Processing I

Image Processing II

1
Biomedical Optics I

Flow velocity measurements using Doppler optical coherence tomography

I. Ellerkamp [1], D. Choi[2], G. Hüttmann[3] and A.K. Ellerbee[4]

[1] Medizinische Ingenieurwissenschaft, Universität zu Lübeck, ellerkam@miw.uni-luebeck.de
[2] Stanford Hospital and Clinics, choid@stanford.edu
[3] Institute of Biomedical Optics, Universität zu Lübeck, huettmann@bmo.uni-luebeck.de
[4] E.L. Ginzton Laboratory, Stanford University, audrey@ee.stanford.edu

Abstract

Doppler optical coherence tomography (DOCT) was used to estimate the flow velocity in a phantom and in human anterior segment in-vivo. The flow was measured qualitatively using phase difference, power of the phase difference and speckle variance. For quantitative velocity measurements the angle between measuring beam and velocity vector was calculated. Flow velocities from 0 to -42.3 mm/s were measured in the phantom with a standard deviation from 0.1 mm/s to 2.4 mm/s. In human corneo-scleral limbus the DOCT system was capable to visualize different biological structures. It was possible to measure blood flow in episcleral vessels. The velocities in two vessels were evaluated to be 20.9 mm/s and 37.7 mm/s. However the DOCT system's solution is not sufficient to resolve conjunctival vessels.

1 Introduction

After cataract, glaucoma is the second leading cause of visual disability globally [1]. It describes a variety of ocular eye disorders, all resulting in optic nerve damage that leads to loss to the field of vision. In extreme cases this may result in total loss of vision [2]. Development of glaucoma is encouraged by an increased intraocular pressure (IOP) which is determined by production of liquid aqueous humour in the ciliary processes of the eye, and its drainage through the trabecular meshwork.
Treatment of Glaucoma aims to reduce the IOP. This is typically accomplished by lowering the production of aqueous or increasing the drainage of aqueous e.g. by use of medication, usually eye drops, or by surgery. The most common conventional surgery performed for glaucoma is the trabeculectomy, where an iatrogenic fistula is created between the trabecular meshwork and the conjunctiva of the anterior chamber in order to drainage aqueous humor. More recently the minimally invasive glaucoma surgery (MIGS) has come up as a new method. It aims to use the eye's normal distribution system and enhancing it. Small implants are placed so the aqeous in the anterior chamber will have direct access to the Schlemm's canal bypassing the trabecular meshwork [4]. However the MIGS surgery have not been efficacious on all patients. One hypothesis is that there is some compromise to flow distal to the trabecular meshwork that affects the effectiveness of the implant. Therefore it is important to visualize the structure of the aqueous outflow pathways and to quantify the flow in the conjunctiva vessels in order to find better locations for placing the stent. Currently there are several methods that can image the anterior segment of the eye, such as gonioskopy, ultrasound biomicroscopy and confocal microscopy. These techniques require contact with the eye and carry the risk of contact abrasions and infections. Therefore, there is the need of a method capable of non-invasively image the anterior segment that is able to quantify flow velocities and image the microstructure and microvasculature in the anterior segment.
Optical coherence tomography (OCT) is a non-invasive image modality based on white light interferometry [5]. Standard OCT imaging uses backscattered intensity as contrast mechanism for displaying the structure of the sample. However the intensity contrast has some limits regarding displaying tissue physiology. Recently functional extensions of OCT such as polarization sensitive OCT and Doppler OCT came into the focus of research. Doppler OCT aims to visualize and quantify flow velocities. Nowadays phase-sensitive detection techniques are most widely used to extract flow from tissue and determine its velocity. In Doppler OCT depth resolved phase differences between adjacent A-lines at all lateral positions are measured. Measurement of the phase difference between two adjacent A-Scans yields a quantitive value for the velociy [6]:

$$v(z) = \frac{\lambda \Delta\phi}{4n\pi T \cos\alpha}, \qquad (1)$$

where λ describes the central wavelenght of the light source, $\Delta\phi$ the phase difference between adjacent A-scans, n the refraction index, T the time between adjacent A-lines and α the angle between measuring beam and velocity vector (fig. 1(a)).
In this paper we present quantitative and qualitative Doppler OCT measurements by use of a commercial OCT-system.

We use a flowphantom to show the feasibility of estimating flow velocities for anterior segment imaging. Furthermore we test the capability of that system to be appropriate for anterior segment imaging.

2 Material and Methods

All measurements were performed with a commercial OCT system (Telesto, Thorlabs). The Telesto system is working at a central wavelength of 1325 nm with an axial scan frequency of 5.5, 28 and 91 kHZ. For calculating flow velocities in a flow phantom, a glass tube (inner diameter: 500 µm) embedded in a PDMS (Polydimethylsiloxane) phantom was filled with Intralipid 20%. A syringe pump generated various flow velocity from 0 to 42.3 mm/s to verify the potential velocity caluculations. Measurements were performed at 28 kHz.

In order to image human eyes *in-vivo*, the Telesto probe was mounted to a head- and chinrest. Power output was measured at 1.3 mW which is well below the ANSI-level for extended beam exposure [7]. To correct motion artifacts a histogram based method for removing bulk motion and an edge based motion correction technique was implemented.

2.1 Quantitative methods

For unambiguous velocity determination the phase difference $\Delta\phi$ needs to be confined to $[-\pi\ \pi]$. If the phase difference exceeds this interval the velocity componente cannot be extracted unambigously anymore. Therefore maximal measurable speed is

$$v_{max}(z) = \frac{\lambda}{4nT\cos(\alpha)} \tag{2}$$

For phantom measurements, performed at 28 kHz, this leads to a maximal detectable velocity of 74.7 mm/s at an angle of 84.7° and a refraction index of 1.35. The minimal detectable velocity is limited by the phase noise of the system. To determine this we used a mirror as a sample and calculated a histogram showing the phase differences of adjacent A-Scans. Fitting a gauss curve to this histogram yields a FWHM of 0.06 rad resulting in a minimal velocity of 7.4 mm/s according to equation (1).

For image processing the received spectral interferogram $I(k)$ was transformed from k-space in spatial domain by a fast Fouriertransform (FFT). For obtaining the intensity information the absolute value was obtained and scaled logarithmically. The phase $\phi(z)$ does not convey any morphologic information by itself. However the phase difference $\Delta\phi(z)$ between adjacent A-lines contains very exact information about morphological changes or flowage in nanometer range.

For angle determination a modified form of the dual plane scanning method was used [6]. Out of the measured volume data two B-scans S_1 and S_2 were extracted to have a small displacement Δy between those scans. If the OCT plane is defined as the x- and z-plane, the y-axis is the direction of

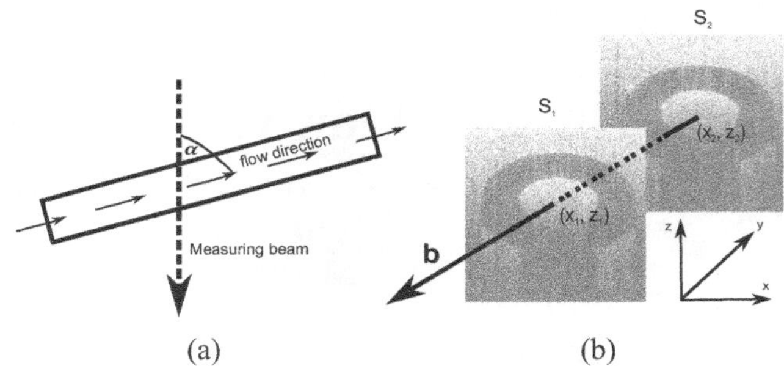

Figure 1: (a) Measuring beam scanning across a vessel - α is the angle between measuring beam and flow velocity vector. (b) Three dimensional diagram of the scanning pattern

the displacement. Fig. 1 (b) illustrates this scanning pattern. With this displacement the center of the blood vessel in those two extracted planes can be described as (x_1, z_1) for B-scan S_1 and (x_2, z_2) for B-scan S_2. Therefore the vector of the blood vessel can be computed by:

$$\vec{b} = [x_2 - x_1, y_2 - y_1, z_2 - z_1] = [\Delta x, \Delta y, \Delta z] \tag{3}$$

Calculating the norm out of the blood vessel vector $\vec{b}$, that indicates the lenght of this vector, allows us to determine the angle α:

$$\cos\alpha = \frac{\Delta z}{\sqrt{\Delta x^2 + \Delta y^2 + \Delta z^2}} \tag{4}$$

To obtain an averaged velocity value for each measurement the peak velocity was extracted from the Doppler image and averaged within a 10 x 10 pixel area.

2.2 Qualitative methods

To qualitatively visualize flow in tissue phase and intensity based methods were used. Speckle fluctuation in the intensity image was calculated from the interframe variance from the structural OCT-signal:

$$SV(j,k) = \frac{1}{N}\sum_{i=1}^{N}\left(I_i(j,k) - \frac{1}{N}\sum_{i=1}^{N} I_i(j,k)\right)^2 \tag{5}$$

where N is the number of B-Scans set in the calculation, and i, j, k are indices for the frame, transverse and axial pixels respectively. Also the phase difference between adjacent A-Scans

$$\Delta\phi(z) = \phi(z)_{k+1} - \phi(z)_k \tag{6}$$

can show flow. The respective A-Scans is referred by index k. To improve the contrast between high phase differences and small phase differences the power of the phase difference can be calculated:

$$PD = |\Delta\phi(z)|^2 \tag{7}$$

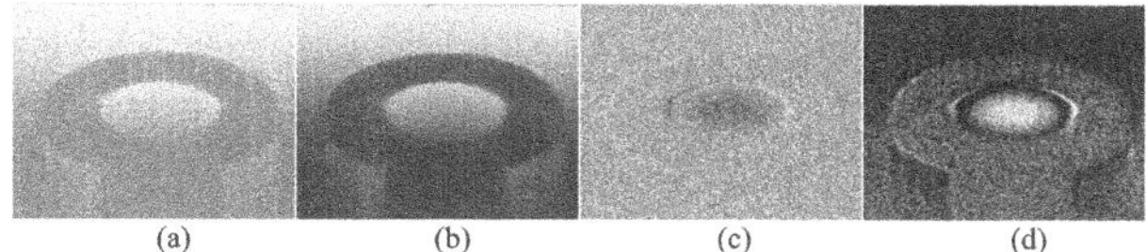

Figure 2: Flow phantom (a) Intensity image (b) Speckle variance (c) Phase difference (d) Power of phase difference

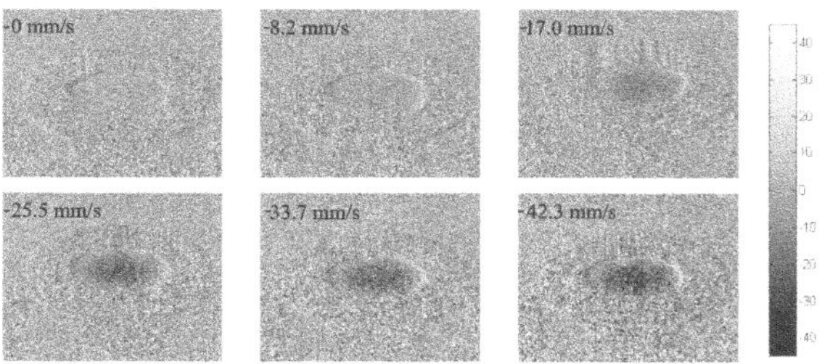

Figure 3: Doppler velocity images of flowing Intralipid in a glass capillary tube at an angle of approx. 84.7 degree. The average flow velocities are 0, -8.2, -17, -25.5, -33.7 and -42.3 mm/s. Doppler images are scaled in mm/s.

3 Results and Discussion

3.1 Flow phantom

Evaluation of qualitative flow measurements

Fig. 2 (a) shows a typical cross sectional scan of the flow phantom in the XZ-plane. Here the Intralipid solution flows at 20.4 mm/s. Fig. 2 (b) shows the logarithmized speckle variance image. The contrast between glass tube and the sourrounding phantom is higher than in the intensitiy image in (a). This can help to create higher contrasts *in-vivo* between blood vessels and circumjacent tissue. Fig. 2 (c) presents a phase difference image. Inside the tube a parabolic flow profile is visible compared to a static phase around the glass tube. A higher contrast between the moving fluid and the static phantom can be received by taking the power of the phase difference (fig. 2 (d)).

Evaluation of quantitative flow measurements

Fig. 3 shows the Doppler velocity images from 0 mm/s to -42.3 mm/s. In the Doppler velocity image the stationary Intralipid does not show any significant Doppler shift. Increasing the flow velocity of Intralipid solution leads to a larger Doppler shift inside the glass tube forming a parabolic flow profile. The tube has a random phase profile while the PDMS phantom does not show significant phase change. Since Intralipid was flowing from right to left, a negative frequency shift occurs and leads to negative flow velocities. That means that Doppler OCT is also useful for determining flow directions. Fig. 4 shows the relation between the averaged velocity measured by DOCT system and the flow velocity set by the syringe pump. Measurements were performed 15 times at each set flow velocity.

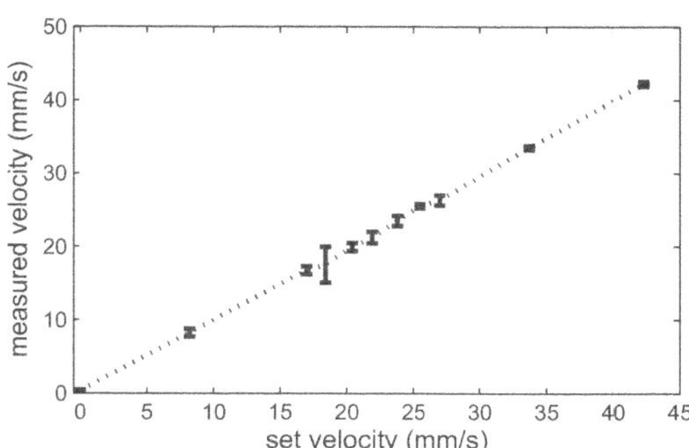

Figure 4: Plots between the absolute averaged velocity measured by DOCT and the set flow velocity. 15 measurements were performed at each set flow velocity. Each data point corresponds to a mean value, and the size of the error bar at each measurement point represents the standard deviation.

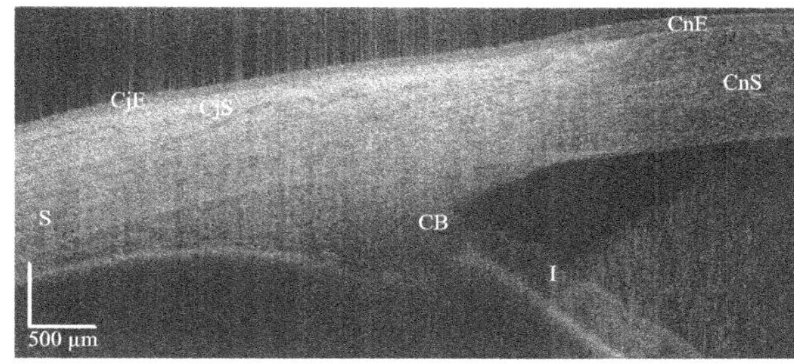

Figure 5: *In vivo* image of the human corneo-scleral limbus. CnE: corneal epithelium; CnS: corneal stroma; CjS: conjunctival stroma; CjE: conjunctival epithelium; S: sclera; CB: ciliary body; I: Iris

Each data point correspondends to a mean value and the error bar represents the standard deviation of the absolue measured velocity. Variation of the average measured velocity lie within the same range other groups have calculated.

3.2 In vivo anterior segment imaging

In vivo OCT intensity image obtained with healthy subjects allowed to identify several biological components in the limbal area. Fig. 5 shows an OCT cross sectional image of the corneo-scleral limbus aquired from a temporal location. In the corneal region, the corneal epithelium (CnE) and the corneal stroma (CnS) can be seen. In the limbal area, that is between the cornea, conjunctiva and sclera, the CnE changes to the more optically opaque conjunctival epithelium (CjE). Beneath the CjE the conjunctival stroma (CjS) can be identified. That is the fist layer of vasculature. The Iris (I) and the ciliary body (CB) appear darker. The structure across the CB is known as the sclera (S). The conjunctival vessels, the trabecular meshwork and Schlemm's canal cannot be discerned in this structural image which makes it difficult to establish this system in the described minimal invasive glaucoma surgeries.

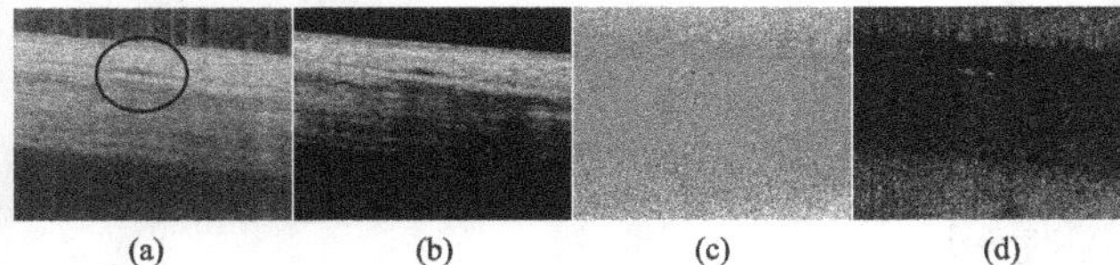

Figure 6: Episcleral vessel in different representation (a) intensity image (b) speckle variance (d) phase difference (e) power of phase difference

Qualitative flow measurements

Fig. 6 shows an episcleral vessel in different representations. Fig. 6 (a) shows a cross-sectional intensity image. The vessel appears darker as the circumjacent tissue but the contrast between them is not very high. The speckle variance image show higher contrast between the vessel and the surrounding tissue that allows easier identification of vessels. However a shadow from the blood vessel can be recognized. Fig. 6 (c) and (d) use phase information. In (c) the phase difference between adjacent A-Scans is shown. The gray colour stands for a phase shift of zero. Brighter gray values mean a positive phase shift. The vessel in this phase difference image can be identified as bright dot surrounded by tissue that does not show phase changes. To improve the contrast of the phase difference images, the power of the phase difference is used (fig. 6 (d). The blood flow in the vessel appears bright while the tissue does not show any movement. Again the image quality suffers from shadows from the blood vessel. These phase based methods can easily be used to show flow over a broad range of flow rates without knowledge of the angle between measuring beam and velocity vector.

Quantitave flow measurements

The flow velocity in episcleral vessels was calculated in two measurements. Flow velocities could be determined between 20.9 mm/s and 37.2 mm/s. This matches the results of a video angiography method conducted by [8]. The flow for episcleral vessels in that study was calculated between 1.6 mm/s and 100 mm/s.

4 Conclusion

We showed qualitative and quantitative flow measurements in a flow phantom and in human anterior segment. Qualitative flow methods conducted by phase difference, the power of the phase difference or speckle variance allowed an angle-independent visualization of flow in tissue. Quantitative Doppler methods allowed to determine the flow velocity in a flow phantom and also in human episcleral vessels without exogenous contrast agents. However shadows from blood vessels influence the image quality especially from blood flow at increasing depth. This situation can be improved by increasing the axial resolution. Since the current system is not able to resolve the conjunctiva vessels as shown in fig. 5 it is not suitable for establishing it in searching locations for MIGS-surgeries. Also an increase of resolution can help to image these smaller vessels. The vessels in the episclera are significantly larger so they can be resolved with the system discussed and flow calculations can be executed as shown. Since glaucoma is often recognized when the disease has progressed e.g. by loss of field of vision an early diagnosis is important. Therefore imaging the episcleral vessels might be useful, because an indication for glaucoma can be associated with idiopathic dilated episcleral vessels as discussed in [9]. Further examination of this feature might lead to support early diagnosis. However for imaging the conjunctiva vessels a different system with higher resolution is needed.

Acknowledgement

The work has been carried out at Stanford University. We would like to thank Jennifer T. Smith and Michael Leung for their assistance.

5 References

[1] S. Resnikoff et al., *Global Data on visual impairment in the year 2002,* Bulletin of the World Health Organization 82: 844–51, 2004

[2] R. Lim and I. Goldberg, *Glaucoma in the Twenty-First Century* The Glaucoma Book pp. 3-21, edited by P. Schacknow and J. Samples, Springer 2010

[3] M. Johnston, A. Jamil, E. Martin, *Aqueous veins and open angle Glaucoma* The Glaucoma Book pp. 65-78, edited by Schacknow P. and Samples, J., Springer 2010

[4] T. W. Samuelson, *Microinvasive glaucoma surgery - Coming of age* Journal of Cataract and Refractive Surgery, August 2014; 1253-1254

[5] D. Huang et al. *Optical Coherence Tomography* Science. 1991;254:1178–1181.

[6] S.Yazdanfar, A. M. Rollins, and J. A. Izatt, *In vivo imaging of human retinal flow dynamics by color Doppler optical coherence tomography* Arch. Ophthalmol. 121(2), 235–239 (2003).

[7] A.N.S.I. *American National Standard for Safe Use of Lasers: ANSI Z136.1–2007* Laser Institute of America, 2007.

[8] P. Meyer, *Patterns of Blood Flow in Episcleral Vessels Studied by Low-Dose Fluorescein Videoangiography.* Eye (1988(2), 533-546.

[9] R. A. Stock et al., *Idiopathic dilated episcleral vessels (Radius-Maumenee syndrome): case report* Arq. Bras. Oftalmol. vol.76 no.1 São Paulo Jan./Feb. 2013

Characterization of a micro machined deformable membrane mirror using optical coherence tomography

C. Pfäffle[1], H. Sudkamp[2], and G. Hüttmann[3]

[1] Medizinische Ingenieurwissenschaft, Universität zu Lübeck, clara.pfaeffle@miw.uni-luebeck.de
[2] Institute of Biomedical Optics, Universität zu Lübeck, sudkamp@bmo.uni-luebeck.de
[3] Institute of Biomedical Optics, Universität zu Lübeck and Medical Laser Center Lübeck GmbH, Lübeck, Germany, huettmann@bmo.uni-luebeck.de

Abstract

The performance of a micro machined deformable mirror (MMDM) system with 37 actuators (OKO Technologies) is studied in order to characterize its utility as an adaptive optic element. The deformation of the mirror surface was measured by optical coherence tomography (OCT) and compared to results taken with a Shack-Hartmann wavefront sensor (SHS). Therefore, the first 20 Zernike polynomials were applied to the surface of the deformable mirror. The acquired images were decomposed into Zernike coefficients and compared with simulations. The OCT system thereby enabled a direct measurement of the surface displacement and was therefore insensitive to aberrations of the setup. This results in a precise measurement of the mirror performance with a maximum error of $\pm$ 30 nm, which was way below the error of the SHS.

1 Introduction

The performance of microscopes and other optical systems is often compromised by aberrations, which lead to a reduction of image- and signal quality. Therefore the effects of aberrations in many different optical systems like confocal microscopy, two-photon microscopy and many other systems were investigated in the past [1]-[4]. Aberrations are deviations of the original flat wavefront and are a result of differences in the optical path lengths of the beam. These differences are caused by reflections on uneven surfaces or by propagation through non-uniform mediums. The aim of adaptive optics is to compensate these aberrations by using modifiable optical elements. Its principle can be divided into two distinct steps. First, the aberration of the wavefront caused by the optical system is measured. An adaptive element such as a deformable mirror is then used to introduce the inverse of the measured aberration into the system, in order to compensate the original with the artificial aberration [1]. For good results it is important to characterize the performance of the adaptive elements. In this paper optical coherence tomography (OCT) is used to characterize the performance of a deformable mirror and to investigate the quality of a Shack-Hartmann wavefront sensor (SHS), which is a common device for the characterization of such adaptive elements. A SHS measures the wavefront aberration caused by the mirror while OCT measures the deformation of the mirror surface and therefore avoids errors caused by the optical system. Besides OCT has higher spatial resolution and therefore should provide more reliable results. Since the OCT device used needs around 3 minutes to measure one configuration of the mirror it provides no real-time measurements like the SHS does and is therefore only suited for the characterization. Optical aberrations are commonly described mathematically using a set of basis functions

$$\phi(r,\theta) = \sum_m \sum_n a_n^m \psi_n^m(r,\theta) \qquad \forall n,m \in \mathbb{N} \vee n \leq m \tag{1}$$

where a_n^m is the modal coefficient, r is the normalized radial distance and $\psi_n^m(r,\theta)$ is an appropriate set of basis modes [1]. A widely used set of such basis functions are the Zernike polynomials [5]. They are a sequence of orthogonal polynomials, which are defined on the unit disk. These functions can be divided into even

$$\psi_n^m(r,\theta) = R_n^m(r)cos(m\theta), \tag{2}$$

and uneven

$$\psi_n^{-m}(r,\theta) = R_n^m(r)sin(m\theta) \tag{3}$$

$$R_m^n = \sum_{k=0}^{(n-m/2)} \frac{(-1)^k(n-k)!}{k!((n+m)/2-k)!((n-m)/2-k)!} r^{n-2k} \tag{4}$$

polynomials, where n and m are the frequency and the order of the Zernike polynomial and R_n^m are radial polynomials. For the normalized Zernike polynomials the modal coefficients are equal to the maximum value of each polynomial.

2 Material and Methods

The 37-channel micromachined deformable membrane mirror (MMDM) system (OKO Technologies) used consists of an gold-coated silicon nitride membrane. 37 electrostatic electrodes underneath the membrane pull down the surface and thereby modulate the shape of the mirror surface [8]. The center of the surface can be deformed as much as 7 µm [6],[7]. The mirror has a circular aperture of 15 mm in diameter. However, since the edge of the membrane is fixed on the casing, only a central part is fully deformable. For our investigations we determined a central diameter of 10.05 mm as the active aperture where the applied deformation appropriately describes the desired Zernike polynomials. This is similar to earlier assumption of the active aperture of these device [6]-[9]. For investigating the Zernike polynomials the MiZer-software was used to apply Zernike polynomials on the mirror surface. For the wavefront measurement a Shack-Hartmann sensor (Thorlabs, WSF300-14AR) and for the OCT measurement a spectral-domain OCT system (Thorlabs, Telesto) with a field of view of $15\,\text{mm} \times 15\,\text{mm}$ were used.

2.1 OCT-measurement

OCT is an interferometric technique, which uses the spectral information of broad bandwidth radiation to achieve a micrometer depth resolution of scattering tissue. The depth resolved intensity profile of one lateral point is called A-scan while a two-dimensional image of the sample consisting of many A-scans is called a B-scan. The surface of the mirror, which can be seen as the same as the aberrations the mirror imposes on the wavefront, was measured using B-scans of different lateral positions. The measured spectral interference patterns of each lateral point were zero-padded in frequency domain so that its inverse Fourier transform yields an interpolated depth-resolved scattering intensity profile. For surface-detection, a square function was fitted to this profile for each A-scan. The maximum of each function was determined and taken as an axial coordinate for the mirror surface. For each deflection applied to the mirror, a reference image was taken of its relaxed state. The surface profile detected in the reference measurement was subtracted from the profile measured during a deflection of the surface to obtain the depth-information of the deformation. This way, the aberrations caused by the system, such as field of curvature, did not influence the measured profiles. With this method a axial resolution of several nanometers could be achieved, which is an increase of two magnitudes compared with common devices like SHS.

To minimize the error caused by the OCT scanner, several scanning modes were tested by taking 180 B-scans at the same place and calculating the variance. The best trade-off between image quality and imaging time were achieved using a A-scan rate of 5.5 kHz at 2048 A-scans per B-scan. This yields a maximum error of $\pm$ 30 nm. For higher scanning speeds the error increases up to $\pm$ 300 nm.

2.2 Zernike-decomposition

To investigate the maximum deflection the highest voltage allowed for the deformation of the mirror for each Zernike polynomial is applied in positive and negative direction. For each image the mirror surface was decomposed into the 20 first Zernike polynomials with their corresponding coefficients. To evaluate the precision of this decomposition, the calculated coefficients were used to create a reconstruction of the mirror surface. The root-mean-square error of the difference of this reconstructed image and the measured mirror surface were calculated as a scale of precision.

3 Results and Discussion

Fig. 1 shows astigmatism, coma and the ψ_3^5-polynomial measured by the OCT system compared with an image reconstructed with the calculated 20 first Zernike coefficients and the ideal polynomial. The reconstructions match well with all measured images. The difference between the reconstructed images and the measured mirror surfaces had a (RMSE) between $\pm$ 11 nm and $\pm$ 36 nm, which is in the error margin of the OCT-device. Therefore the decomposition into the first 20 Zernike polynomials is a suitable approximating the real mirror surface and the calculated coefficients are a good parameter for the mirror performance. The RMS of the measured surface and the reconstructed image increases with the order of the Zernike polynomial applied. Astigmatism has a root mean square error of $\pm$ 11 nm and is therefore one of the best described images while Zernike polynomial ψ_3^5 already has a RMSE of $\pm$ 28 nm. In Fig. 2 (a) the calculated coefficients of all applied Zernike polynomial are shown for the highest allowed voltage in positive and negative direction. The ratio of the calculated coefficient of the applied Zernike polynomial the sum of all calculated coefficients is shown in Fig. 2(b). However, the polynomials piston, tip, tilt ,and defocus are omitted since they are aberrations which can easily be removed without adaptive optics and therefore were not of interest for our investigations. The two measurements provide results which differ. This may be caused by the different methods of measuring. The OCT system provides a direct measurement of the mirror surface itself while the SHS provides a measurement of the wavefront. Therefore the measurement of the SHS also contains aberrations caused by the optical system itself. In addition, the SHS measurements contain the aberration caused by the flat mirror, which were corrected in the OCT measurement by subtracting a reference image. Furthermore, the axial resolution for OCT is approximately two magnitudes above the axial resolution of the SHS and therefore provides more precise results. However, for both measurements the performance and the maximum deflection of the mirror decreases with increasing order of the polynomials. This is a result of the limited number of electrodes, which fail to modulate more complex structures. Therefore, the deviation from the ideal Zernike polynomial gets bigger for higher orders and the mirror is less capable of correcting the higher order optical aberration . To investigate the

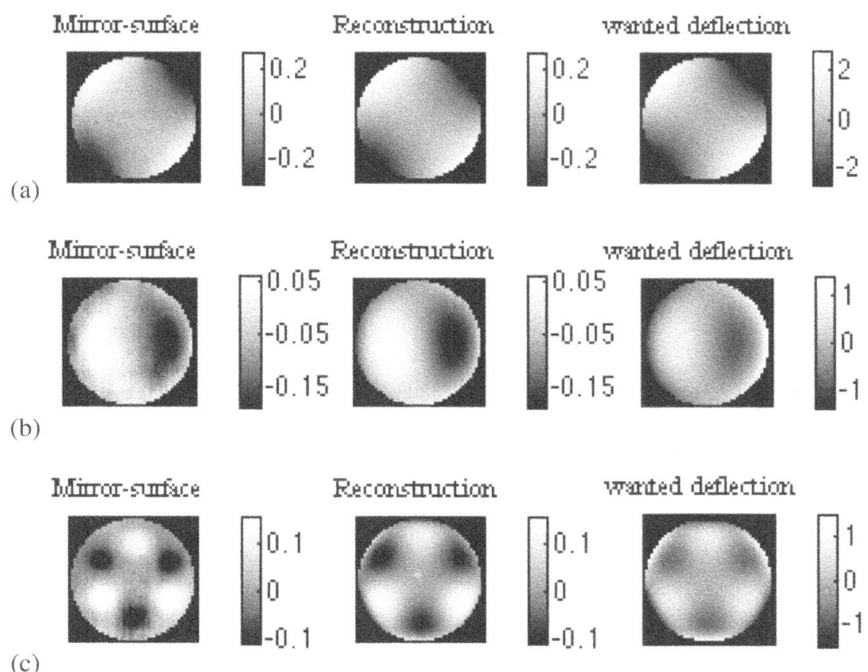

Figure 1: Measured mirror surface using OCT (left), reconstructed mirror surface (middle) and real Zernike polynomial (right) for astigmatism (ψ_2^2) (a), coma (ψ_1^3) (b) and Zernike polynomial ψ_3^5 (c). Colorbars are scaled in µfor the measured surface and the reconstructed images. The real Zernike polynomial are scaled in an arbitrary unit

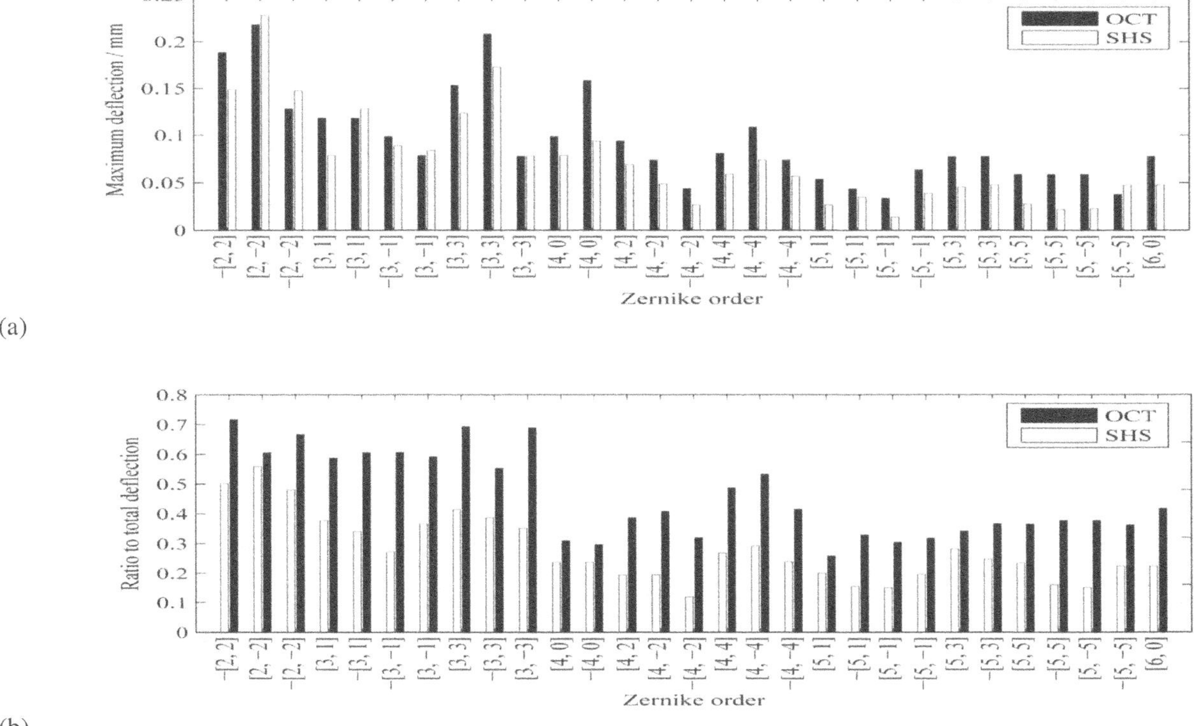

Figure 2: (a) Maximum deflection of different Zernike polynomial measured by OCT (black) and by SHS (white); (b) Ratio of the measured Zernike coefficient of the Zernike polinomial applied to the sum of all Zernike coefficients after decomposition measured by OCT (black) and by the SHS (white)

relation between the unitless values of the MiZer-software and the deflection of the mirror, the measured maximum deflection of the desired polynomial was plotted against the unitless values for several polynomials. In Fig. 3 and 4 this is shown for spherical aberration and astigmatism. An approximately linear relation is visible, which slightly differs for the two different measurement methods. This could be caused by a non optimal chosen diameter for the aperture in one of these measurements, although it was tried to use the same diameter for both measurements.

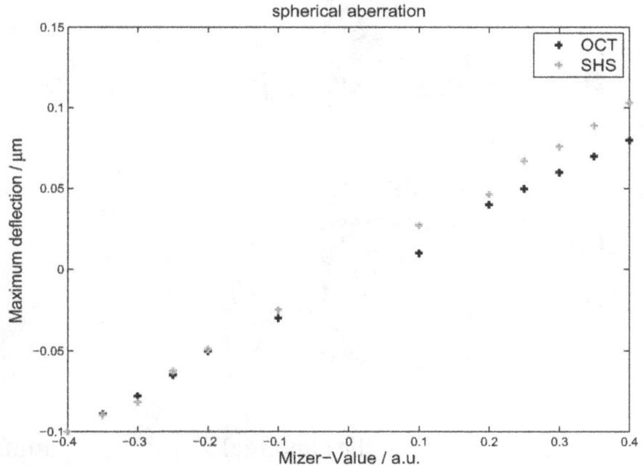

Figure 3: Maximum deflection for spherical aberrations plotted against the applied MiZer-Value for OCT (black) and SHS (gray)

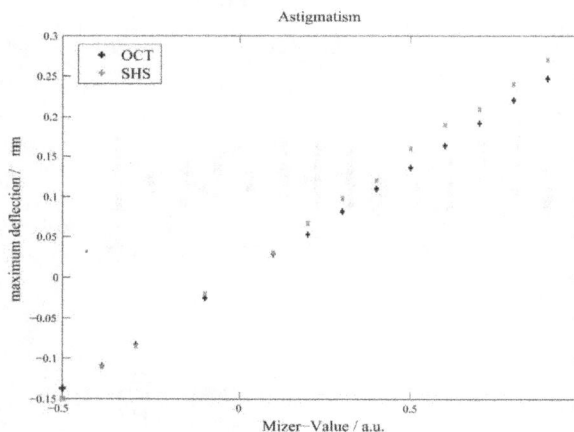

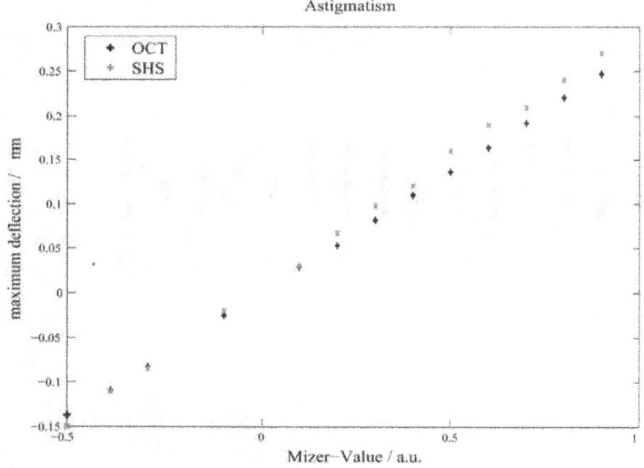

Figure 4: Maximum deflection for astigmatism plotted against the applied MiZer-Value for OCT (black) and SHS (gray)

4 Conclusion

In this paper the characteristics of a 37-channel MMDM system was measured and OCT as a new method to investigate the performance of adaptive elements like deformable mirrors was introduced. We could show that the measurement with the OCT-scanner provides results which are precise enough to characterize a given adaptive element in the limits of its accuracy and therefore yields more reliable results than common measuring methods by means of a Shack-Hartmann sensor. However, this method proved to be very time-consuming and measures the surface of the mirror instead of the real wavefront. Thus, it is only suited to characterize adaptive elements and not suitable for real-time wave-front detection.

Acknowledgement

The work has been carried out at the Universität zu Lübeck at the institute of Biomedical Optic (BMO). In addition I would like to thank Helge Sudkamp and Fred Reinholz for his help and support during this investigation and Dr. Hüttmann for giving me the possibility to work on this project.

5 References

[1] M. J. Booth , *Adaptive Optics in Microscopy*. Springer, Berlin/Heidelberg, 2008.

[2] M. J. Booth, M. A. A. Neil, R.Juskaitis and T. Wilson *Adaptive aberration correction in a confocal microscope*. Applied Pysical Science, 2002

[3] M. J. Booth, M. A. A. Neil, T. Wilson *Aberration correction for confocal imaging in refractive-index-mismatched media*. Journal of Microscopy, Vol. 192 Pt 2, November 1998, pp. 90-88

[4] M. A. A. Neil,R.Juskaitis,M. J. Booth, T. Wilson *Adaptive aberration correction in a two-photon microscope*. Journal of Microscopy, Vol. 200, Pt 2, November 2000, pp. 105-108

[5] J. Liang and D.R. Williams *Aberrations and retinal image quality of the normal human eye*. J.Opt.Soc.Am.A, Vol.14, No. 11, November 1997

[6] E.J. Fernández and P.Artal *Membrane deformable mirror for adaptive optics:performance limits in visual optics*. Optics Express, Vol. 11, No. 9, May 2003

[7] E. Dalimir and C. Dainty *Comparative analysis of deformable mirrors for ocular adaptive optics*. Optics Express, Vol. 13, No. 11, May 2005

[8] L. Zhu, P.-C. Sun,D.-U. Bartsch, W. R: Freeman and Y. Fainman *Wave-front generation of Zernike polynomial modes with a micromachined membrane deformable mirror*. Applied Optics, Vol. 38, No. 28, October 1999

[9] L. Zhu, P.-C. Sun, D.-U. Bartsch, W. R. Freeman and Y. Fainman *Adaptive control of micromachined continuous-membrane deformable mirror for aberration compensation*. Applied Optics, Vol. 38, No. 1, January 1999

Laser Ray Tracing Setup for Measuring the Refractive Index Changes in Bovine Lenses

J. C. Schwarzer [1], E. Vaghefi [2], and R. Birngruber [3]

[1] Medizinische Ingenieurwissenschaft, Universität zu Lübeck, janka.schwarzer@miw.uni-luebeck.de

[2] Institute of Optometrie and Vision Science, Auckland University, e.vaghefi@auckland.ac.nz

[3] Institute of Biomedical Optics, Universität zu Lübeck, birngruber@bmo.uni-luebeck.de

Abstract

Our eyesight is precious, but easily disturbed. To gain a better understanding of the risks and potential therapies for the eye a thorough understanding of the eyes anatomy and function is required. In order to create a refractive model of the eye the refractive index relief of the lens is to be determined. Therefore a setup is developed that is able to perform ray tracing on a bovine lens. During this work an existing camera setup could be improved in accuracy and was enabled to measure a laser beam refracted by a lens and visualize it in a 3D coordinate system. This will allow calculating the lengths and angle of the different parts of the laser beam which is fundamental to ray tracing and therefore a determination of the refractive index distribution inside of the lens.

1 Introduction

The maintenance of the lenses clarity is of crucial importance to the function of the eye. There are several mechanisms inside the lens that aim to maintain the lenses clarity by maintaining a defined refractive index profile with specific refractive indices in different depth of the lens. Since the refractive index is linked to the water concentration in the lens, the gradient has to be maintained actively. Otherwise it would disappear over time due to the flow of water in direction of the gradient [8].

Its transparency is based on the structure and the function of the fibre cells it consists of. Those cells are continuously generated from epithelial cells that elongate while maturing and loosing their organelles and nuclei. To maintain the mature cells nutrients need to be delivered into the lens as well as waste products need to be removed. This is ensured by an internal micro circulation system[5][6].

It is known that certain diseases as diabetes can affect those mechanisms, which leads to a loss of visual function over time [5][6]. To gain a more thorough understanding of the effects taking place, when the environment of the lens is changed the University of Auckland is working on a complete model of the eye lens that is able to simulate the lenses reactions to those changes. As part of that model the changes of the refractive index inside of the lens needs to be determined as exactly as possible.

In order to determine the refractive index profile a setup is needed that is suitable to perform ray tracing. To acquire the needed information for ray tracing a system is required that is able to measure the length and angle of a small laser beam transmitting through a lens. The exit angle and distance to the optical axis of the lens is analysed on triangulation photos with a Matlab code written for the purpose.

A setup meeting parts of the requirements already existed, but was not set up to carry out measurements on lenses. Furthermore the accuracy of the setup was not high enough to gain satisfying results.

1.1 Ray Tracing

Raytracing was first introduced by Chu as a method to determine the refractive index profile of an optical fibre without destroying it [4]. Since then it has been used for a number of different purposes including the refractive index profile of eye lenses and has been modified and further developed to suit the different purposes. The essential idea however remains the same in all of them[1]-[3], [7].

A laser ray falls through the object of interest parallel to its optical axis. The beams distance to the optical axis of the object is measured before it enters the object and at the point where it leaves the object again. At this point the angle of the laser ray to the optical axis is measured as well.

This is repeated for a number of distances to the optical axis right to the edge of the object. The results of those measurements lead to a function of the refractive index profile of the object in relation to the distance to the objects centre.

2 Material and Methods

In order to receive satisfying results the exact knowledge of the setups properties is required, as well a basic knowledge of the properties of the lens under investigation.

2.1 Triangulation

The setup (Fig. 1) consists of two Canon EOS 1100D cameras that are orientated rectangularly to each other. Both take images of the same area in which the measured object is placed. To generate quantitative results the measured object should make use of the most of the cameras' fields of view. The lens to be measured is placed in a silver mount inside a liquid filled cuvette to match its outer refractive index to the surrounding medium and keep the lens moist. For artificial lenses the surrounding medium is water, for bovine lenses a sodium buffer is used.
A laser beam is directed at the lens by a prism, so that

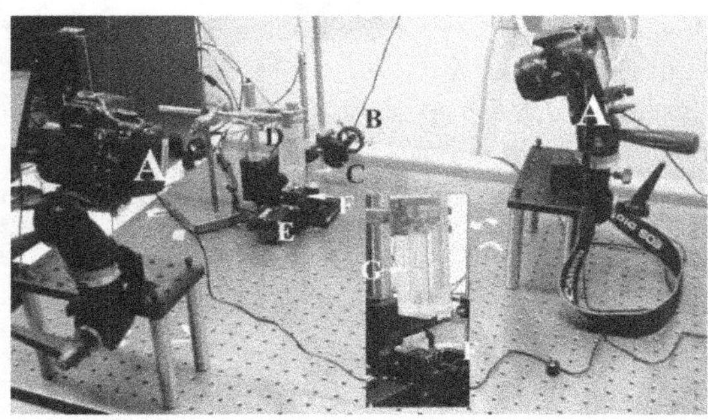

Figure 1: The setup including the lens. A:Cameras, B:Laser, C:Pinhole, D:Cuvett with lens, E:Moveable table, F:Prism, G:Lens

it falls through it parallel to the lenses optical axis. To determine the effects of different wavelengths two different lasers were used (532nm, 633nm).
The prism is mounted on a moveable desk, which allows to move the beam along the length of the lens. The diameter of the laser beam is restricted by a pinhole in front of the laser. The smaller the laser beams diameter is chosen, the more accurate measurements are possible in the course of the experiment, since the rays diameter determines the area the measurement averages. The pinhole used had a changeable diameter to choose the smallest possible diameter for every laser that allowed the beam to be seen on the camera pictures. To increase the detectability of the laser beam inside the water for small light intensities a drop of milk can be added to the water.

2.2 Camera Calibration

For the calculations it is of high importance to receive exact length and angle measurements. The first step to achieve those is the calibration of the camera setup.
To calibrate the setup each camera took 50 pictures of a known checkerboard pattern that was moved across the field of view of the camera (Fig.2). With those pictures the intrinsic parameters of the camera and the distortion of the camera lens could be determined. In order to do that a computer

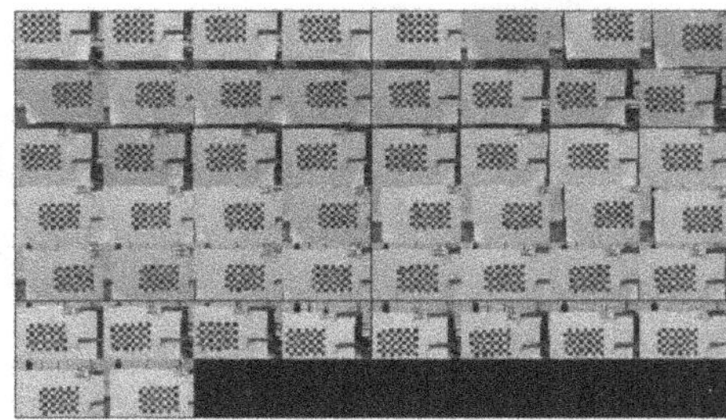

Figure 2: Picture set for single camerea calibration

program detected the checkerboard edges on every picture and distorted the picture to optimize the checkerboard pattern. From the distortion of the single pictures the average distortion of the camera could be received. Together with the information about the size of the checkerboard the pixel information gained by the camera could be transformed into real world information.
In the second step of the calibration 50 pictures of the checkerboard pattern were taken by both cameras at the same time. With the previously gained information about the intrinsic parameters the pictures of both cameras are matched together leading to a transformation function between both camera views. This is recorded as a rotation matrix that gives the position of a point in space.
To validate the camera calibration and the accuracy of the measurements pictures of high precision angle blocks were

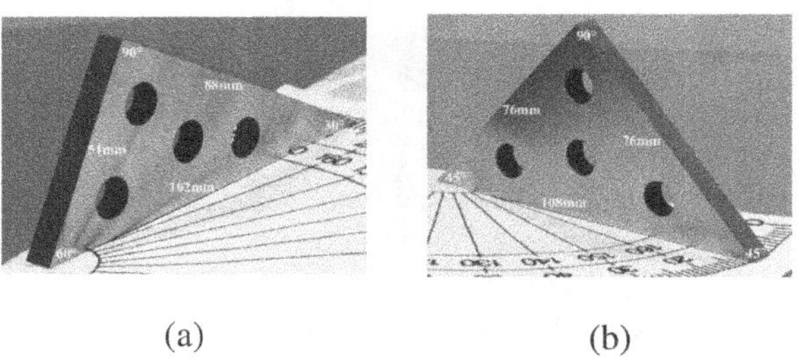

(a) (b)

Figure 3: Angle blocks with different angles and lengths. Used to validate the accuracy of systems measuremaent.

taken (Fig.3). Due to the known length and angles of those blocks the average error of the setup could be determined. Therefore the corners of the angle blocks were selected in the pictures, while a Matlab program, written by Amir HajiRassouliha, calculated the real world lengths and angles from the previously obtained transformations and compare it with the real values.

3 Results and Discussion

The most crucial step was the improvement of the accuracy reached by the length measurement to fit the applications demands and determine the system errors. The system then was modified for the more complex task of a beam falling through a lens.

3.1 Length and Angle Measurements

To determine the accuracy of length and angle measurements pictures are taken from checkerboard patterns of different known sizes and angle blocks with known angles and side lengths. The pictures are processed with a Matlab code that was written for this purpose. The base of the calculation is the manual selection of the edges of the triangle that is to be measured.
The angle and length measurements were performed on two different kinds of phantoms; three differently sized checkerboards (20mm, 25mm and 30mm) and two different angle blocks. The results for the length measurements (Table 1) and angle measurements (Table 2) are rounded to one decimal point.
The angle measurements seem to be more accurate than the length measurements. The error for the measured angles appears to be randomly distributed. The average error is 1.1%, which is about the same value than in earlier measurements. The length measurement appears to generate more exact results than before the optimisation. The average error for the length measurement is 5,5%, which is a big improvement to earlier measurements [9] that had an error of about 10%. The error does not change much between the different phantoms, even though it might be a little smaller for the angle blocks.
Since the error is for the length measurements is always positiv the actual length of a measurement can be determined quite accurately by simply taking 5.5% of the measured value.
To validate the results further length and angle measurements were carried out on the image set used for the stereo camera calibration. The average error over all 50 images was 5.6% for the length measurements and 1.2% for the angle measurements.

Table 1: angle measurements

	measured angle [deg]	actual angle [deg]	total error [deg]	relativ error
Checkerboard 1	44.9	45	-0.1	0.3
	44.2	45	-0.8	1.8
	90.9	90	0.9	1.0
Checkerboard 2	45.1	45	0.1	0.1
	44.1	45	-0.9	1.9
	90.8	90	0.8	0.9
Checkerboard 3	44.4	45	-0.6	1.3
	44.4	45	-0.6	1.3
	91.4	90	1.4	1.6
Angleblock 30/60	30.5	30	0.5	1.8
	59.0	60	1.0	1.7
	90.5	90	0.5	0.5
Angleblock 45	46.0	45	0.9	2.0
	44.6	45	-0.3	0.8
	89.5	90	-0.5	0.6
average error				1.1

Table 2: Length measurements

	measured length [mm]	actual length [mm]	total error [mm]	relativ error
Checkerboard 1	21.2	20.0	1.2	6.0
	20.9	20.0	0.9	4.7
	30.0	28.3	1.8	6.2
Checkerboard 2	26.1	25.0	1.1	4.4
	26.5	25.0	1.5	6.1
	37.5	35.4	2.1	6.0
Checkerboard 3	31.7	30.0	1.7	5.7
	31.6	30.0	1.6	5.3
	45.3	42.4	2.9	6.8
Angleblock 30/60	106.9	102.0	4.9	4.8
	54.3	51.0	3.3	6.5
	91.6	88.0	3.6	4.1
Angleblock 45	113.0	108.0	5.0	4.6
	81.2	76.0	5.2	6.8
	79.4	76.0	3.4	4.5
average error				5.5

3.2 Including a Lens

A first check of the newly optimized setup was done by measuring a glass lens as a pahntom of a bovine lens. The laser beam falling through the phantom lens (Fig.4, Fig.5) is clearly visible, which enables further measurements. The points where the beam enters and leaves the lens are visible in both camera perspectives. To determine points on the beam outside of the lens a grid has been applied to the outside of the cuvette. The green laser proves to have a better visibility than the red laser, which was hard to see with the eye and on camera. The visibility on camera could be improved with changes in the camera settings, but was still poorer than the results for the green laser. The outlines of the lens are visible, which will make it possible to determine its shape for further calculations.
Using real bovine lenses (Fig.6) the visibility of the beam is similar to the glass lens. It might even be improved due to the different solution surrounding the lens. The path inside the lens and the points of entry and exit are more easily to determine then in the glass lens. The outlines of the lens itself are less prominent then with the glass lens, but still clear enough to be seen.
Over all the setup is able to provide the information needed in raytracing.

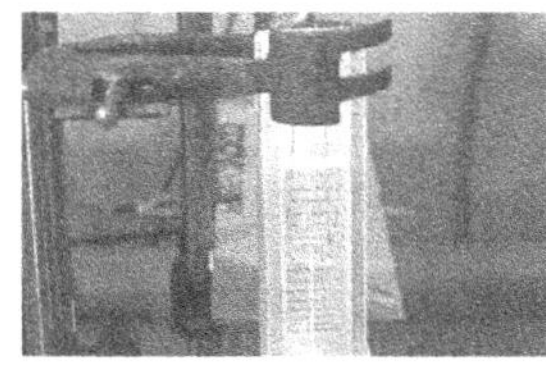

left camera

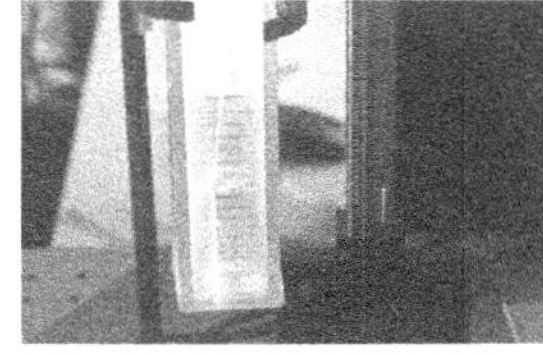

rigth camera

Figure 4: Green laser falling through a glass lens with a changing refractiv index in water.

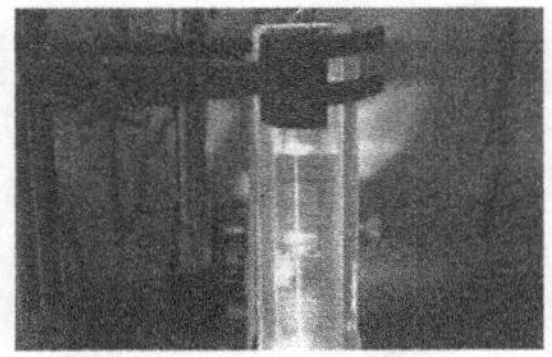

left camera

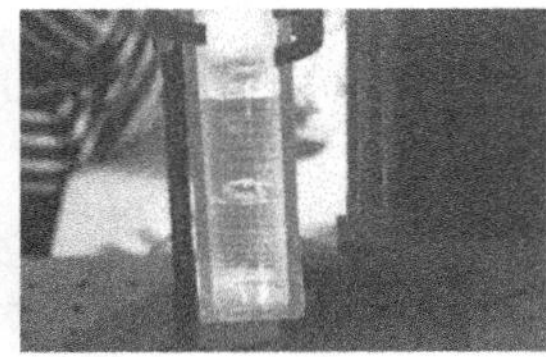

rigth camera

Figure 5: Red laser falling through a glass lens with a changing refractiv index in water.

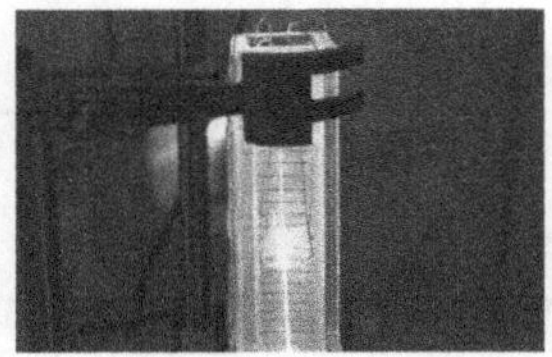

left camera

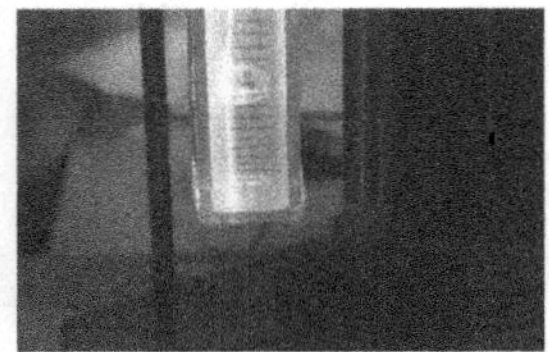

rigth camera

Figure 6: Green laser falling through bovine lens in a sodium buffer.

4 Conclusion

The accuracy of the camera setup could be significantly improved during this work, which now allows to measure distances and angles accurate enough for tha analysis of the optical index profile of the gradient index lens by ray tracing measurements. The setup has further been enabled to accommodate lenses and measure a beam through them in a desired position. There is still room for improvement of the setup to fit the needs of the beam and the lens more precisely and to simplify working with the setup. However a promising base is created for further work on this project. The next step will be the ray tracing measurement of a well known gradient index lens and compare the result with the data from the manufacturer.

Acknowledgement

The work has been carried out at the Department of Optometry and Vision Science, University of Auckland.
Many thanks to Amir HajiRassouliha and Jason Turuwhenua for their help and advice.

5 References

[1] Barrell, K. F., and C. Pask , *Nondestructive index profile measurement of noncircular optical fibre preforms.*Optics communications 27.2 (1978): 230-234.

[2] Campbell, Melanie CW. *Measurement of refractive index in an intact crystalline lens.* Vision research 24.5 (1984): 409-415.

[3] Chan, Derek YC, et al. *Determination and modeling of the 3-D gradient refractive indices in crystalline lenses.* Applied optics 27.5 (1988): 926-931.

[4] Chu, P. L. *Nondestructive measurement of index profile of an optical-fibre preform.* Electronics Letters 13.24 (1977): 736-738.

[5] Donaldson, Paul J., et al. *Functional imaging: new views on lens structure and function.* Clinical and experimental pharmacology and physiology 31.12 (2004): 890-895.

[6] Donaldson, Paul J., et al. *Regulation of lens volume: Implications for lens transparency.* Experimental eye research 88.2 (2009): 144-150.

[7] Sharma, Anurag, D. Vizia Kumar, and Ajoy K. Ghatak. *Tracing rays through graded-index media: a new method.* Applied Optics 21.6 (1982): 984-987.

[8] Vaghefi, Ehsan, et al. *Visualizing ocular lens fluid dynamics using MRI: manipulation of steady state water content and water fluxes.* American Journal of Physiology-Regulatory, Integrative and Comparative Physiology 301.2 (2011): R335-R342.

[9] Zhang, Linda *Camera calibration towards a system for measuring laser deflection using a stereo camera setup.* University of Auckland (2014)

Optically Monitored Selective Laser Trabeculoplasty

A. Shpychak [1], K. Bliedtner [2], E. Seifert [2] and R. Brinkmann [2]
[1] Medical Engineering Science, University of Luebeck, Luebeck, Germany, alexander.shpychak@miw.uni-luebeck.de
[2] Medical Laser Center Luebeck GmbH, Luebeck, Germany, {bliedtner, seifert, brinkmann}@mll.uni-luebeck.de

Abstract

Selective Laser Trabeculoplasty (SLT) has the potential to evolve into a cost-effective first-line treatment for open angle glaucoma as an alternative to medication treatments and argon laser trabeculoplasty (ALT). So far, the irradiation endpoint is the appearance of macroscopic visible bubbles far above the threshold of damage for pigmented trabecular meshwork cells. Here we present an optically monitoring of micro-bubble formation in enucleated porcine eyes to investigate the possibilities of a dosimetry system for SLT. Laser pulses with µs pulse duration are applied on the trabecular meshwork, iris and iris root and the backscattered light is analysed for micro-bubble formation. Macroscopic visible bubbles during irradiation produce strong oscillations in corresponding reflected signals. Furthermore micro-bubble formation could be detected for spots with less applied energy where no macroscopic visible effect was observed. This indicates that this system is capable of monitoring damage below the visible threshold.

1 Introduction

Selective Laser Trabeculoplasty (SLT) is a laser treatment for ocular hypertension or open angle glaucoma. Since glaucoma is often induced by high intraocular pressure, reduction of this pressure is necessary to slow down the progression of the disease. While medication therapy is still first line treatment, laser trabeculoplasty represents a common alternative for cases of open angle glaucoma that are medically uncontrolled. It has evolved into a standard treatment with similar intraocular pressure reduction as the medication therapy. There are two common types of the laser trabeculoplasty, the first one is Argon Laser Trabeculoplasty (ALT) and the second is SLT. Both treatments apply laser spots on the trabecular meshwork (TM). After the absorption of laser light by pigmented structures of the TM, mechanical and biological changes [1][2] induce an increased ocular outflow through the TM, which leads to a reduction of the intraocular pressure. Whereas ALT causes mechanical changes in the TM, SLT induces a biological change to obtain an impact in the eye. ALT is performed with an argon laser with 514 nm, pulse durations of 0.1 s and a pulse energy of 40-60 mJ. The spot size is 50 µm [3]. SLT is preformed with a Q-switched Nd:YAG laser at 523 nm, a pulse duration of 3 ns and pulse energy of 0.2-2.0 mJ [4]. The spot size in SLT is 400 µm [5] and covers the entire anteroposterior TM [6]. In the case of nanosecond pulse application the induced heat does not flow out of the irradiated area to significant amounts during the time of irradiation. The absorbing structures are targeted selectively [7]. Hence, heating of the surrounding tissue is reduced and coagulation can be avoided [4]. Side effects of ALT such as destructiveness and scarring in the TM [1] are not present in the SLT, which makes it safer and repeatable compared to ALT. Since the TM is heated with nanosecond pulses emerging micro-bubbles are the origin of cell damage [8]. This micro-bubbles diameter and lifetime increase with the laser pulse energy [9]. At a certain pulse energy cluster-formation of big micro-bubbles can form a ophthalmoscopically visible macro-bubble. The pulse energy range in which SLT is supposed to achieve selectivity shall be defined from the minimum pulse energy to induce micro-bubbles to the minimum pulse energy to induce ophthalmoscopically visible macro-bubbles. The actual treatment is carried out below the pulse energy threshold to induce macro-bubbles. While lowering the pulse energy is necessary to avoid an over-treatment of the TM, the attending physician has no feedback whether the applied dosage is appropriate. However pigmentation of TM varies, and the risk of over- or undertreatment due to lack of an objective monitoring of achieved damage in the TM is present. The intention of this paper is to evaluate the possibilities of an optical detection of micro-bubble formation during SLT in enucleated porcine eyes as a first step towards an optically monitored dosing system for SLT. This would make SLT even more effective and reduce the treatment time.

2 Material and Methods

2.1 Optical Detection of Bubble Formation

Since micro-bubbles are the origin of selective damage on the TM cells their existence can be used as its indicator. The change in the backscattering properties of the tissue by micro-bubbles lead to micro-bubble correlated characteristics in the acquired signal. An example can be seen in Fig. 3, where an applied pulse and the corresponding backscattered light influenced by bubble formation are shown. When pulse energy is below the threshold of micro-bubble formation, the backscattered light has the same progression as the applied pulse. Above the selective targeting range ophthalmoscopically visible macro-bubbles can be observed. Previous research on this feedback technique [10] lead to the assumption that macro-bubbles will lead to very pronounced oscillations on the backscattered pulse. Thus less pronounced oscillations can be expected within the therapeutic window.

2.2 Optical Setup

The measurement series was carried out with an existing optical setup based on a Q-switched, frequency doubled Nd:YLF laser at 527 nm (LU-LQ 527-12, Monochrom) with a pulse duration of 1.7 µs and a repetition rate of 100 Hz. This long pulse duration compared to common SLT treatments is necessary to illuminate the formation of bubbles for reflectometry purpose. The laser beam passes a shutter (SR475 Laser Shutter, SRS), which is programmed to open for 30 ms and an acousto-optic modulator (AOM, R23080-3LTD, Goooch & Housego), which is used to control the applied energy. Directly after the AOM a photodiode (photodiode 1) is used to acquire the applied pulse, so that the energy applied to the target can be calculated via calibrated functions. Through a dichroic mirror a second laser is coupled into the beam path. This laser has a wavelength of 632 nm and is used as a pilot laser, which continuously illuminates the treated spot and has the same beam diameter as the treatment laser. The beam is then coupled into a fiber (50 µm core diameter, NA=0.11). The fiber is coupled to an optical zoom system designed to image the fiber tip to the treatment plane. The zoom system allows to change the spot size to 50, 100, 200, 500 and 1000 µm. Through the slit lamp the area to be treated can be observed. Through a gonioscopic lens (Ocular Latina 5 Bar SLT, Ocular Instruments) the laser pulse is guided to the eye and a part is scattered back from the target area. The backscattered light entering the laser link again and a beam splitter ensures it is guided to a second photodiode (photodiode 2, APD 110A/M, Thorlabs). In order to synchronize the acquisition a LabVIEW routine has been used. It also was utilized for data collection and processing tasks. The recorded signals from photodiode 2 could be used to calculate a reflectometry value for each treatment pulse. This feedback value represents the amount of micro-bubble correlated characteristics (oscillations) on the backscattered pulse. A principle drawing of the optical setup that was used for the measurements can be viewed in Fig. 1.

2.3 Series of Measurements

To evaluate the possibilities of an optical detection of micro-bubbles, measurements with enucleated porcine eyes were performed. Pig eyes were used because they have similar volume and size compared to human eyes, especially in the anterior chamber. Furthermore the corneoscleral trabecular tissue looks similar, with identical size, shape and lamellar structure [11]. During the measurements the pulse energy, spot size and the irradiated area have been varied. Besides the trabecular meshwork, also the iris root, and the iris, that are more pigmented then TM, have been irradiated. These regions of higher pigmentation near to the TM have been irradiated to ensure to reach the point of macro-bubble formation even with the low pulse energy of the available laser. Each structure was irradiated with three different spot sizes: 50 µm, 100 µm and 200 µm. For each structure and spot size the pulse energies of 100%, 80%, 60%, 40% and 20% were applied regarding a maximum energy of 159 µJ.

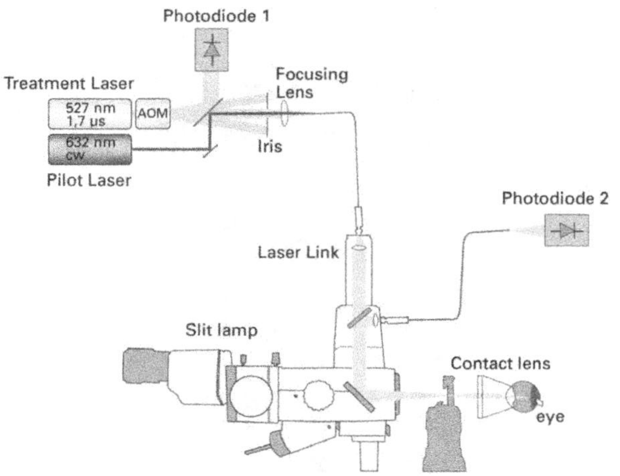

Figure 1: Experimental setup with important parts for irradiation and detection.

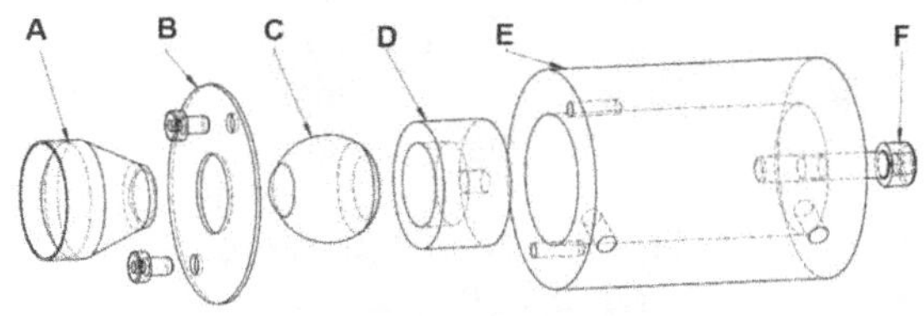

Figure 2: Schematic drawing of the eye mounting with the principle parts. A: contact lens, B: anchor ring, C: eye, D: eye support, E: cylinder, F: fixation screw

To get a good view of the iridocorneal angle an eye mount that allows the eye to be rotated and tilted has been developed. A sketch of the mount is shown in Fig. 2. The mounting allows to influence the pressure on the eye and enabled a variable connection of the eye and the SLT contact lens that was attached in front of the slit lamp.

3 Results and Discussion

To evaluate the optical feedback algorithm for all structures and spot sizes each applied pulse was associated with

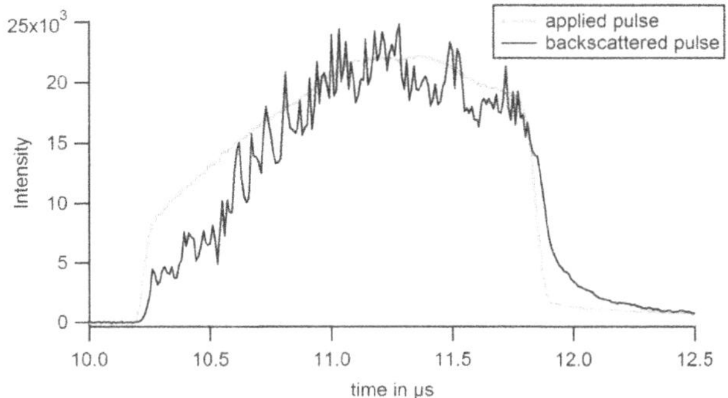

Figure 3: Applied laser pulse with 159 µJ and the detected backscattered light during irradiation.

the respective ophthalmoscopically visible effect. Every pulse with macroscopic bubble formation was categorized as "bubbles". An indication of tissue alteration below the threshold of macroscopic bubble formation could be observed on the basis of modulations of the backscattered light during irradiation. These pulses were categorized as "modulation". When no damage effect was observed, the pulse was categorized as "invisible". The calculated reflectometry values of each pulse could now be linked with the classified damage effects. In Fig. 4 three different scatter plots that depict applied energy versus calculated feedback value are shown as an example. Each scatter plot displays the applied 200 µm pulses for a different structure. The shape of each point represents the visibility of each spot. It is apparent that with rising energy the feedback values increase as well. Reduction of the spot size also led to higher feedback values which follows from the fact that irradiation decreases with rising spot size. While for 50 µm spot size an energy of 159 µJ results in 80.98 mJ/mm², for a spot size of 200 µm the same energy leads to an irradiation of 5.061 mJ/mm². Another fact that stands out is that the more the structure is pigmented the more bubble formation could be observed. For spot size of 200 µm 47 spots led to bubble formation on the iris root, for the less pigmented TM no macroscopic bubbles could be generated. A comparison over all spot sizes shows that 75% of all pulses applied on the iris root led to bubble formation, whereas on the TM only 1.5% of the applied pulses led to ophthalmoscopically visible bubble formation. The separation of the observed effects using the calculated feedback value works well for structures that are more pigmented. Less pigmented structures have a wider spreading of calculated values, which makes an exact separation difficult. It is also notable that for higher pulse energies spreading increases which indicates a broader range of achieved damage.

A LabVIEW program has been developed to perform statistical analysis of the acquired data. The performance measure of the monitoring system is the dependent probability to make a correct assignment of a spot to a tissue-response category. The probability to correctly assign a spot of selective cell damage is called sensitivity. Likewise the probability to correctly assign an invisible spot is called specificity. The algorithm calculates for every possible threshold with

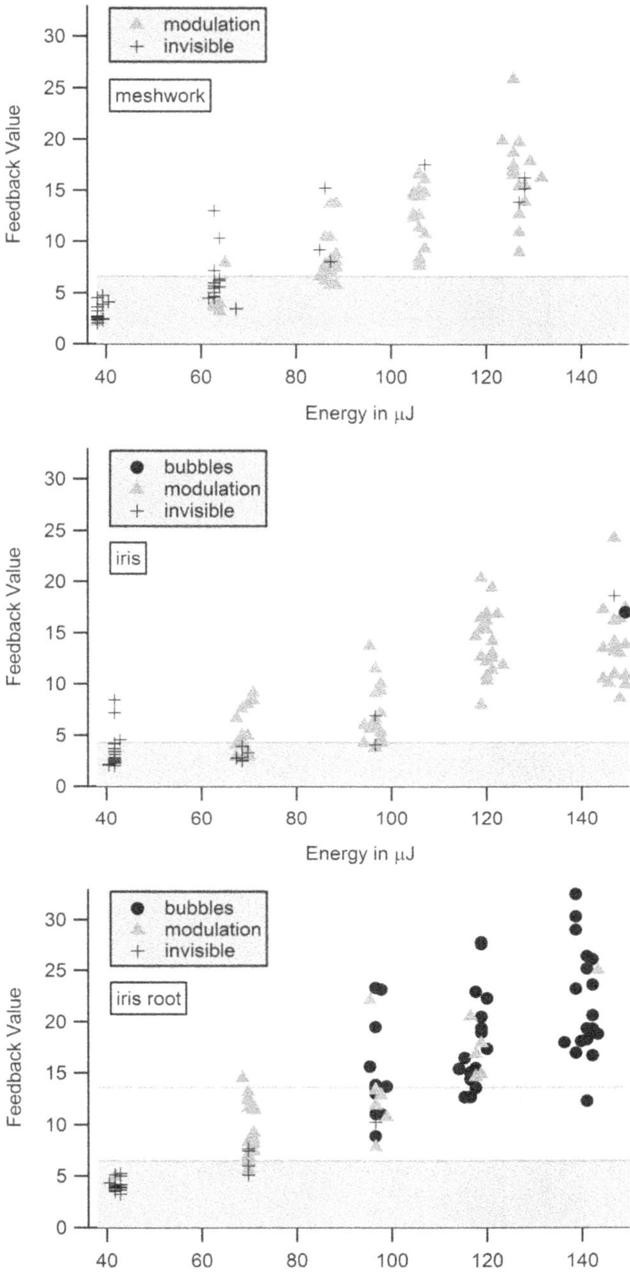

Figure 4: Scatter plots for treatments of the TM (top), iris (middle) and iris root (bottom) with a spot size of 200 µm. The dark grey background represents the lower threshold and the light grey background the threshold for macroscopic bubble formation.

the corresponding sensitivity and specificity a Youden's index. The closer the Youden's index is to one, the precisely the respective threshold can differentiate between both categories. To visualize the quality of the classification the receiver operating characteristic (ROC) graph for the pulses of 200 µm spot size are shown in Fig. 5 as an example. In favour of a better distinction this was realized for two different thresholds. The lower threshold differentiates if a macroscopic effect was visible (modulations, bubbles) or

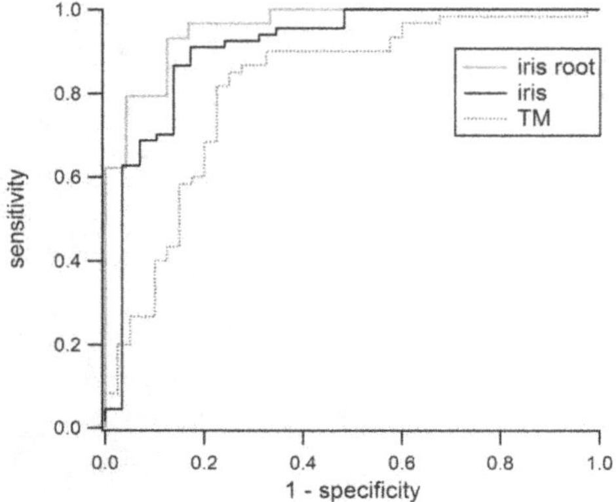

Figure 5: ROC plots of all three irradiated structures. The curves represent a validation whether the ophthalmoscopically visible effects (bubbles, modulations) during treatment correlate with the classification by the algorithm.

not. The upper threshold differentiates if bubbles were visible. The scatter plot in Fig.4 shows the thresholds coloured in the background. While for treatment of the iris root both thresholds are shown, for pulses on the TM no visible bubbles could be observed. Therefore no upper threshold could be calculated by the algorithm. The best Youden's index for the treatment of the iris is 0.738 for the treatments of the iris root the calculated Youden's index is 0.806. The calculated Youden's index for spots on the TM is 0.6. This is due to the fact that TM is less pigmented, so less energy is absorbed by the pigmented TM cells in comparison to the other irradiated structures. Thereby the range of possible damage caused to the structure is narrow and used algorithms have difficulties to resolve the detected damage value. Another fact is that only a small amount of treatment spots led to bubble formation. However this is important for a proper statistical evaluation. To achieve a presentable outcome the applied maximum energy has to be increased. This would raise the absorbed energy for the TM cells and in turn deliver more damage to the target structure.

4 Conclusion

This project investigated whether a controlled damage feedback for SLT can be realized. Therefore measurement series on differently pigmented structure in the iridocorneal angle of enucleated porcine eyes were carried out. It has been found that the principle method of detecting the backscattered treatment light and analysing it for oscillations caused by micro-bubble formation could be utilized to develop optically monitored SLT. The applied algorithms for detection and categorization perform well for heavily pigmented structures like the iris and the iris root. Due to lesser pigmentation of the TM it was rarely possible to achieve macroscopic visible bubbles with the available pulse energy. However this is indispensable for a proper statistical evaluation. For the future a new calculation of the feedback value should be implemented. A laser with higher energies included in the setup would make a greater damage range possible. Another important step would be a better reference for actual structural or cellular damage since the ophthalmoscopical observed effect depends on the subjectivity of the treating individual. A possible opportunity for a matching reference could be optical coherence tomography (OCT). A high resolution would be necessary to visualize created damage. Other possibilities as a reference could be vitality assays or histology. Proper histological section could improve the detection of damage below macroscopic bubble formation and lead to more accurate results.

Acknowledgement

The work has been carried out at the Medical Laser Center Luebeck GmbH, Luebeck, Germany and the Institute of Biomedical Optics, University of Luebeck, Luebeck, Germany.

5 References

[1] J.B. Wise and S.L. Witter, *Argon laser therapy for open angle glaucoma: A pilot study.* Arch Ophthalmol 97:319–322 (1979)

[2] K. F. Damji, *Selective Laser Trabeculoplasty: A better alternative.* Survey of Ophthalmology 53(6):646-651 (2008)

[3] U.P. Best, H. Domack and V. Schmidt, *Pressure reduction after selective laser trabeculoplasty with two different laser systems and after argon laser trabeculoplasty - A controlled prospective clinical trial on 284 eyes.* Klin Monatsbl Augenheilkd 224 (3):173–179 (2007)

[4] M.A. Latina and J.M. de Leon, *Selective Laser Trabeculoplasty.* Ophthalmol Clin North Am 18:409–419 (2005)

[5] T. Wacker and S. Eckert, *Laser trabeculoplasty: therapeutic options and adverse effects.* Ophthalmologe 2010-107:13–17 (2010)

[6] M.A. Latina, S.A. Sibaya, D.H. Shin, R.J. Noecker and G. Marcellino, *Q-switched 532nm Nd:YAG laser trabeculoplasty (selective laser trabeculoplasty): A multicenter, pilot, clinical study.* Ophthalmology 105(11):2082-2090 (1998)

[7] R.R. Anderson and J.A. Perrish, *Selective Photothermolysis: Precise Microsurgery by Selective Absorption of Pulsed Radiation.* Science 220, 524-527 (1983)

[8] J. Neumann and R. Brinkmann, *Cell disintegration by laser-induced transient microbubbles and its simultaneous monitoring by interferometry.* Journal of Biomedical Optics 11(4), 041112 (2006)

[9] A. Fritz, L. Ptaszynski, H. Stoehr and R. Brinkmann, *Dynamics and Detection of Laser Induced Micro Bubbles in the Retinal Pigment Epithelium (RPE).* SPIE-OSA Vol. 66321C-10 (2007)

[10] E. Seifert, *Automatic irradiation control by an optical feedback technique for selective retina treatment (SRT) in a rabbit model*, Proc. of OSA-SPIE Vol. 8803 880303-3 (2013)

[11] P.G. McMenamin and R.J. Steptoe, *Normal anatomy of the aqueous humour outflow system in the domestic pig eye.* Journal of anatomy 178:65 (1991)

2
Biomedical Optics II

Development of standardized tissue phantoms for evaluation of Holographic Photoacoustic Tomography

B. Schmarbeck [1], M. Muenter [2], J. Horstmann [3], C. Buj[2] and R. Brinkmann [3]

[1] Medizinische Ingenieurwissenschaft, Universität zu Lübeck: benedikt.schmarbeck@miw.uni-luebeck.de
[2] Institute of Biomedical Optics, Universität zu Lübeck, Luebeck, Germany, M.Muenter@outlook.de and buj@bmo.uni-luebeck.de
[3] Institute of Biomedical Optics, Universität zu Lübeck, Luebeck, Germany and the Medical Laser Center Lübeck GmbH, Luebeck, Germany, horstmann@mll.uni-luebeck.de and brinkmann@bmo.uni-luebeck.de

Abstract

Photoacoustic imaging is a growing field in science. In biomedicine it allows imaging of tissue chromophores with a high contrast and a high penetration depth. At present, no standardized tissue phantom for photoacoustic imaging exists, which is optically close to human skin. In this work, the production of phantoms made of silicone for a holographic photoacoustic tomograph (HPAT) is explained. The variation of optical properties through additives, measurement of this modified properties is described and the possibility of the HPAT to acquire reliable data of these phantoms is investigated. The created phantoms have optical properties like human skin for the used wavelength, are reproducible and suitable for co-evaluation. The results of the measurement with the HPAT show, that the system is capable of detecting photoacoustic signals from the produced phantoms. Furthermore, the impact of a temporal filtering to the acquired data and a high noise suppression without signal-loss is investigated.

1 Introduction

Photoacoustic imaging is a rising new imaging technique which is based on the emission of ultrasonic waves after the absorption of light, which leads to a pressure rise followed by thermoelastic expansion. This expansion results in emission of ultrasonic waves which propagate through the tissue and can be detected at the surface. From the data, the absorbing structures can be reconstructed.
The benefits of this data acquisition are the high specific absorption of biological chromophores, which are used as contrast agents, and the lower attenuation of acoustic waves compared to photons in scattering media. This allows a higher imaging depth compared to conventional optical imaging methods.
The most photoacoustic (PA) systems are based on detecting PA pressure by piezoelectric transducers. Disadvantages of this detection are shading of the excitation through the transducer and a limited bandwidth of the transducers. To overcome these limitations in current transducer based photoacoustic approaches, the Medical Laser Center Lübeck developed a non-contact full field holographic photoacoustic tomography (HPAT). An important step in development of the mentioned system, before experiments on ex vivo tissue or in vivo animal and humans, is to proof the possibility of data acquisition of phantoms which are reproducible, well defined in optical properties and comparable to tissue. Physical phantoms for photoacoustic imaging need to:

- offer defined properties such as optical scattering and absorption coefficient and speed of sound.
- provide a defined position of emitting structures.
- be suitable for co-evaluation.

A difficulty is that there is no standardized phantom for PA imaging, especially in terms of surface deformation measurement. The purpose of this work was to fabricate and examine phantoms enabling the measurement of deformation by PA pressure waves. It is important to clarify whether the mentioned system provides reliable data for the measurements of these phantoms.

2 Material and Methods

In literature, different approaches for manufacturing phantoms are mentioned, but there are no standardized phantoms for photoacoustic imaging [1],[2]. The use of standardized phantoms would facilitate the comparison between the results of different working groups in PA.

2.1 Holographic photoacoustic tomography

HPAT is based on speckle interferometry which uses diffuse reflected light from the surface of the object to detect surface displacement caused by emitted acoustic waves from the chromophores. This approach provides a sensitivity regarding the axial deformation of ± 1nm in a field of view of

7.7 mm^2 with a lateral resolution of 40 μm. The temporal resolution of the setting is 25 ns. This results in a sampling rate of 40 MHz. To acquire this high recording speed, a high speed camera (Photron, SA3) and a detection laser (Spectra, Explorer) with 532 nm wavelength are used. An excitation laser (Edgewave, BX60-2-G) with 1064 nm wavelength and a pulse duration under 10 ns is used to excite chromophores for emission of acoustic waves under stress confinement. The radiant exposure of the excitation is 16 mJ/cm^2, which is below the maximum permissible exposure of 20 mJ/cm^2 [3], limited by the excitation parameter of the HPAT. Further specifications of the system are given at Horstmann et al [4], a sketch of the basic principle of the system is shown in Fig.1.

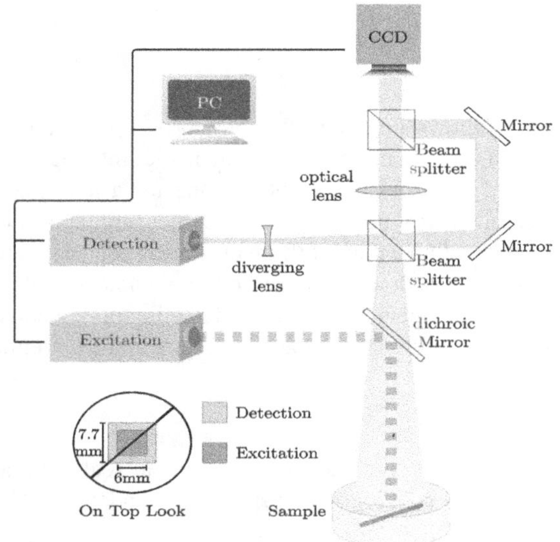

Fig 1: HPAT system. Use of interference from backscattered light of the phantom-surface and reference light to measure deformation on a nanometer scale.

2.2 Material for the phantoms

The main material for the construction of the phantoms was a two-component silicone (Wacker, Elastosil RT 604 A/B). This silicone consists of silicone oil and hardens by combining both parts. The transparent silicone can be varied in optical properties by additives to enhance scattering or absorption. As a result, the silicone provides an advantageous variability in its characteristics. The phantoms should have different optical properties. On the one hand, the absorbent structure should provide an optical absorption coefficient μ_a in the range of oxy-haemoglobin, $\mu_a = 3$ cm^{-1} at 1064 nm, which is often used as contrast agent in human tissue. On the other hand, a surrounding carrier matrix with an optical scattering coefficient μ_s near to human skin, $\mu_s = 10$ cm^{-1} at 1064 nm [5], is needed.

In order to vary optical features different additives were used. To simulate the oxy-haemoglobin, a part of the silicone (Wacker, Elastosil RT 604 A) was blended with graphite powder (pureness: 99.7%, particle size: 55 μm) to enhance the absorption. The carrier matrix was made of both parts of silicone oil. To vary μ_s, the silicone was mixed with barium sulfate $BaSO_4$ (pureness: 99.4%). An advantage in the use of $BaSO_4$ is the high x-ray density. This allows a co-evaluation using a μ-CT, which shows advantage compared to the reconstruction. The accuracy of reconstructed data can then be determined, through an comparison of the reconstructed data.

2.3 Manufacturing of the phantoms

As a first step in producing phantoms, the silicone was blended with barium sulfate. In order to achieve a homogeneous distribution of the scattering bodies, the mixture was blended for 30 minutes with a magnetic stirrer. The mixture was filled out in Petri dishes. The Petri dishes were prepared with two holes on opposite sides, to place needles to them. The needles had different diameter from 0.6 mm to 1.8 mm. They are used as a reservation of space for a absorbing fluid within the surrounding matrix. In order to reduce the acoustic scattering through air the filled Petri dishes were evacuated. After evacuation the mixture was heated up in an oven to 50 degree for 45 minutes to speed up the hardening. After cool down of the medium, the needles were removed and replaced by a silicone graphite mixture. To prevent the leak of fluid from holes, they were sealed with tape.

2.4 Adding doubling method

The adding doubling method is an approach to determine the scattering and absorption coefficient of a sample by measuring the transmittance and reflection for a specific thickness of the sample. Important for this calculation is the homogeneity of the sample with respect to the scattering and that the reflectance and transmittance is high enough. The first approximation is for a thin slice of the sample whose scattering would be single scattering. After calculating the scattering of a thin slice, the diameter of the sample is mathematically doubled and the new transmittance and reflectance is determined. These steps are repeated until the thickness in calculation and the sample are matching.

To measure transmittance and reflectance integrated spheres are often used. These spheres are coated with a high reflective material like barium sulfate ($BaSO_4$). The reflectance of barium sulfate is about 96%, so there is just a little loss of light at the surface of the spheres but this can be considered by a reference measurement. In total there are 3 measurements necessary to estimate the scattering coefficient. A zero measurement to compensate the loss of light without a sample and the measurements of transmittance and reflectance [6]. The different measurements are shown in Fig.2.

2.5 Signal evaluation and temporal filtering

The data acquisition by the HPAT system is based on speckle interferometry. Speckles are local spots in which the reflection of coherent light sources at optical rough surfaces leads to a constructive interference. Caused by the

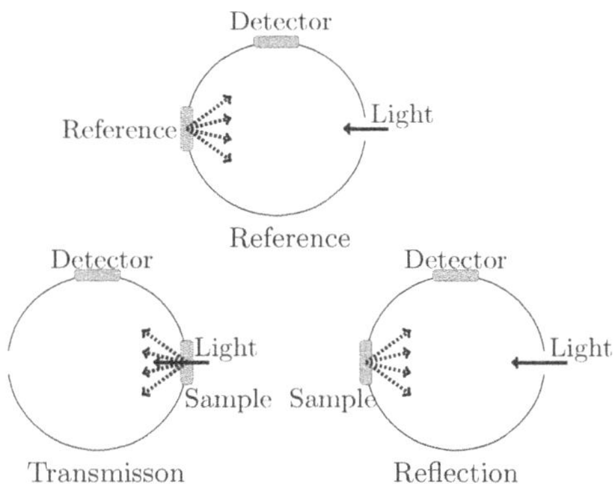

Fig 2: Different arrangements of the sample in a sphere for the acquisition of data for the adding doubling method

constructive interference, the phase within a speckle is constant. By using the static phase and the interference with reference light, information about the relative phase, between surface and camera, within a speckle can be acquired. To detect a displacement, the relative phase of a speckle at the deformed interface has to be compared to the relative phase of the initial undeformed surface. Each phase calculation at pixels which are not part of a speckle are calculated wrong and are randomly distributed. The calculated displacement of a pixel within and a pixel outside of a speckle, while there was no deformation through excitation, is shown in Fig.3.

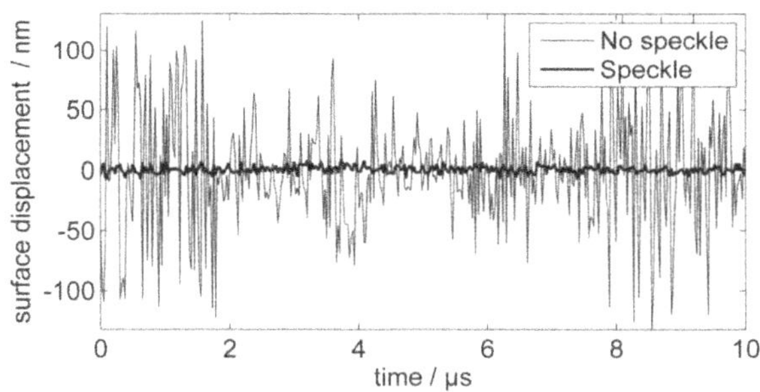

Fig 3: Calculated surface displacement, without excitation, from a pixel which is part of a speckle and a pixel which isn't part of a speckle.

The fluctuations of the calculated deformation show a high noise amplitude in regions outside a speckle, where no information can be revealed. The noise values are covering the complete dynamic range of the measurement and have the highest sampled frequency. In regions within a speckle, the noise is substancially lower and mainly caused by photon noise. In order to separate the high frequency, high amplitude noise in the space between speckles and the true photoacoustic signal, a temporal low-pass filter can be used.

3 Results and Discussion

3.1 Optical properties of the phantoms

To calculate the needed concentration of barium sulfate in silicone for optical scattering comparable to human skin, different concentrations were measured and the scattering coefficients were calculated [1]. The results are shown in Fig.4.

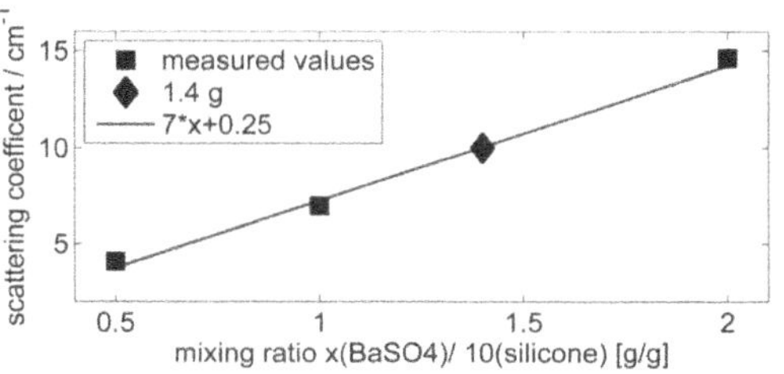

Fig 4: Concentration of barium sulfate in silicone and the resulting scattering coefficient. The squares represent the measured values and the diamond the needed concentration to reach an optical scattering coefficient like skin.

After determination of the scattering coefficient of the different concentrations, a nearly linear dependence between concentration and scattering would be recognised. To investigate the concentration which is needed to reach a $\mu_s = 10\text{cm}^{-1}$ a regression line of the measured values was constructed. The calculated mixing ratio out of the regression line is 1.4 g barium sulfate on 10 g silicone.
To simulate oxy-haemoglobin as a contrast agent a mixture from one part of the silicone and graphite powder was prepared. The mixing ratio to achieve a μ_a like oxy-haemoglobin was $0.3\ g/10\ g$.

3.2 Photoacoustic measurement of the phantoms

The sketch at Fig.5 illustrates the shape and position of the absorbent structure within the produced phantoms.

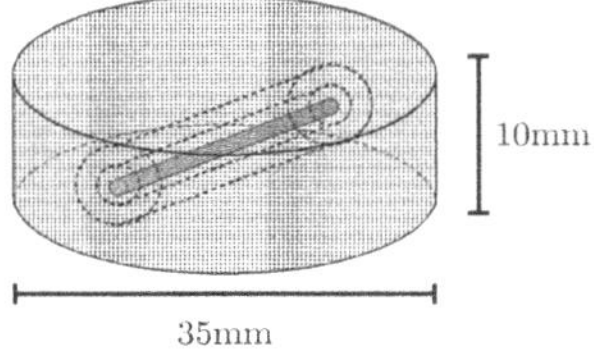

Fig 5: Shape of the produced phantom and position of the absorbent structure within the phantoms.

The different produced phantoms were adjusted in the HPAT set-up to study the surface displacement triggered by the PA ultrasound emission. A region of interest (ROI) for each phantom with a size of 300 μm^2 was defined and the temporal conduct of the mean value of this ROI was examined. From the delay between the excitation pulse and

[1] http://omlc.org/software/iad/index.html

the time of arrival, the depth was determined. To calculate the depths, the delay has to be multiplied by the velocity of sound, within the phantom. The results and expected distance between the absorbing structures and the surface are shown in table 1.

Table 1: Variation in the size of absorbing structures and distances to the surface. The measured depth is based on time of displacement peak and the velocity of sound, which is determined with 900 m/s.

Phantom No.	absorber diameter [mm]	estimated depth [mm]	measured depth [mm]	variance [mm]
1	0.6	1.7	1.2	0.5
2	0.6	2.8	2.5	0.3
3	1.0	1.7	1.6	0.1
4	1.0	3	2.9	0.1
5	1.8	2.5	1.9	0.6
6	1.8	4	4.2	0.2

The differences between the estimated and measured depths are in a sub-millimeter scale. The results fit the expected data very well and shows that the acquisition of data from absorbing structure with a diameter of 1.8 mm in depths up to 4 mm is possible.

3.3 Effect of the temporal filtering

In order to investigate and compare the impact of the temporal filtering, the mean values and the standard deviation in an ROI of 300 μm^2 before and after filtering with a cut-off frequency of 2 MHz have to be compared. The cut-off frequency was higher then the expected maximum signal frequency of 1.5 MHz. The mean values are shown in Fig 6.

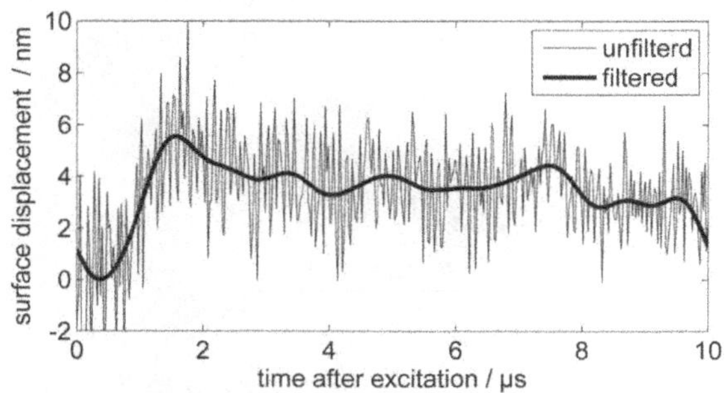

Fig 6: Difference between original data and the 2 MHz low-pass filtered data from an cylindrical absorber in a ROI of 300 μm^2.

The result of the filtering is a reduction of the standard deviation, from 2.0 nm unfiltered to 1.14 nm filtered, with a small effect to the mean value, 3.44 nm to 3.45 nm. The small effect on the average illustrates the random but uniformly distributed values which are not speckle. The use of the filter provides a good suppression of local artefacts with a high frequency and a low influence of the correctly recorded data.

4 Conclusion

We developed a reproducible and well defined tissue phantom made of silicone. The use of transparent two component silicone provides the advantage to vary and adjust properties like optical scattering μ_s and absorption coefficients μ_a. The mixing ratio from barium sulfate and silicone of about $1.4/10$ was determined to get optical scattering like human skin at 1064 nm. Furthermore the mixing ratio of graphite powder and liquid silicone oil from $0.3/10$ was defined to simulate blood. The possibility of the HPAT system to collect data from an object which is similar too skin with a radiation exposure below the maximum radiant exposure for human skin could also be examined. In addition, the benefit of a temporal filter was investigated to suppress the noise of local artefacts without a large impact on the acquired data which is correctly calculated. In summary, well defined phamtoms were developed, which are suitable for further investigations at HPAT.

Acknowledgement

The work has been carried out at the Medical Laser Center Lübeck GmbH, Luebeck, Germany and the Institute of Biomedical Optics, Universität zu Lübeck, Luebeck, Germany.

5 References

[1] G. M. Spirou, A. A. Oraevsky, I. A. Vitkin, and W. M. Whelan, "Optical and acoustic properties at 1064 nm of polyvinyl chloride-plastisol for use as a tissue phantom in biomedical optoacoustics," *Physics in Medicine and Biology*, vol. 50, no. 14, p. N141, 2005.

[2] S. E. Bohndiek, S. Bodapati, D. Van De Sompel, S.-R. Kothapalli, and S. S. Gambhir, "Development and application of stable phantoms for the evaluation of photoacoustic imaging instruments," *PloS one*, vol. 8, no. 9, p. e75533, 2013.

[3] A. Standard, "Z136. 1. american national standard for the safe use of lasers. american national standards institute," *Inc., New York*, 2000.

[4] J. Horstmann and R. Brinkmann, "Non-contact photoacoustic tomography using holographic full field detection," vol. 8800, pp. 880007–880007–6, 2013. 10.1117/12.2033599.

[5] S. L. Jacques, "Skin optics," *Oregon Medical Laser Center News*, vol. 1998, no. 1, pp. 1–9, 1998.

[6] S. A. Prahl, "The adding-doubling method," in *Optical-thermal response of laser-irradiated tissue*, pp. 101–129, Springer, 1995.

Investigation of the influence of pulse variations on photoacoustic response and damage thresholds for laser induced bubble formation at the fundus of the eye

G. Vogel [1], K. Schlott [2], and R. Brinkmann [2]

[1] Medizinische Ingenieurwissenschaft, Universität zu Lübeck, vogel@miw.uni-luebeck.de
[2] Medizinisches Laserzentrum Lübeck GmbH, {schlott,brinkmann}@bmo.uni-luebeck.de

Abstract

Selective retina therapy is a gentle method of treatment for certain retinal diseases. It is conducted under conservation of the photoreceptors. For therapeutic purposes, it is important to know the damage threshold in dependence of laser energy. A pulsed laser was used in this work. The temporal laser pulse shape changes with the pulse energy. To attenuate energy without changing the shape of the pulse, optical filters were used to investigate the influence of the pulse shape independently from the energy. Porcine eyes were radiated, which were examined for laser induced damage using a fluorescence microscope. Two contact lenses with built-in ultrasound transducers were employed to examine their suitability for detecting ultrasonic waves emitted by laser induced micro bubbles. The resulting transients were analyzed with respect to visible fluctuations and by using a mathematically algorithm. As a result of this work, an energy threshold for visible damage generation was evaluated.

1 Introduction

The strongly absorbing property of the retinal pigment epithelium (RPE) of the fundus of the human eye is used by selective retina therapy (SRT). The RPE is a heavily pigmented monocellular layer between the retina and the choroid and serves the metabolism and the regulation of fluid content between the two layers [1]. In contrast to the conventional laser photocoagulation , in which a continuous wave laser is used, short laser pulses in the range of microseconds are applied in this work [2], [3]. By the pulses, the temperature increase is limited to the cells of the RPE without an influence of heat conduction. This approach with pulsed light is advantageous to treat degenerative diseases like age-related macular degeneration and macular edema, because it leads to a recovering effect on the RPE, resulting in an increase of metabolism [4], [5], [6]. By the short pulses, the increase in temperature is limited to the RPE, leading to laser-induced micro bubble formation. The bubbles are acoustically detectable because they emit ultrasound waves. These acoustic transients can be detected by an piezoelectric ultrasound microphon which is embedded into a contact lens placed on the cornea.
There are special requirements to the design and frequency domain of the transducer. In this paper, there are described two different contact lenses with built-in ultrasound-transducers, which came to use for the irradiation of enucleated porcine eyes. The resulting transients were analyzed mathematically and visually with respect to differences between supraliminal and subliminal laser treatment due to bubble formation.
The second focus of this project is the contemplation of the impact of changes in the pulse length and pulse shape with increasing energy on the effect of bubble formation and the visible damage to the explant. Increasing energy leads to pulse elongation. Two energy ranges were investigated separately in order to determine the influence on bubble formation. It is also assumed that pulse variations have an influence on the acoustic signal and the predictability of a tissue damage.
Threshold value criteria were considered, for example the energy and an optoacoustic value (OA-value), which was calculated to distinguish the transients to predict micro bubble formation reliably. Because the bubble formation and the resulting damage is not visible for the attending physician without optoacoustic feedback, the damage was examined microscopically.

2 Material and Methods

For the experiments, a frequency-doubled ND: YAG therapy laser (modified Visulas 532, Carl Zeiss Meditec AG) was used. The laser emits green light with a wavelength of 532 nm. It can be used in a continuous wave mode and a pulsed mode. 30 pulses were applicated for each lesion, leading to 30 optoacoustic transients for each pulse sequence. The pulse rate was set to 100 Hz. The laser pulses were coupled into a square fiber which couples the signal into a slitlamp. The irradiation beam diameter can be set

from 70 μm to 1000 μm on the slitlamp. In this work, 70 μm was chosen.
The fundus explant was placed into a cuvette at a distance of about 23 mm to the contact lens, which corresponds to the average axial length of the human eye. During the irradiation, the cuvette was filled with *physiological saline solution* (NaCl 0.9 %) at room temperature. For each measurement series, a square sample of the fundus of porcine eyes was extracted. The retina was removed under use of *Ringer's solution* to avoid disturbance of the measurement by uncontrolled detachment. The eyes were stored in *Dulbecco's modified eagle's medium* (DMEM) (D6046, Sigma-Aldrich, Co.) in the refrigerator. To full setup is shown in Fig. 1.

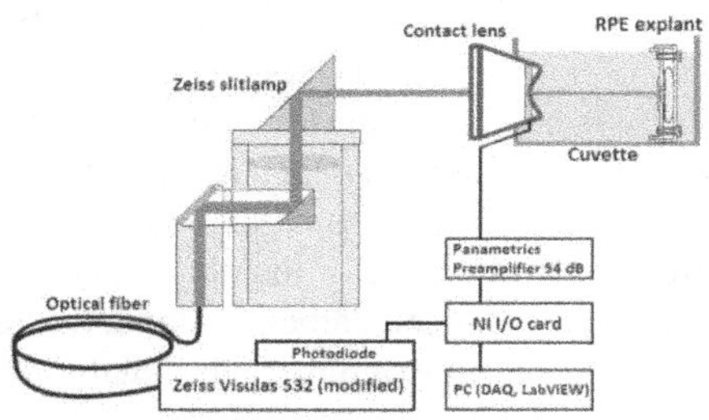

Figure 1: Optical setup for SRT. For the measurements with the Zeiss contact lens, the preamplifier was not required due to a built-in preamplifier in the contact lens.

The first series of measurements were performed using a contact lens by Zeiss with an integrated amplifier. It has the optics of a Mainster contact lens and a resonance frequency of 1 MHz. A series of 21 explants were irradiated. The laser spot was focused on the explant in the cuvette using the red pilot laser spot. The laser energy was adjusted from a minimum of 5 μJ up to a maximum of 58 μJ. The lesions were applied in a grid to the tissue, considering an approximately straight beam path trough the contact lens. This procedure resulted in 12 lesions per sample. Marker lesions were applied for visible orientation. To determine the damage threshold, all explants were examined by using the fluorescent dye Calcein immediately after irradiation. The 30 transients for each pulse sequence were recorded digitally using a data acquisition card (GaGe) and the data was evaluated, visualized and stored by a LabVIEW (National Instruments) routine.
Further measurements were performed with a contact lens of different properties (Mainster). It was operated with a preamplifier (Panametrics), which was set to 54 dB. The laser parameters were the same as those of the measurements with the Zeiss contact lens to obtain a direct comparison between the two contact lenses. 16 explants were irradiated. The intention of the measurement series with the Mainster contact lens was it to separate the energy range of the laser into two sections depending on the shape of the temporal laser pulse to obtain a series of equidistant energy values but two fixed pulse shapes. This was achieved by using optical filters with different optical density. The two

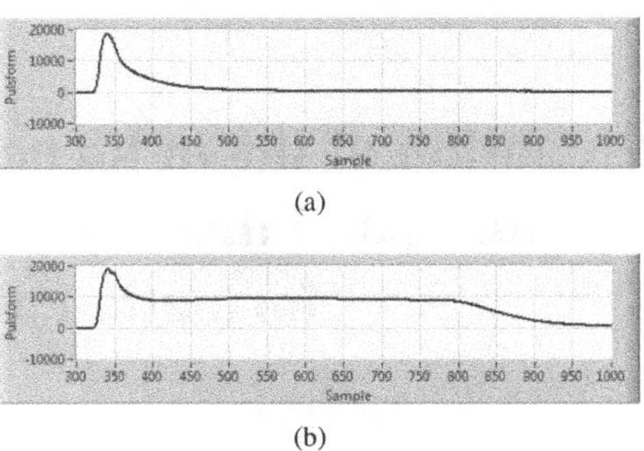

Figure 2: Shape of the laser pulse with increasing energy: (a) 15 μJ (Shape 1) and (b) 30 μJ (Shape 2). This graphic is a representation of the temporal development of the laser pulses for different energies. Both axis are sectioned in arbitrary units. The y-axis corresponds to the measured voltage by the photodiode, the x-axis is proportional to the time elapsed. One sample-unit correlates to a time frame of about 0.05 μs. The energy (area beneath the curve) grows into a shoulder region of the curve when a particular threshold value of energy is exceeded, and the amplitude of the first peak (length = 5 μs, approximately) is no longer increased. The threshold is defined with a value greater than 15 μJ. The length of the pulse has a maximum of about 30 μs.

defined pulse shapes can be seen in Fig. 2. If the energy is attenuated by the laser control panel, the shape of the laser-pulse for each energy value changes. Furthermore, from an energy of about 15 μJ, the amplitude of the first peak is no longer increased, instead the pulse developes a shoulder region. These two cases were considered separately. The development of the laser pulse with increasing energy was obtained by using LabVIEW. The pulse was detected by a photodiode, which is built into the laser.
To define nearly equidistant energy intervals, first the maximum value for each pulse shape was considered. For the case in which increasing pulse energy leads to an increased peak of the laser pulse, a maximum of 15 μJ is defined. In the other case, in which the increasing energy leads to a temporal extension of the pulse without an increase of the peak, a maximum of 55 μJ was defined. To attenuate the energy in 5 μJ steps, two optical filters were used, one with an optical density of 0.3 and another filter with an optical density of 0.15. The filters were used individually and in combination and were mounted in front of the contact lens. This procedure was an attempt to reduce the change in the pulse shape for each energy sector as possible.

2.1 Evaluation of the optoacoustic transients

To define a threshold criterion with respect to the tissue damage, the recorded transients were evaluated. After each lesion and thus after each pulse sequence, the resulting 30 transients were displayed superimposed by the SRT measuring program. The bubble formation was evaluated visually based on the fluctuations of the superimposed transients

to each other. Large amplitude- and phase differences between the curves indicate the formation of micro bubbles in the RPE cells. Fig. 3 shows two images of superimposed transients for two energy values. To obtain a reliable criterion, the transients were analyzed mathematically by using an algorithm whose basic structure was implemented as a part of a doctoral thesis in LabVIEW at the Medical Laser Center Lübeck (MLL) [7]. The algorithm provides a dimensionless value (OA-value) by which a threshold is to be defined and was developed to distinguish purely thermoelastic transients and thermoelastic transients with micro bubble formation. The basic structure of the algorithm is explained in the following.
From the $n = 30$ measured transients $P_j(t)$ the average transient $\bar{P}(t)$ is calculated:

$$\bar{P}(t) = \frac{1}{n}\sum_{j=1}^{n} P_j(t) \tag{1}$$

In the following, the averaged transient $\bar{P}(t)$ of all measured transients $P_j(t)$ is subtracted. This results in the deviation $D_j(t)$ of the transients $P_j(t)$ from the average transient $\bar{P}(t)$:

$$\bar{D}_j(t) = P_j(t) - \bar{P}(t). \tag{2}$$

The magnitude of the deviations D_j is then integrated over a time interval $[t_1, t_2]$:

$$E_j = \int_{t_1}^{t_2} |D_j(t)| dt \tag{3}$$

The value $E_j(t)$ describes the deviation of the transient $P_j(t)$ from the average transient $\bar{P}_j(t)$. The maximum value of the deviations $E_j(t)$ is defined as the OA-value:

$$OA \ \ value = max[E_j], \quad j = 1...n. \tag{4}$$

This value is a measure of the maximum pressure differences of a pulse train in a predetermined time range [7].

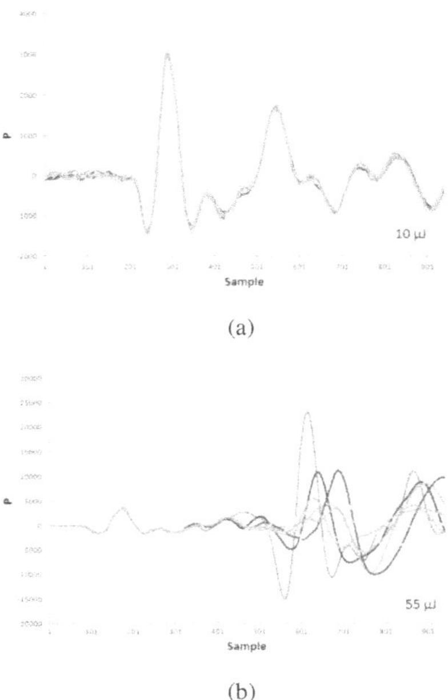

(a)

(b)

Figure 3: Exemplary transients detected with the Mainster contact lens: (a) Subliminal irradiation (Pulse shape 1) without micro bubble formation and (b) above threshold irradiation (Pulse shape 2) with micro bubble formation. The bubble formation is evaluated based on the fluctuations of the transients with respect to differences in amplitude and phase. Large fluctuations indicate micro bubble formation in the melanin granules. The units of the axes are arbitrary units.P is proportional to the detected voltage by the transducer. The x-axis describes the time elapsed. One sample unit corresponds approximately to 0.005 μs. The transit time trough the cuvette is cut off, the transients arise only after the laser pulses have reached the RPE explant. The images are an illustration of the transients and their ratio to each other.

3 Results and Discussion

The contact lenses were evaluated and compared with respect to their suitability for detecting evaluable transients. The OA-values and energies were assigned to the visibilities of the lesions.

3.1 Measurements with the Zeiss contact lens

Fig. 4 shows the distribution of OA-values and energies with respect to the visibility of tissue damage under the fluorescence microscope. Considering the energies, there is an overlap in the range of 20 μJ and 40 μJ. Despite this, the energy threshold for bubble formation can be defined with 45 μJ (Fig. 4a). The distribution of OA-values is not distinct, the values for energies corresponding to a subliminal irradiation are concentrated in a range of less than 100 (Fig 4b). The values for visible lesions are spread over the entire range of OA-values, resulting in an overlap. Hence an absolute threshold can not be defined. Furthermore, the threshold value with the Zeiss contact lens above which micro bubble formation can be verified is defined with $OA > 989.784$.

3.2 Measurements with the Mainster contact lens and optical filters

Fig. 5 shows the distribution of OA-values and energies with respect to the visibility of tissue damage. To vary the energy values, optical filters were used. These measurements were performed to evaluate the dependence of the micro bubble formation of the two pulse shapes. Considering the energy distribution, there is a larger overlap than in the measurements with the Zeiss contact lens (Fig. 5a). The energy threshold for this measurements can be defined with 55 μJ. The OA-threshold value is considered with $OA > 6608.76$ (Fig. 5b). Furthermore, the results show that bubble formation only occurs under irradation with pulse shape 2 ($E > 15\,\mu$J), exept for one lesion (15 μJ).

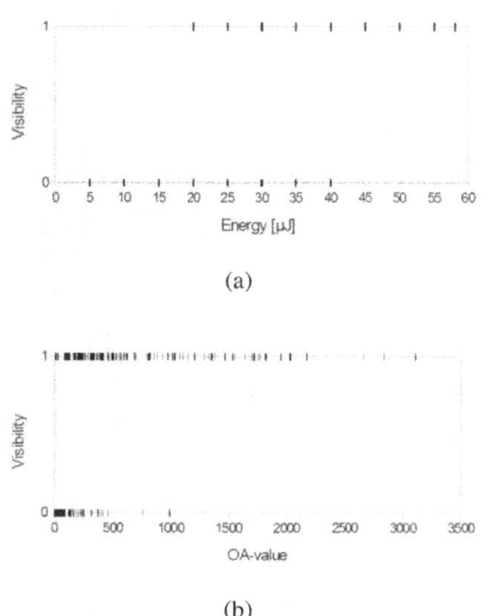

Figure 4: Visibilities of tissue damage by use of the Zeiss contact lens (0: no visible damage of the RPE, 1: visible damage of the RPE): (a) Applied energy and associated visibility (b) Calculated OA-values and corresponding visibility.

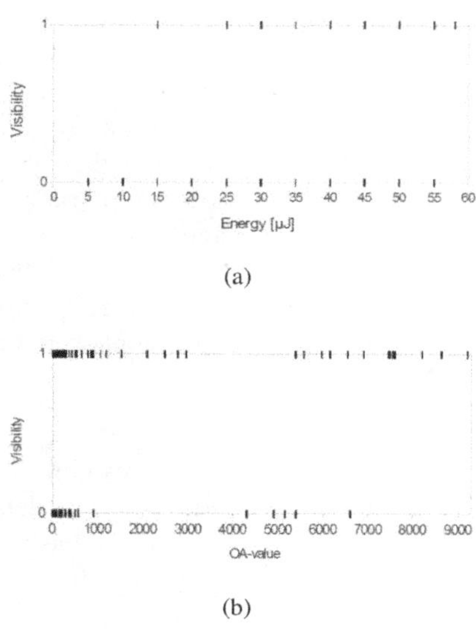

Figure 5: Visibilities of tissue damage by use of the Mainster contact lens (0: no visible damage of the RPE, 1: visible damage of the RPE): (a) Applied energy and associated visibility (b) Calculated OA-values and associated visibility.

4 Conclusion

For the explants irradiated in this work, it has been shown that the shape of the laser pulse has an influence of micro bubble formation. It has been proved, that micro bubbles in RPE cells can be generated above a certain energy by the modified laser used in this work. Threshold energies for tissue damage for the use of two contact lenses could be defined. Despite a wide scattering, a threshold for bubble formation from the OA-values was defined. The threshold values determined in this work describe the maximum energy und OA-values, at which no damage is visible. Despite this, the minimum values for the energy and the OA-values at which a damage is visible, are beneath the maximum values. This results in an overlap, which must be reduced for a reliable predictability of micro bubble formation.

The algorithm has to be modified in order to distinguish transients more clearly with respect to micro bubble formation, because the overlap can not be reduced with further measurements. Furthermore, the contact lenses could be varied in order to investigate different frequency responses of the embedded transducers and their influence on the detected transients. For further statements regarding the tissue damage, the period between irradiation and evaluation of the damage should be varied. With respect to a clinical use of the laser system, further in-vivo and in-vitro measurements are necessary.

Acknowledgement

The work has been carried out at the Medical Laser Center Lübeck (MLL) GmbH, Lübeck.

5 References

[1] R. Brinkmann and R. Birngruber, *Selektive Retina Therapie (SRT).* in: Z.Med.Phys., Elsevier, vol. 17, no. 1, pp. 6–22, 2007.

[2] H. Elsner et al., *Selective retina therapy in patients with central serous chorioretinopathy.* Graefe's Arch Clin Exp Opthalmol 244, Springer Verlag, pp. 1638–1645, 2006.

[3] C. Framme, G. Schuele, J. Roider, R. Birngruber and R. Brinkmann, *Influence of pulse duration and pulse number in selective RPE laser treatment.* in: Laser in Surgery and Medicine, Wiley-Liss, Inc., vol. 34, no. 3, pp. 206–215, 2004.

[4] P. Prahs et al., *Selective retina therapy (SRT) in patients with geographic atrophy due to age-related macular degeneration.* Graefe's Arch Clin Exp Opthalmol 248, Springer Verlag, vol. 248, no. 5, pp. 651–658, 2010.

[5] J. Roider et al, *Selective retina therapy (SRT) for clinically significant diabetic macula edema.* in: Lasers in Surgery and Medicine, Wiley-Liss, Inc., vol. 248, no. 9, pp. 206–215, 2004.

[6] R. Brinkmann, J. Roider, R. Birngruber, *Selective Retina Therapy (SRT): A review on methods, techniques, preclinical and first clinical results.* in Bull. Soc. belge Opthalmol, vol. 302, pp. 51–69, 2006.

[7] G. Schüle, *Mechanismen und On-line Dosimetrie bei selektiver RPE Therapie.* PhD Thesis, Universität zu Lübeck, 2002.

Development of a new, non-invasive, laser-assisted experimental model for Fuchs Endothelial Dystrophy

A. Pahl [1], S. Grisanti [2], M. Ranjbar [2], A. Vogel [3], F. Reinholz [3]

[1] Medizinische Ingenieurwissenschaft, Universität zu Lübeck, pahl@miw.uni-luebeck.de

[2] Department of Ophthalmology, Universitätsklinikum Schleswig-Holstein, {salvatore.grisanti, mahdy.ranjbar}@uksh.de

[3] Institute of Biomedical Optics, Universität zu Lübeck, {vogel, reinholz}@bmo.uni-luebeck.de

Abstract

Fuchs endothelial corneal dystrophy is characterized by progressive lesions of the corneal endothelium leading to the formation of a corneal edema. Current treatment methods aim at replacing the affected cornea through allogeneic transplantation. Drug therapies that prevent disease progression or induce healing in early stages do not exist yet. To explore such approaches, it is necessary to develop suitable experimental models that simulate these particular early stages of the disease. Therefore, it was investigated whether single endothelial cell defects can be caused by a Nd:YAG laser in porcine corneas. In addition, the usage of light and multi-photon microscopy for quantification of the laser-induced lesions was evaluated. The experiments showed that laser pulses in a small, centrally circumscribed area of the cornea provide the best results. In order to develop a model for the early form of Fuchs endothelial dystrophy the chosen parameters still need to be optimized.

1 Introduction

Fuchs endothelial corneal dystrophy (FECD) is a progressive, degenerative disease of the cornea, in which the back side of the cornea, the endothelium, is affected. This monolayer of hexagonal cells regulates the hydration state of the cornea by means of active pumping processes resulting in its transparency. Throughout life, the number of endothelial cells decreases. The physiological cell loss from postnatal to adult is about 3.000 cells per mm^2 and can be compensated by adjustment processes of the remaining cells [1]. However, a regeneration of the post-mitotic tissue is not possible. If the density falls below 500 cells per mm^2 due to pathogenic processes, corneal problems are the result [2]. In 1910, Ernst Fuchs reported pathological changes in the cornea that characterize the clinical picture of FECD. In addition to the thickening of Descemet's membrane, the basal membrane of the endothelium, and the formation of the so-called cornea guttata [cf. Fig. 1] by collagen deposits, a dilution and excessive loss of endothelial cells happen [3]. Due to increasing lesions in the endothelial cell layer and the associated reduced pumping capacity of the remaining endothelium, intraocular fluid is able to enter the corneal stroma resulting in corneal edema. The uniform structure of the cornea is changed and blurring occurs, which reduces the visual acuity. A highly advanced stage of the disease results in a complete loss of eyesight.

The exact cause for the development of FECD is still unknown and subject of research. Gene mutations are considered to be responsible for the onset of the disease [4].

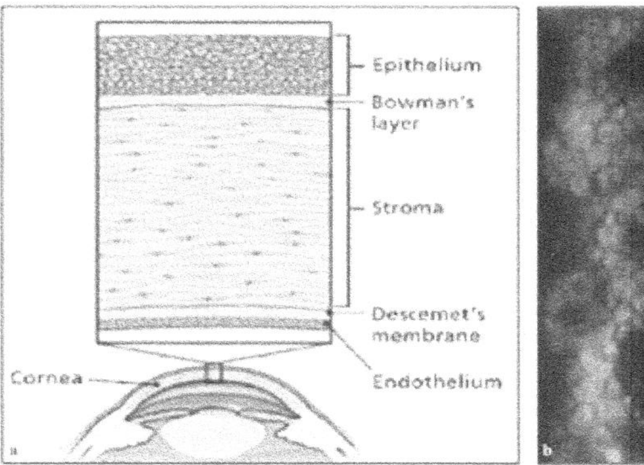

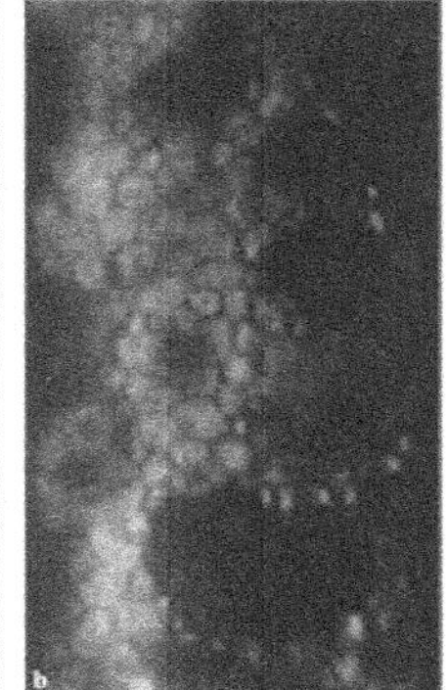

Figure 1: a: Cornea structure [7]. b: Microscopic photograph of a cornea guttata [8]

There are different options for therapy dependent on the stage of the disease. In early stages hypertonic eye drops or therapeutic contact lenses are applied to temporarily dehydrate the cornea. In late stages corneal transplantation is needed [5].

All those therapies have been tested in experimental models, which simulate the disease, beforehand. These models are based on the use of Benzalkonium- Chloride to damage the endothelium chemically. Normally however, this causes widespread toxically induced lesions that are characteristic to late stages of the disease. Furthermore, inflammatory alterations of different tissues like the iris, lens and other corneal layers can emerge that are not pathognomonic

for FECD [6]. In order to develop a model for early stage FECD it is necessary to consider a different approach for damaging single endothelial cells.
The aim of this investigation was to explore whether endothelial cells of porcine corneas could be damaged mechanically through treatment with a laser. During that investigation several questions arose, which had to be answered:

1. Are whole eye bulbs or corneal flaps the better specimen for the chosen type of imaging?
2. How does intracamerally injected Methocel affect the preparation of corneal flaps?
3. How should the laser pulses be arranged in order to produce proper data?
4. How many laser pulses does it take to produce visible, circumscribed endothelial defects?
5. What pulse energy has to be used to produce the smallest lesions possible?

2 Material and Methods

2.1 Preparation

Porcine eyes were used for the experiments, because of the comparable anatomy to human eyes. They were freshly enucleated and at the time of the experiments not older than 5 hours. Until their use they were stored at around 5 degrees Celsius to stop enzymatic processes and prevent the early decomposition of cells. In a first step the eyes were cleaned of excessive tissue (muscles, fat, optic nerve) so that the pure eye bulb remained. The eye bulbs were rinsed and stored in Phosphate buffered saline (PBS). The adjusted PBS solution represents an environment similar to that of the lacrimal fluid. Therefore, it protects the cornea from dehydration.

2.2 Laser treatment

Table 1: Parameters of laser treatment

laser area	1x10 mm	3x4 mm	1x4 mm
laser points per area	10	5	8
pulse energy [mJ]	4.3	4.3	2.6
laser area	1x4 mm	1x2 mm	1x2 mm
laser points per area	4	1	1
pulse energy [mJ]	2.6	2.6	1.3

Damaging of the endothelial cells was performed with the slit lamp-laser-unit visuLAS YAG II plus from ZEISS.

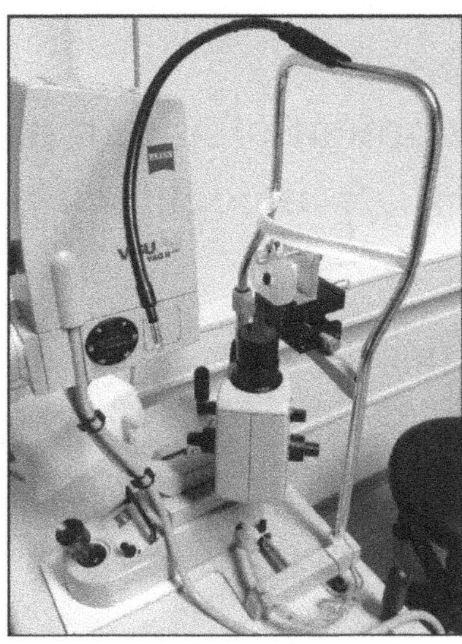

Figure 2: Fixated eye bulb in slit lamp-laser-unit.

The Nd:YAG laser has a wavelength of 1064 nm. The beam diameter in air is 10 microns.
The eye bulb was inserted in a specially designed holder that can be fastened on the chin rest of the slit lamp [Figure 2]. Thus, rotation of the eyeball was avoided and the cornea was accessible. A 12x magnification function of the slit-lamp was used. The illumination unit was deflected to visualize the individual corneal layers in an optical section. The focusing beam was positioned so that a water jet was produced in the anterior chamber. In the best case, this induced defects in the corneal endothelium by ejecting cells out of the tissue. For marking the region of interest on the cornea a cutting punch was used. These areas differed depending on location and size.
Also, the number of laser points per field and the energy of the individual laser pulses was varied. Table 1 lists the six different experiments. Four eyes were treated for each experiment, summing up to 24 eyes.

2.3 Cornea preparation

Methocel (0.2 ml) was injected into the anterior chamber via a clear-cornea small incision to stabilize the eye during the trepanation process. The corneal flap was produced by a punch with a diameter of 10 mm.

2.4 Imaging

For visualization a multi-photon microscope (MPM) including a standard bright field mode of operation was used. Via transmission mode a rough impression of the sample was obtained. To achieve this, lenses with 4- and 16-fold magnification were used. The MPM was then used for a more detailed inspection.
The MPM consisted of a TriM Scope II microscope. The light source was a mode-coupled 80 MHz Titanium-Sapphire Laser: the MaiTai HP with a tuning band of 690 up to 1040 nm. The average optical power was more than

2.5 W. The laser was controlled via a computer. The sample carrier table was adjustable in all three axes. An immersion lens from Olympus with a 25-fold magnification, a Numerical Aperture of 1.05 and a working distance of 2 mm was used. Methocel served as immersion medium.
The sample was excited with pulses of 100 to 220 fs at a wavelength of 740 nm and an averaged optical power of about 20 mW. This caused auto-fluorescence in the tissue, which could be detected via 4 false color channels (grey, red, green, blue) by a photo-multiplier. Before the start of the actual series of experiments the imaging method was tested in untreated eye bulbs and cornea flaps with or without prior Methocel injection.
For fixation and positioning of the eye bulb a special support receptacle was used. The flap is put onto a microscope slide, which had a cavity on the top to avoid slipping of the sample. The endothelium was pointing upwards.

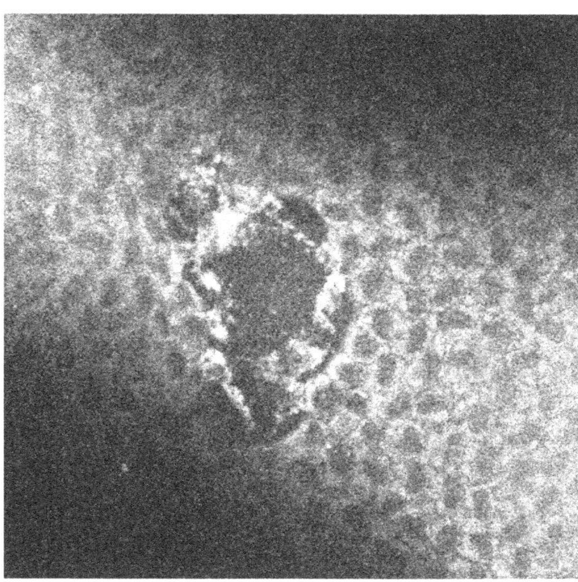

Figure 3: Laser-induced peripheral defect of endothelial cells with pulse energy of 2.6 mJ.

3 Results and Discussion

3.1 Preparation of samples

In the examination of the eye bulbs with transmitted light microscopy the endothelial tissue layers were hardly recognizable. The MPM showed only details of the epithelium and stroma. Despite the excellent transparency of the cornea the penetration depth of the MPM was not sufficient. Therefore, it was necessary to prepare cornea flaps before imaging to examine and analyze potential endothelial defects. They had to be placed in the cavity of the slide with the endothelial side pointing upwards. This was the only way to obtain clear auto-fluorescence images of endothelial cells in the MPM.

3.2 Influence of Methocel injection

Cornea flaps without prior injection of Methocel showed very disturbing, dotted artifacts. When they were limited to a small area, the endothelial structures could barely be seen. The artifacts were caused by iris pigment coming from the high tension induced on the cornea. If the back surface of the cornea touches the iris during the trepanation procedure small particles adhered. In the chosen wavelength band their autofluorescence is much higher than that of the endothelium because of their high amount of pigmented fluorophores. In order to generate MPM pictures that are suitable for analysis the cornea flap had to be punched with the smallest amount of force possible. Injecting Methocel supported the integrity of the tissue and prevented a collapse of the anterior chamber while punching.

3.3 Imaging

Due to the 2-photon excitation of the sample with infrared light (740 nm) tissue autofluorescence was generated. This was best detected in the green (495 - 560 nm) and blue (435 - 495 nm) color channel.
However, the natural curvature of the cornea decreased the field of view significantly. The MPM provided a maximum field of 400 x 400 μm but only one strip of cells could be recognized clearly. To get an overview of the film of endothelial cells the measurement depths for one scan had to be adjusted continuously. Before each shot this depth area had to be estimated and adjusted. The microscopic examination of the flaps showed clear endothelial structures and could consequently be used as an aid in orientation for the experimental measurements.

3.4 Verification of damaged endothelial cells

The ten laser shots in the 10 mm area were nearly unrecognizable. Endothelial defects that were anticipated from light microscopy could not be verified with the MPM. The areas that could presumably contain defects were too big for the small field of view of MPM.
By using the smaller 4 mm markings the orientation improved. Light microscopy showed laser-induced lesions, but it was difficult to estimate in which tissue layer they were exactly located. Near the peripheral range of the markings single endothelial cells could be seen and discriminated. However, this could not be applied for a continuous field of cells. No cells were visible in the center. The MPM showed distinct laserinduced holes in the Descemet's membrane, but no endothelial cells. Thus, it can be assumed that the pulse energy of 4.3 mJ and the production of 5 laser dots each completely destroyed the endothelial layer in the corresponding marked areas.
Examination of the cornea with central laser dots and a pulse energy of 2.6 mJ provided similar results. Light microscopy showed laser-induced defects. The images taken with the MPM however showed small lesions in the peripheral area of the markings. The field of endothelial cells was

preserved. Only single cells had been torn out of the mosaic as seen in Figure 3. The whole endothelial cell structure was destroyed in the center of the sample like before.
The extent of damage of a single laser dot with energy of 2.6 mJ could easily be recognized in light microscopy. Thus, no cellular imaging with the MPM was deemed necessary. A distinct area without endothelial cells was spotted that covered the whole center of the marking. In the periphery smaller defects in transition into an intact field of endothelial cells were observed. More subtle defects could be produced utilizing smaller laser energy levels.
The expected extent of damage of a central laser dot with energy of 1.3 mJ could not be verified because all of the four punched cornea flaps showed intense structural damage. Yet, this experiment should be repeated eventually.

3.5 General observations

No comment could be made as to if eventual diseases or damages of the cornea were preexisting, because the endothelial layer could only be examined after trepanation. Also it had to be considered that the force of the punch might create damage to the endothelium. Those damages were expected in the peripheral area of the 10 mm punch, but a central impact could not be excluded. The consistency of the eye bulbs was not the same every time. So it could be that some eyes were taken from older animals than others and therefore had differences in structure. Soft eyes were more difficult to punch, so that despite support through intracameral Methocel iris pigment was attached to the endothelium. The evaluation was more complicated or not possible at all. Finally, the cornea is a small and light sample. It has to be considered that it might move during the application of an immersion lens. This again contributes to the difficulty of taking the images and analyzing them.

4 Conclusion

In summary, it can be stated that laser induced mechanical damage of endothelial cells of porcine eyes is possible.
To obtain meaningful data for developing a new model for FECD it is important to induce small, single laser pulses with energies $\leq$ 2.6 mJ. Yet, the settings of parameters to generate single cell lesions still need to be improved. Therefore, investigations related to the effect of small changes in the laser focus and the related change in distance to the endothelium should be performed.
To carry out before-after-comparisons of the examined eyes it can be recommended to image eyes of smaller animals. In this way the penetration depth of the MPM will suffice when a complete eye bulb is used. Moreover, the hazard of damaging the cornea by trepanation could thereby be eliminated. Finally, if porcine eyes shall be subject of these experiments again, another trepanation method based on a vacuumassisted trephine could be used.

Acknowledgement

This work has been carried out at the Department of Ophthalmology and the Institute of Biomedical Optics, Universität zu Lübeck.

5 References

[1] H. F. Edelhauser, *"The Balance between Corneal Transparency and Edema The Proctor Lecture"*, Invest. Ophthalmol. Vis. Sci., pp. 1755–1767, May 2006.

[2] M. Valtnik, M. Nitschke, T. Götze, K. Engelmann, C. Werner, *"Kultivierung transplantierbarer Zellverbände aus cornealem Endothel"*, Wiss. Z. Tech. Univ. Dresd., pp. 31–37, 2008.

[3] A. O. Eghrari and J. D. Gottsch, *"Fuchs' corneal dystrophy"*, Expert Rev Ophthalmol Author Manuscr., pp. 147–159, 2011.

[4] J. Teichmann, *"Tissue Engineering des Humanen Cornealen Endothels"*, 2013.

[5] L. H. Suh, V. Vaughn Emerson, A. S. Jun, *"Cornea and External Eye Disease Fuchs Endothelial Dystrophy: Pathogenesis and Management"*, 2008

[6] L. Bredow, J. Schwartzkopff, and T. Reinhard, *"Regeneration of corneal endothelial cells following keratoplasty in rats with bullous keratopathy"*, Mol. Vis., pp. 683–690, May 2014.

[7] S. A. Wilson and A. Last, *"Management of Corneal Abrasion"*, Am. Fam. Physician, pp. 123– 128, Jul. 2004.

[8] C. Akimune et al., *"Corneal guttata associated with the corneal dystrophy resulting from a beta-ig-h3 R124H mutation"*, vol. British Journal of Opthamology, pp. 67–71, 2000.

FT-IR investigation of the nonlinear optical crystal CLBO

O. Ragulina [1], R. Brinkmann [2] R. von Elm [3], and J. Lawrenz [3]

[1] Medizinische Ingeniuerwissenschaft, Universität zu Lübeck, ragulina@miw.uni-luebeck.de

[2] Institut für Biomedizinische Optik, Universität zu Lübeck, brinkmann@bmo.uni-luebeck.de

[3] Coherent LaserSystems GmbH & Co. KG, Lübeck, {ruediger.vonelm, joerg.lawrenz}@coherent.com

Abstract

This paper reports the investigation of the nonlinear optical crystals for the laser induced nonlinear frequency conversion like cesium lithium borate (CLBO) with dimensions of 5 mm x 5 mm x 10 mm, which is very sensitive on ambient atmosphere. Depending on the atmospheric condition the CLBO can absorb or desorb the humidity. We estimated the change of OH content in the crystal at different air humidity and temperature by using non-polarized Fourier transform infrared spectrometer (FT-IR). It was proved that the water or OH groups content in the crystal had risen with the increasing humidity in the air at room temperature. We found that a balance develops between humidity in CLBO sample and in the air. That is why at 175°C in dry atmosphere the concentration of OH group in the crystal does not completely eliminate.

1 Introduction

With expanding development in medicine, industry and research the requirements for use of UV and deep UV- light sources increase as well. In comparison to the conventional excimer laser the solid- state laser generates an improved radiation quality and requires less maintenance [1]. The quality of radiation by solid-state laser depends on the nonlinear optical crystal (NLO), in which the short wave is developed through frequent conversion from long wavelength. In particular, NLO crystals like CLBO is suitable for the fourth (266 nm) and fifth (213 nm) harmonic generation of the 1064 nm Nd:YAG laser with output pulse energies from 500 mJ at 266 nm, corresponding to a 50 % conversion efficiency of the second harmonic input energy and 230 mJ at 213 nm with a conversion efficiency of 10,4 % from the fundamental input energy [2]. This is due to CLBO crystals provides good nonlinear properties, having a small walk-off, a larger angular matching phase and high optical damage threshold in comparison to other NLO crystals like BBO, LBO and CBO. Thus a high conversion coefficient and improved radiation quality of harmonic can be reached with CLBO [1], [2].

The application of CLBO crystal is limited due to its hygroscopic properties. Depending on the ambient atmosphere the CLBO can absorb or desorb the humidity. The inclusion and accumulation of ambient humidity can lead to a change in refraction indices, worsening of output parameters and even to an irreversible damage of the crystal (> 45% humidity) [3]. Hence the handling from production until mounting and use of the laser has to occur under stringent humidity control.

CLBO crystal belongs to a non-symmetrical tetragonal space group I-42d with a 3- dimensional borate network [4]. The network consist of $(B_3O_7)^{5-}$ rings, which are located similarly parallel to each other and therefore form the channels. Alternate in these channels lie cesium and lithium cations. The bond length between cations and borate anionic frame is so large that the foreign molecules - among other, water molecules, - can diffuse through channels into the CLBO crystal and strong bonds with atoms of crystal are formed [5]. The presence of water in the inside of the CLBO crystal has been first reported by Kovacs, K. Lengyel, A. Peter, K. Polgar and A. Beran [6]. This was evidenced by occurrence of the absorption bands at around 3400 and 3600 cm^{-1} in IR spectrum of CLBO, which attributes to the symmetric and asymmetric OH- stretch of water molecule. These bands were also seen by Kovacs, K. Lengyel, A. Peter, K. Polgar and A. Beran in dry atmosphere, which attributes to the strong bonds of water molecule in CLBO. Seroytkin, Ekaterina A. Fomina and Lyudmila I. Isaenko investigated CLBO (less 1 mm^{-1}) hydration at the different air humidity using thermogravimetry [7]. They revealed the dependence of the hydration rate on the environmental humidity and indicated that the water content in the crystal increases linear with time when CLBO is kept in the moistende air for the first time.

To understand the dependence of water or OH groups content in CLBO (5 x 5 x 10 mm^3) on different ambient atmosphere better, we present more measures using FT-IR spectrometry in this paper. Through the change of OH absorption bands we will draw a conclusion about the increase and decrease of the humidity in the crystal.

2 Material and Methods

The interaction humidity with the CLBO crystal is investigated by a Bruker APLHA Fourier transform infrared (FT-

IR) spectrometer. The IR absorption spectra were measured with a range of 3000 – 7500 cm^{-1}. The spectral resolution was 2 cm^{-1}. From the beginning of the experiment the CLBO crystal with dimensions of 5 mm x 5 mm x 10 mm was kept in a reservoir with a desiccant "Molecular Sieve" for several months to reduce the water impurity in the sample.

The IR transmittance spectra were measured first in dry (dew-point of -60°C) and then in humid atmosphere (dew-point of 12°C) at the room temperature. In comparison IR transmittance spectra of air were also detected at the same condition. During the measuring the sample chamber was purged by dry air with a rate of about 2 ml/min. To the humidity treatment some moisturized air was added, in order to reach the certain humidity with dew-point of 12°C. The time between measuring was several minutes and the CLBO crystal was in the sample chamber for the whole time. The reason for that was to avoid the contact of the crystal with the surrounding outside of the sample chamber. By comparing the intensity of the IR spectra during humidification we assessed the change the water content in the NLO crystal. Then we adjusted the humidity to the -60°C DP and increased the temperature up to 175°C using integrated furnace around the crystal. Under these conditions we measured IR transmittance spectra for 10 days. Thus it was investigated the temporal trend of change of humidity in the CLBO sample.

3 Results and Discussion

3.1 The behaviour of the CLBO sample at different humidity

In Fig.1 the dependence of IR transmittance spectrum from CLBO on the wave number at room temperature in dry (a) and humid (b) atmosphere is shown. Also the IR absorption spectra of air are demonstrated under the same condition. At dry atmosphere (-60°C DP) the IR transmittance of air was maximum above the wave number range. In contrast, in the CLBO sample lower transmittance of IR- radiation at around 3400 and 3600 cm^{-1} is observed, which results, as it was pointed out by Kovacs *et al.*, from the water content in the sample [6]. The presence of these OH absorption bands means that the CLBO crystal was not anhydrous. This proved the strong bond of water molecules with atoms of crystal as Kovacs *et al.* reported [6]. We also conclude that the desiccant "Molecular Sieve" does not create an anhydrous crystal, but helps avoiding CLBO from cracking and allows keeping the CLBO above long time. Furthermore it should be noted that the shape of absorption bands depend on the thermal history of the desiccant "Molecular Sieve". The other bands at around 3800 and 4100 cm^{-1} are the typical for most oxide crystals and therefore they are not used for estimation of humidity in the crystal.

If the humidity in the sample chamber was increased, the IR transmittance spectrum decreased for air as well as for CLBO crystal. This change in the IR spectra of crystal is not stronger than in the spectra of air. Furthermore the OH absorption bands in the spectrum of air and crystal have different positions (Fig.1 (b)). Through the interaction between OH groups and atoms of CLBO it leads to the shifting of band maximum in the direction of the weak wave number and to reduction of the band intensity in the crystal. In addi-

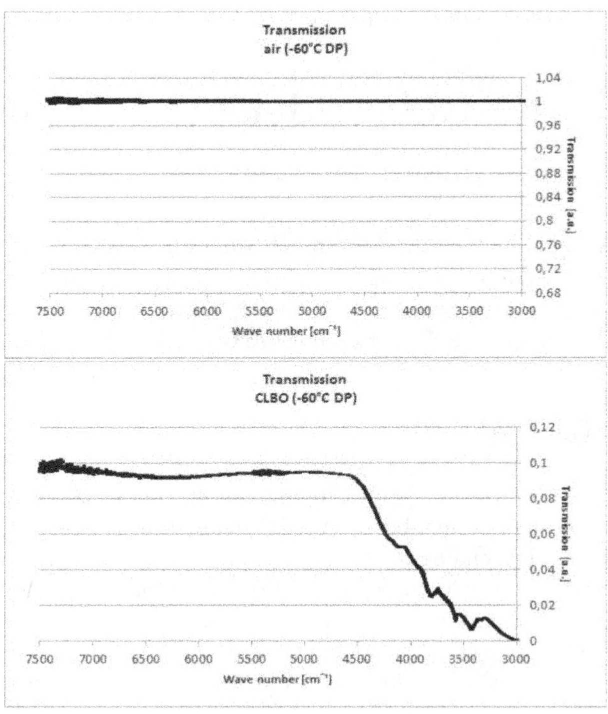

a)

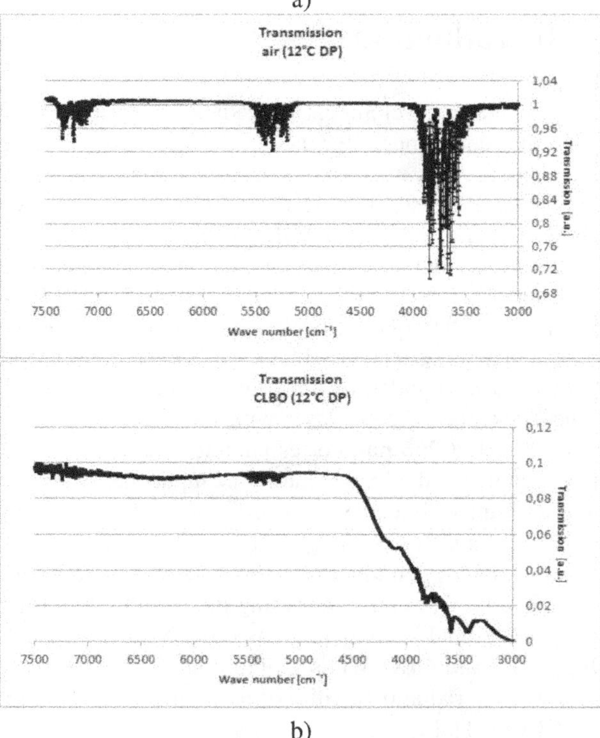

b)

Figure 1: IR transmittance spectra of air and CLBO (5 x 5 x 10 mm^3) in the range of 3000 - 7500 cm^{-1} wave number in dry (a) and humid (b) atmosphere

tion to the absorption bands at around 3400 and 3600 cm^{-1} the bands appear at around 5500 and 5020 cm^{-1} (Fig.1 (a)), which reveal in the air as well as in CLBO IR spectra. Kovacs *et al.* attributed these to the first overtones of the fundamental vibrations of H_2O and they can be seen if there is a high amount of water in the CLBO sample [6].
In Fig.2 the IR transmittances of CLBO in dry (-60°C DP) and humid (12°C DP) atmosphere were shown. We can clearly see the difference between the spectra of crystal in dry and humid atmosphere. With higher humidity the bands are more shaped and intense. This proves the dependence of water content in the crystal sample on humidity. This result also shows that there was a notable change in the absorption bands despite of the short stay of just several minutes in the humid atmosphere. This coincides with the theory, where the dry crystal absorbs the water with higher rate for the first time, when it was placed in humid atmosphere [7].

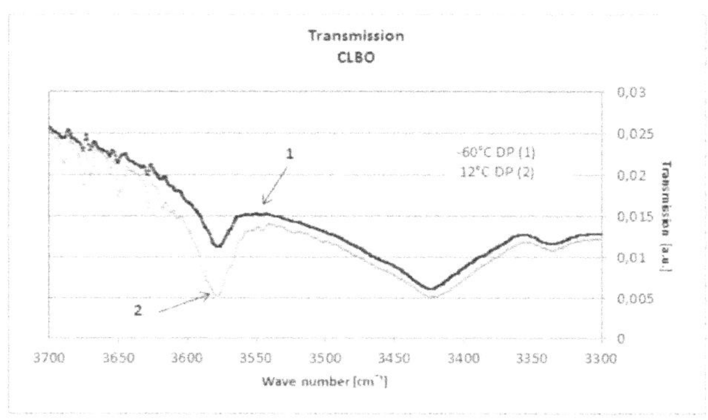

Figure 2: IR transmittance spectra of CLBO crystal in the range of 3300 - 3700 cm^{-1} wave number in dry (1) and in humid (2) atmosphere

Beside of the OH absorption band at around 3400 cm^{-1} several weak bands can also be seen in IR spectra of CLBO sample. We suppose that these weak bands from water vapor in the air. Before the IR radiation reaches a detector, the IR ray covers a certain distance in the humid air. The bands of these molecules, which from IR ray are stimulated on this distance, are visible in CLBO spectra. If comparing the spectra of humid air and crystal, it can be seen the same structure of the OH groups, as shown in Fig.3.

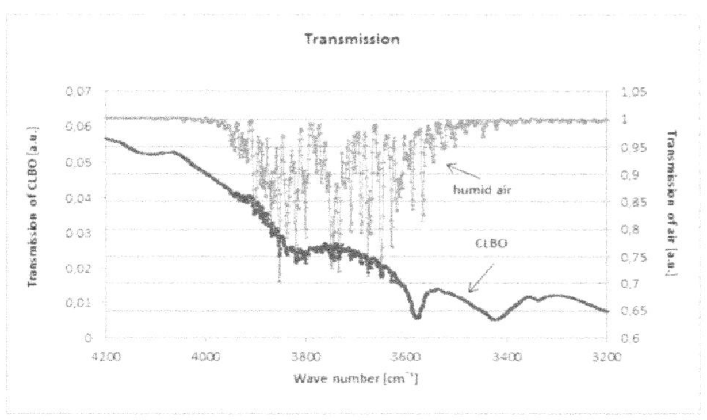

Figure 3: IR transmittance spectra of humid air and CLBO crystal in the range of 3200 - 4000 cm^{-1} wave number

3.2 The behaviuor of the CLBO crystal during heating

Fig.4 (a) demonstrates the change of the IR transmittance spectra with time at room temperature of about 175°C and humidity of -60°C DP for 10 days. It is visible that the first scan had very low IR transmittance at around 3400 and 3600 cm^{-1}. This indicates higher moisture content in the crystal. With time the IR transmittance increases by this wave number, which is an evidence for the loss of water. Therefore the heating is the effective way to avoid crystal hydration.

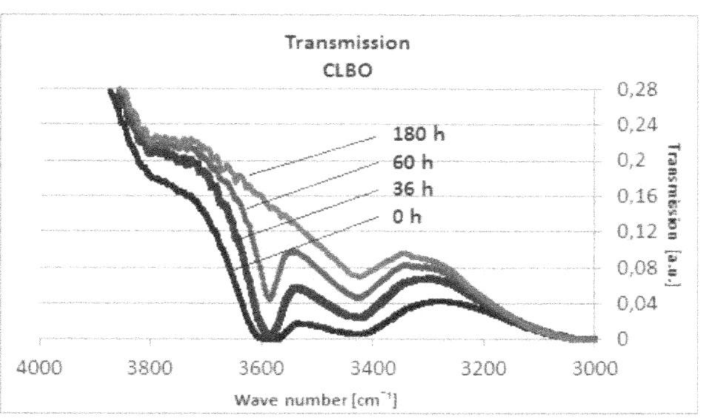

a)

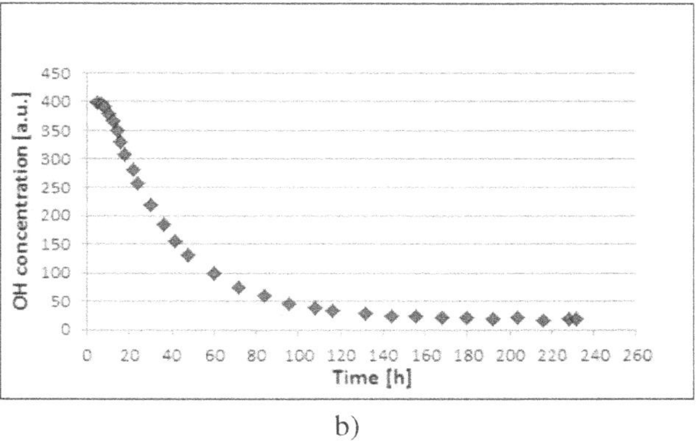

b)

Figure 4: IR transmittance spectra of the CLBO crystal in the range of 3000 - 4000 cm^{-1} kept for 10 days in dry atmosphere at 175°C. In (b) the change of the water concentration in the CLBO sample as function of the heating duration.

Fig.4 (b) shows the concentration of the OH groups in the CLBO crystal during heating. The concentration was calculated from the peak-surface of absorption bands (3400 and 3600 cm^{-1}). We can see the rapid fall of water concentration in the initial stage of the heating. We suggest that the H_2O molecules of the surface and the weak bond in the crystal leave the sample in this time essentially. The strong bonded water molecules in CLBO sample are responsible for the rest of the time, when an anhydration with lower rate than at the first stage takes place. These water molecules take essentially more time to leave the crystal. After 10 days the saturation was reached. The water concentration did not decrease to 0. We assumed that a balance between the moisture in the sample and in the air was reached and for this reason no more water exchange took place at this ambient condition.

4 Conclusion

The interaction between ambient atmosphere and CLBO using FT-IR spectrometry was investigated. The IR spectra of crystal, which were registered at room temperature in dry atmosphere, include the OH absorption bands at around 3400 and 3600 cm^{-1}. These OH absorption bands get stronger with the increasing humid air and this shows that the hydration of crystal with humidity in air is extreme. With the increase of the temperature (175°C and -60°C DP) the moisture in the crystal first sinks rapidly and then with a lower rate. Due to the developed balance between the humidity in CLBO and in the air, complete water elimination by this condition is not reached. Whether the present of the OH group in the crystal under these conditions has an influence on the UV properties, the aim is the next investigations.
All results show that the humidity as well as the temperature by application of the solid-state laser with CLBO crystal should be strictly controlled to avoid the water vapor absorption in the crystal and thus increase its application time.

Acknowledgement

The work has been carried out at Coherent LaserSystems GmbH & Co. KG. I would like to thank all people who have helped and supported me during my investigation there.

5 References

[1] Y. Mori, Y. K. Yap, T. Kamimura, M. Yoshimura and T. Sasak *Recent development of nonlinear optical borate crystals for UV generation.* Optical Materials 19 (2002) 1-5

[2] Y. K. Yap, M. Inagaki, S. Nakajima, Y. Mori and T. Sasaki *High-power fourth- and fifth-harmonic generation of a Nd:YAG laser by means of a* $CsLiB_6O_{10}$ Opt. Lett. 21 (1996) 1348-1350

[3] A. Taguchi, A. Miyamoto, Y. Mori, S. Haramura, T. Inoue, K. Nishijima, Y. Kagebayashi, H. Sakai, Y. K. Yap and T. Sasaki *Effects of the moisture on CLBO.* OSA TOPS Advanced Solid State Lasers, 10 (1997)

[4] T. Sasaki, Y. Mori, I. Kuroda, S. Nakajima, K. Yamaguchi and S. Watanabe *Acta Cryst.* C 51 (1995) 2222

[5] F. Pan, X. Wang, G. Shen, D. Shen *Cracking mechanism in CLBO crystals at room temperature.* J. Cryst. Growth 24 (2002) 129

[6] L. Kovacs, K. Lengyel, A. Peter, K. Polgar and A. Beran *IR absorption spectroscopy of water in* CLB_6O_{10} *crystals.* Opt. Mater. 24 (2003) 457-463

[7] Yurii V. Seryotkin, Ekaterina A. Fomina and Lyudmila I. Isaenko *Humidity effect on hydration of* $CsLiB_6O_{10}$ *nonlinear optical crystal: X-ray diffraction study.* Opt. Mater. 35 (2013) 1646-1651

[8] Y. Morimoto, S. Miyazawa and Y. Kagebayashi *Water-associated surfage degration of* CLB_6O_{10} *crystal during harmonic generation in the ultraviolet region.* J. Mater: Res. 16 (2001) 2082-2090

[9] Y. Mori, I. Kuroda, S. Nakajima, T. Sasaki and S. Nakai *New nonlinear optical crystal: Cesium lithium borate.* Appl. Phys. Lett. 67 (1995) 13

[10] T. Kawamura, M. Yoshimura, Y. Honda, M. Nishioka, Y. Shimizu, Y. Kitaoka, Y. Mori, T. Sasaki *Effect of water impurity in* $CsLiB_6O_{10}$ *crystals on bulk laser-induced damage threshold and transmittance in the ultraviolet region,* Appl.Opt. 48 (2009) 9

3
Biochemical Physics

LED-based Illumination Set-up for *In Vitro* Photodynamic Therapy

S. A. Abedi [1], A. Rodewald [2], K. Scheffler [1] and R. Rahmanzadeh [2]
[1] Medizinische Ingenieurwissenschaft, Universität zu Lübeck, {ebadi, scheffle}@miw.uni-luebeck.de
[2] Institute of Biomedical Optics, Universität zu Lübeck, {rodewald, rahmanzadeh}@bmo.uni-luebeck.de.

Abstract

Photodynamic therapy (PDT) is a treatment modolity, based on the light activation of a photosensitizer (PS) to cure cancer and diseases characterized by uncontrolled cell proliferation. In this work, a special *in vitro* illumination set-up for PDT was designed, constructed and characterized. Different light-emitting diodes (LED) with emission wavelengths of 650 nm and 690 nm are used as light sources and their beam profiles was characterized before and after collimation. Culture experiments with cervixcarcinom cells HeLa and BPD as photosensitizer demonstrated the functionally of the illumination set-up. In view of the technical properties, the illumination set-up leads to reproducible cell irradiation experiments.

1 Introduction

Photodynamic therapy (PDT) is a clinically approved emerging, minimally invasive treatment and already used for the therapy of cancer and other diseases [1]. PDT is based on three components: A photosensitizer (PS), light at the specific wavelength and tissue oxygen. A PS is a light sensitive molecule and upon light irradiation produces reactive oxygen species (ROS) which lead to selective damage of cells. The PS absorbs photons at a specific wavelength and the emission of the light source should correspond with the absorption of the PS. The absorption of a photon brings the PS from ground singlet state (S0) to an excited singlet state (S1). Lifetime of S1 state is short. From the excited singlet state, the PS can either emit a photon (fluorescence) and go back to its ground state or may transfer to an excited triplet state (T1) via intersystem crossing. From here two types of reactions are possible. Type I is an electron transfer from the PS to surrounding molecules, whereas Type II is an energy transfer where energy is transferred to molecular oxygen, finally producing singlet oxygen $^1O_2$. Singlet oxygen is cytotoxic and leads to damage of the surrounding cells. For PDT type II mechanism is preferred because the PS can be activated many times. PDT can induce direct cytotoxic reactions on cells, deterioration of vasculature in tumors or inflammatory reactions [1],[2].
Another technique where this irradiation set-up is applied for is Photochemical internalization (PCI), which is an approach for the release of macromolecules from lysosomal and endosomal vesicles. The PCI method is based on PDT and has the similar mechanisms to destroy membranes. The photosensitizer is localized in lysosomal and endosomal vesicles. After irradiation vesicles membranes are finally destroyed, and the loading of the vesicles is released. PS concentration and light energy are in PCI much lower than in PDT. PCI can deliver proteins, nucleic acid, chemotherapeutics agents, etc.

Incoherent and coherent light sources are used already in PDT and both of them are effective. Deep tissue penetration with light is possible with wavelengths in between the optical window of tissue between 600 and 1200 nm. Wavelength lower than 600 nm are absorbed by biological tissue and wavelength longer than 800 nm have not enough energy to produce ROS [3]. The choice of the light source depends on the application of PDT. The effectiveness of PDT depends on many factors, such as structure and the dose of PS, light exposure, its dose and fluence rate plus oxygen concentration in tissue. The Benzoporphyrin derivative (BPD), Amphinex and FITC are PSs widely used in the PDT.

In this study an illumination system with defined emission spectrum is used for photo activation of the PS in *in vitro* experiments. Wideband light, laser and LED are already used PDT. The choice of light source depends on many parameters. Emission spectrum of light must be appropriated to the absorption spectrum of PS. Further the optical power should be sufficient to produce of ROS. A laser light source has enough optical power, but disadvantage of laser is the narrow beam and high costs. A wideband light generate heat during the irradiation, which is a possible disturbance factor and is not wavelength specific. LEDs produce low heating and are small in comparison with other light sources, with the lifetime up to 10000 h. Moreover, have a narrow-band emission spectrum ($\pm$ 20 nm at FWHM). In this work is an illumination system based on LED characterized, designed, constructed and finally checked for functionality.

2 Material and Methods

2.1 Characterization of the illumination system

Two illumination systems for 96-well plate (353075, Falcon) and petri-dish (627870, Greiner Bio-One) are constructed, both based on high power LEDs. As only a single well should be exposed for a specific irradiation, a single light source was proposed for the 96-well plate. The optical power should be variable and the beam profile homogeneous and constant, for achieving reliable and comparable results.

2.2 Construction

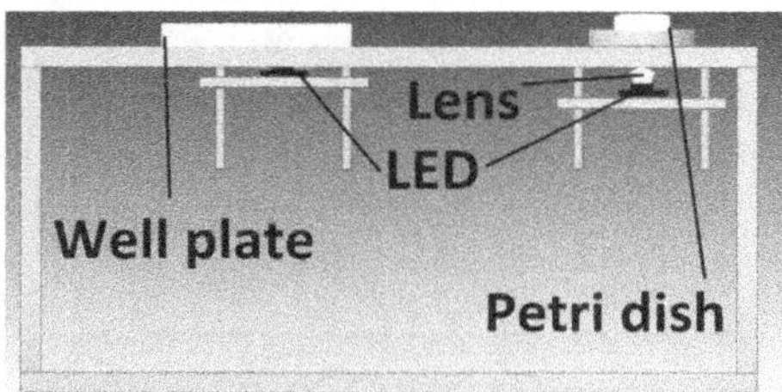

Figure 1: Schematic diagram of the illumination system

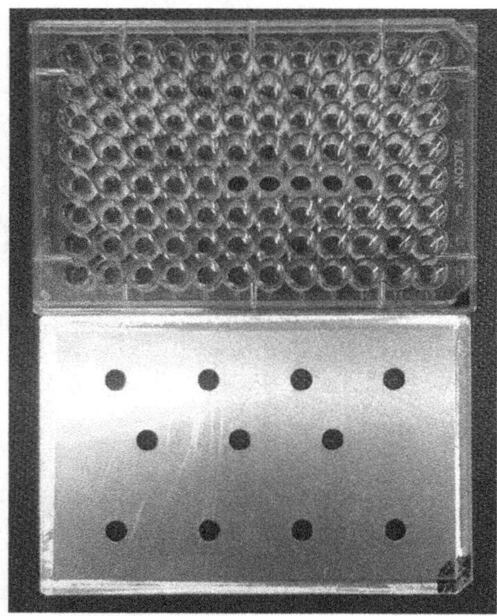

Figure 2: Aperture with 11 holes for reduction of the light scattering.

Fig. 1 shows the schematic diagram of the irradiation system. There are two set-ups for different wavelengths, 650 and 690 nm (H2A1-H650, optical power 40 mW; H2A1-H690, optical power 60 mW, High Power single chip LED, ROITHNER LASERTECHNICK GmbH, Vienna, Austria). Each set-up consists of two LED with similar wavelengths. The choice of the LEDs was dependent on the PS used for the experiments. The optical power is regulated with the Laser diode driver (NEWPORT, Model 505 Laser diode driver). Cells in the 96-well plate were exposed directly, as the LED diameter (6.61 mm) is almost the same as the well diameter (6.9 mm). With the help of a 15 ° half angle collimator lens (10017, ROITHNER LASERTECHNICK GmbH, Vienna, Austria) The beam was collimated from $\pm 75°$ to $\pm 15°$. for illumination of the petri-dishes. Fig. 2 shows an aperture plate for reduction of the light scattering. The aperture plate fits perfectly between the 96-well plate and illumination system. The aperture plate has 11 holes and is used for irradiating the wells always at the same position.

2.3 LED spectrum measurement

The spectral emission for all LEDs was verified with a spectrometer (AvaSpec-USB2, OSC-UB, Avantes 7.6, Netherlands). The spectrometer had a spectral range between 330 nm and 800 nm and a resolution nearly 0.17 nm.

2.4 Measurement of the optical power

The optical power was recorded with a high-sensitivity optical sensor (RoHS) (LM-2 VIS, FieldMaster GS Power/Energy Analyzer, Coharent, USA) with a 7.9 mm active area diameter, power resolution 1 nW and 5% calibration uncertainty.

2.5 Measurement of beam profiles

To record the beam profiles for the different optics, a beam profiling camera (Wincam-XHR, 1/2", CMOS, ND-4 C-mount Neutral Density filters, DataRay Inc., Bella Vista, CA 96008, USA) was used. The camera had 3,1 MPixels (2048 × 1538) with a CMOS sensor active area 6.5 × 4.9 mm and all data was processed with software provided by the manufacturer (DATARay Inc. v7.1, Bella Vista, CA).

2.6 Measurement of temperature

The temperature was measured during irradiation and recorded with a thermocouple (hypo-33-1-t-g-60-smpw-m, MiniHypodermic Probe, type T thermocouple, OMEGA). To illustrate the temperature change in the well during irradiation the cells, the wells were filled with 200 μL Phosphate Buffered Saline (PBS) with Mg and Ca and irradiated at 690 nm with 44 mW/cm^2 for 20 min.

2.7 Measurement of absorption spectrum of 96-well plate

The absorption spectrum of the 96-well plate (Falcon) was characterized with the Spectrometer (SpectraMax M4 MultiMode Microplate Reader, Molecular Devices LLC). Absorption was measured within in the range of wavelengths between 350 and 750 nm, in 1 nm steps.

2.8 Cell culture

HeLa cells are epithelial cells, that were derived in 1951 from a human cervical cancer.
HeLa cells (ATCC, Nr. ACC 57) were cultured in Dulbecco's Modified Eagle's Medium (DMEM), supplemented with 10 % fetal calf serum (FCS), (PAA) and 1 % Penicillin-Streptomycin (10.000 units Penicillin and 10 mg/mL Streptomycin) in a 5 % CO_2-humidified atmosphere at 37 °C. Cells were cultivated in 25 cm^2 cell culture flasks and passaged two times weekly.

2.9 *In vitro* PDT experiment

For PDT, cells were seeded with BPD in DMEM medium (200 nmol/L) supplemented with 10 % FCS into a 96-well plate (Falcon) at a density of 6000 cells per well and incubated for 20 h at 37 °C. After incubation, the cells are rinsed twice with 200 μL Dulbecco's Phosphate Buffered Saline with $MgCl_2$ and $CaCl_2$ (DPBS+) (Sigma-Aldrich). Cells were then exposed for 120 s at 690 ±20 nm and a total light dose of 6 J/cm^2 and 10.5 J/cm^2. After irradiation DPBS+ was replaced with 200 μL DMEM and cells were incubated for 48 h at 37 °C.

3 Results and Discussion

3.1 Spectrum of the LED

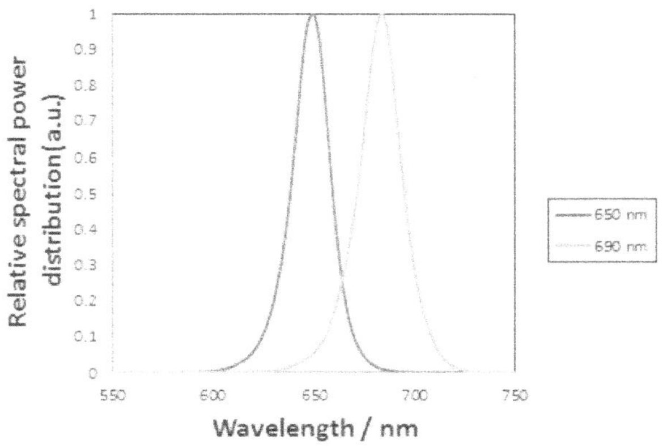

Figure 3: Normalized output power vs. wavelength by 650 and 690 nm LED's

Fig. 3 shows the spectral emission of the 690 nm LED and the maximum peak at 683.6 nm. The full width at half maximum (FWHM) is 23.4 nm. Also the 650 nm LED had FWHM value of 24.5 nm. The maximum peak was recorded at 649.4 nm.
To investigate the beam, optical power was measured during irradiation for 15 min. The sampling frequency was 2 Hz. For example the 690 nm LED with a power of 19.6 mW had a maximum value of 19.8 mW and a minimum 19.6 mW the mean of power was 19.6 mW. Standard deviation from 43 μW shows the stability of the LED during irradiation. Other LEDs show similar results and was therefore proved for use.

3.2 Beam profile

With a beam profiling camera, the distribution of light can be illustrated. An equal light distributions is necessary for reproducible cell experiments.

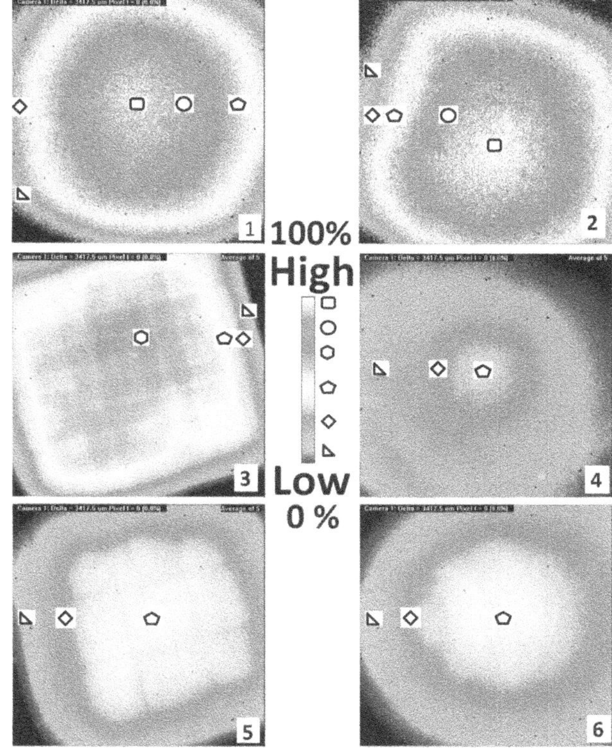

Figure 4: Beam profiles: 1) 650 nm LED without optical elements, 2) 690 nm LED without optical elements, 3) 690 nm LED + special optic for fiber coupling, 4) 690 nm LED + ± 6 ° reflector 5) 690 nm LED + ±5 ° half angle collimator, 6) 690 nm LED + ±15 ° half anlge collimator

Table 1: Beam profiles

No.	Wavelenght	Optic	Power [mW]	Power loss [%]
1)	650 nm	no	12	0
2)	690 nm	no	20	0
3)	690 nm	fiber coupling	17	15
4)	690 nm	6 ° reflector	0.88	95.6
5)	690 nm	± 4 ° collimator	8.04	59.8
6)	690 nm	± 15 ° collimator	11.5	42.5

Fig 4 shows the beam profile of 650 and 690 nm LEDs, in combination with different optical elements. Beam profiles (1) and (2) had almost intensity distribution; because LEDs had the same construction design and emitting surface. The optic for fasercoupling (3) had the best homogeneity under the profiles, but also an optical power loss of 3 mW (15 % of the total power) (Table 1). The reflector (4) led to power loss up to 95.6 % and therefore the focused beam was undesirable. The $\pm 15^\circ$ Collimator would be chosen for the irradiation of the petri dishes, because the power loss was lower than $\pm 4^\circ$ Collimator.

3.3 Measurement of the temperature change during irradiation

Measurements of temperature changes during irradiation were conducted, in order to exclude photo-thermal effects e.g. to kill cells. The irradiation, the multiwell plate and thermocouple were left at room temperature for 1 hour. The measurement shows a temperature increase of only $0.5\,^\circ$C during irradiation.

3.4 Absorption spectrum of 96-well plate

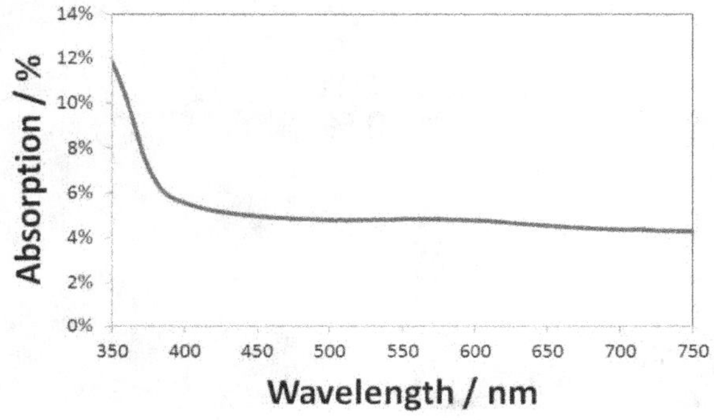

Figure 5: Absorption spectrum of 96-well plate (Falcon)

Fig. 5 shows that the absorption spectrum between 650 nm and 690 nm is approximately 4%. The absorption is strongly dependent on the wavelength and drops when the wavelength increases.

3.5 Cells after irradiation

For the measurement of cell viability, the activity of mitochondrial succinate dehydrogenase was tested in a MTT-assay. The result shows (Fig.6) that, as expected, cell viability is decreased when cells are incubated with BPD and irradiated at 690 nm. [4]

4 Conclusion

In this study we showed the successful design and characterization of a LED-based illumination set up for PDT. The optical power can be set in a range from 0 to 20 mW with an accuracy of ± 0.1 mW wich means an irradiance of 40 mW/cm^2 for well-plate and 7 mW/cm^2 for petri dishes. The functionality was proven with cell culture experiments,

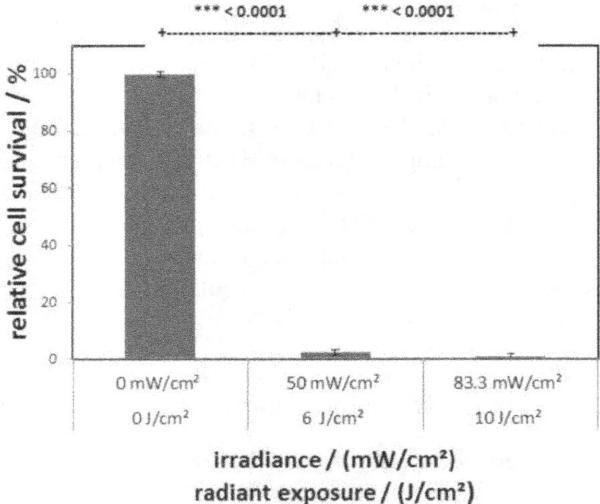

Figure 6: HeLa cells in combination with BPD in a concentration of 200 nmol/L after an irradiation of 2 minutes by 690 $\pm$20 nm. Error bars indicate the standard deviation, significances were calculated using the t-test.

where the expected decease in cell viability after PDT was observed.

Acknowledgement

The work has been carried out at Institute of Biomedical Optics, Universität zu Lübeck.

5 References

[1] D. E. Dolmans, D. Fukumura, R. K. Jain, *Photodynamic therapy for cancer*, Nature Reviews Cancer vol. 3, pp.380–387, 2003.

[2] A. P. Castano, P. Morz, M. R. Hamblin,*Photodynamic therapy and antitumour immunity*, Nature Reviews Cancer vol. 6, pp.535-545, 2006.

[3] A. Juzeniene, K. p. Nielsen, J. Moan, *Biophysical aspects of photodynamic therapy* J Environ Pathol Toxicol Oncol. Vol. 25 , pp.7-28, 2006.

[4] T. Mosmann, *Rapid Colorimetric Assay for Cellular Growth and Survival: Application to Proliferation and Cytotoxicity Assays*, Journal of Immunological Methods 65, pp. 55–63, 1983.

Construction and implementation of a simple stopped-flow apparatus for the investigation of rapid kinetics using confocal fluorescence microscopy

H. Müller [1] and C. G. Hübner [2]
[1] Medizinische Ingenieurwissenschaft, Universität zu Lübeck, mueller@physik.uni-luebeck.de
[2] Physics Institute, Universität zu Lübeck, huebner@physik.uni-luebeck.de

Abstract

The observation of conformational changes of molecular structures, the identification of reaction intermediates and the determination of rate constants of state transitions is of great interest in biophysics and life sciences. One method to study the mentioned processes is the stopped-flow method. In this work, the construction and basic testing of a stopped-flow apparatus with a confocal fluorescence microscope is described. The driving part of a discarded quenched-flow apparatus was combined with a polymer-chip based fluidic micromixer. First fluorescence measurements inside the mixer were carried out with fluorescein. The basic test reaction was denaturation of green fluorescent protein (GFP) using sodium dodecyl sulfate (SDS). It is shown that reaction processes can be observed in real time using our stopped-flow apparatus. Further testing, characterisation and improvement of the device have yet to be done to enable the production of valid scientific data.

1 Introduction

The study of fast conformational changes in molecular structures, the identification of intermediate states as well as the rate constants of the transitions between these different states is a broad field in biophysics and life science. Some of these transitions are extremely fast and thereby hard to observe. After inducing refolding of an unfolded protein, by changing the physical parameters or the chemical environment, it is assumed that the hydrophobic collapse occurs within the first $100\,\mu s$ [1].
The rate constant of a chemical reaction is an expression of the time dependency of reactant concentrations. As described in [2], for a first order reaction the time dependence is the solution of the differential equation

$$-\frac{dc}{dt} = k \cdot c \tag{1}$$

which is

$$c(t) = c_0 \cdot e^{-k \cdot t} \tag{2}$$

where $c(t)$, c_0, k denote the time dependent reactant concentration, the initial reactant concentration and the rate constant of the reaction, respectively.
Several methods such as quenched-flow (QF), continuous-flow (CF) or stopped-flow (SF) have been developed and used to examine the kinetics of fast reactions. Each of these methods have advantages and disadvantages over each other making them suitable for different types of reactions and analytical methods.

In this work the construction of a SF apparatus from a discarded QF apparatus using a polymer-chip based fluidic micromixer for use with confocal fluorescence microscopy (CFM) is presented. The apparatus was tested with two reactions: The quenching of fluorescein by a pH drop and the denaturation of green fluorescent protein (GFP) using sodium dodecyl sulfate (SDS).

2 Material and Methods

2.1 The stopped-flow method

The SF method is a technique for the investigation of fast reaction kinetics such as for example conformational changes in protein structures, enzyme activity or chemical reactions. Two or more reactants are mixed and afterwards sent into an observation-chamber [3]. The reaction can then be observed in real-time mainly by optical (e.g. absorption and fluorescence measurements) or electro-chemical (e.g. conductivity measurement) methods [4].
The time between contact of the reactants and the mixed solution getting stopped in the observation chamber is called dead-time. Commercially available SF apparatus allow for reactions with a reaction rate of $3500\,s^{-1}$ to be observed (BioLogic, Claix, France). The mixed solution can be observed for any period of time without further sample consumption. Thereby this method has a high 'dynamic time range' even though the time of first observation is limited by the dead-time. Also detection is carried out in one sample volume achieving time resolution depending on sampling

rate, enabling scanning free single point detection such as a simple spectral photometer.

2.2 Setup

To perform a SF experiment, the reagents designated for mixing must be driven through the channel and mixing system. It is important that the amount of reagents used and the drive time as well as the volumetric flow rate can be adjusted and is delivered precisely as it is set. Even though a steady, non pulsed flow is not as important for SF as it is for CF applications, precise shot control is highly appreciable. To achieve this goal, a discarded QF apparatus (QFM-5, BioLogic SAS; Claix, France) was modified to serve as the driving system for the experimental SF apparatus which can be seen in Fig.1.
The QFM-5 consists of a lower driving part containing the stepping motors and electronics as well as an upper mixing head, containing the fluid-system including valves, mixer and syringes. The syringes are vertically oriented and the syringes plungers are connected to the stepping motors by steel rods and screws. The mixing head and the lower driving part are screwed together. An external power-supply (MPS-52) provides the required power for running the stepping motors and facilitates low- to mid-level motor control. The MPS-52 in turn can be controlled by a PC via an RS-232 serial interface. The software for creating and downloading mixing sequences to the MPS-52 as well as triggering their execution is provided by BioLogic (BioKine v4.72). Unfortunately this software utilises no interface for external control e.g. via LabView. Attempts to create an own control software failed due to BioLogic refusing to disclose the control sequences for programming the MPS-52 as well as a lack of knowledge about reverse engineering by the author.
The mixing head of the QFM-5 was disassembled for studying its construction. The syringes are loaded through female slip-Luer ports on top of the QFM-5. One mechanical 3-way valve per syringe can be set in load- and shot-position. In shot-position, the fluid can enter the mixing-core of the QFM-5. It contains 3 mixer and 2 ports for delay lines in the order: mixer 1 $\rightarrow$ delay-line 1 $\rightarrow$ mixer 2 $\rightarrow$ delay-line 2 $\rightarrow$ mixer 3.
The first idea was to utilise mixer 1 and creating an exit port through the port for delay-line 1 by inserting a custom made "fake delay-line". It failed due to missing delay-lines, the unavailability of replacements from BioLogic and the refusal to release information about the outer dimensioning of these parts by BioLogic.
Instead of using the mixing head of the QFM-5, two of its syringes for fluid driving were connected to an external mixer by using the flange fittings of the QFM-5 with new tubing, hplc flange fittings and custom made slip-Luer-to-M6-adapters (see below).
The mixer used was a herringbone mixer on an object slide sized polymer-chip based fluidic micromixer (microfluidic ChipShop GmbH; Jena, Germany). The chip is made from Zeonor (Zeonex). It consists of two inlet channels (rectangular cross-section, width 300 µm, height 200 µm) which are joined in a y-junction into a main channel (rectangular cross-section, width 600 µm, height 200 µm) with the herringbone structure, leading to one outlet. The channels are located at the bottom of a carrier plate and covered by a lid (thickness 188 µm) for optical access. Female slip-Luer connectors are attached at the two inlets and the outlet. Three of these mixers are arranged at one chip.
Instead of using an external observation chamber, the optically accessible exit channel of the mixer was used for observation. Due to this exit channel our apparatus is in principle capable of CF application.
ETFE tubing (ID 0.5 mm, OD 1.8 mm, GE Healthcare) with fittings (PP/PEEK, GE Healthcare) were flanged and used to connect the syringes and the mixer. The slip-Luer-to-M6-adapters used for the connection between the tubing and the mixer were made from Delrin (DuPont). The top end is a female M6 thread, the bottom end a male slip-Luer connector with an 0.5 mm through-hole (See Fig. 1, bottom right).
The slip-Luer-to-M6 (Delrin) adapters were bonded to the female slip-Luer connector on the mixer-chip (Zeonor) using two component epoxy resign glue (UHU plus, endfest 300) and cured over night. Even though bonding with surface treatment using oxygen plasma would be more resistant, this bonding provides enough halt for flow rates of $0.2\,\mathrm{mL\,s^{-1}}$ per port.
The system used for fluorescence intensity measurement and imaging was a confocal fluorescence scanning microscope utilizing an avalanche-photo-detector (APD) (SPCM-AQ14, Perkin-Elmer). The bin-time was set to 500 µs. The excitation light source was a Coherent Sapphire 488. The detection channel was filtered by a bandpass filter (ET 525/50, Chroma). Measurements were carried out using a Nikon microscope objective (Plan, 10x/0.25).
The mixer was mounted on top of a cross table using an custom made aluminium clamp.

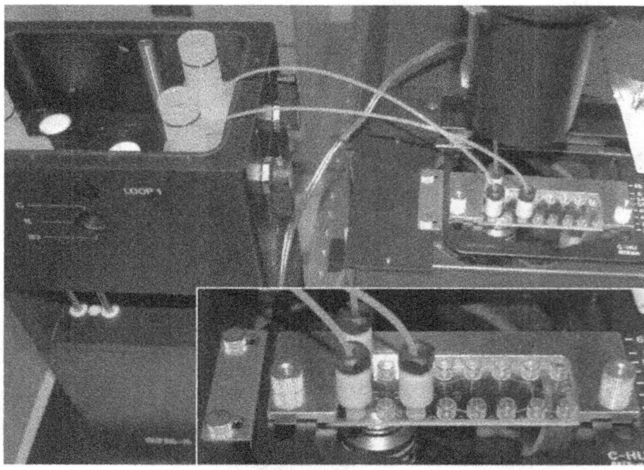

Figure 1: The current setup. The QFM-5 driving section and two syringes (left) are connected to the mixer by tubing and custom made connectors (right). The mixer is mounted on a cross table with an aluminium clamp.

2.3 Dead-time estimation

The estimation of the dead-time of a SF apparatus is an important evaluation to be carried out to determine the age of the mixed solution at the time of the first usable sampling point. Rate constants of reactions that reach equilibrium state shortly after the dead time can only be estimated with relatively high possible error as only a small segment of the exponential waveform can be used for fitting. Reactions that reach equilibrium state within the dead-time cannot be observed at all [3][5].

The driving system of the QFM-5 provides a maximum volumetric flow-rate of $4.5\,\mathrm{mL\,s^{-1}}$ per syringe. The tubing connections however are tight at flow-rates of $0.2\,\mathrm{mL\,s^{-1}}$ per syringe. A practicable safe flow-rate is e.g. $0.1\,\mathrm{mL\,s^{-1}}$ per syringe which means a total flow-rate $0.2\,\mathrm{mL\,s^{-1}}$ in the mixing channel. The distance of the point of first contact to the observation point behind the herringbone structure is $l = 15\,\mathrm{mm}$. The channel dimensions are height $h = 0.2\,\mathrm{mm}$ and width $w = 0.6\,\mathrm{mm}$. The dead-time can be estimated as

$$t = \frac{V}{\dot{V}} = \frac{l \cdot h \cdot w}{\dot{V}} = \frac{1.8\,\mathrm{mm}^3}{200\,\mathrm{mm}^3\mathrm{s}^{-1}} = 0.009\,\mathrm{s} \qquad (3)$$

where V and $\dot{V}$ denote the volume of the relevant channel area and the volumetric flow-rate respectively [6].

This value gives the theoretical minimal possible dead-time at the given flow rate and with the present mixer.

2.4 pH-quenching of fluoresceine

Fluorescein is a widely used fluorescent dye with an excitation maximum at a wavelength around $490\,\mathrm{nm}$ and an emission maximum at around $520\,\mathrm{nm}$. The intensity of fluorescence is pH dependent and quenched below pH 4 [7]. For performing first fluorescence measurements in the SF apparatus, a diluted fluorescein solution (pH neutral) was mixed with acidic solution (HCl in desalinated water, pH ~ 2). Fluorescein isothiocyanate isomer I (Sigma-Aldrich, F7250, $\lambda_{ex,max}$ $492\,\mathrm{nm}$, $\lambda_{em,max}$ $518\,\mathrm{nm}$) was used. The actual excitation wavelength used was $488\,\mathrm{nm}$. Measurements were carried out in front of the herringbone structure to test the measurement of fluorescence inside the channels of the mixer. Measurement points were distributed across the channel width and the two fluids were mixed at $0.3\,\mathrm{mL\,s^{-1}}$ total flow rate for a duration of 2 seconds.

2.5 Unfolding of GFP using SDS

GFP is a very stable protein originally isolated from a jellyfish (Aequorea Victoria) [8]. It is frequently used for protein labelling and for analysing metabolism pathways in living organisms. As described in [9], GFP is vulnerable to denaturation by SDS at a pH of 6.5. Due to the unfolding caused by SDS, the GFP looses its fluorescence within a minute. This slow reaction is suitable for first testing of our SF apparatus.

GFP ($0.66\,\mathrm{\mu M}$ in $50\,\mathrm{mM}$ TRIS, pH 6.5) was mixed with SDS (0.67% in $50\,\mathrm{mM}$ TRIS, pH 6.5) in a ratio of 1 to 1 ($10\,\mathrm{\mu L}$ each) to a final concentration of $0.33\,\mathrm{\mu M}$ GFP + 0.34% SDS. The total volumetric flow rate was $0.2\,\mathrm{mL\,s^{-1}}$. The pH was adjusted using 1 M HCl. The excitation power was $100\,\mathrm{\mu W}$.

2.6 Data analysis

Curve fitting (double exponential) and visualisation was performed with Igor Pro (WaveMetrics).

3 Results and Discussion

The pH-drop induced quenching of fluorescein right after the t-junction of the inlet channels showed a decreasing fluorescence level across the channel width (see Fig. 2) during 2 s shots and an almost immediate loss of fluorescence after stopping the flow (results not shown). The variations in the fluorescence level show that the y-junction in front of the herringbone structure does not mix the fluids sufficiently at the applied flow speed. The fast quenching after stopping the flow can be explained by fast proton diffusion and the protonation of fluorescein, occuring within one bin-time [7].

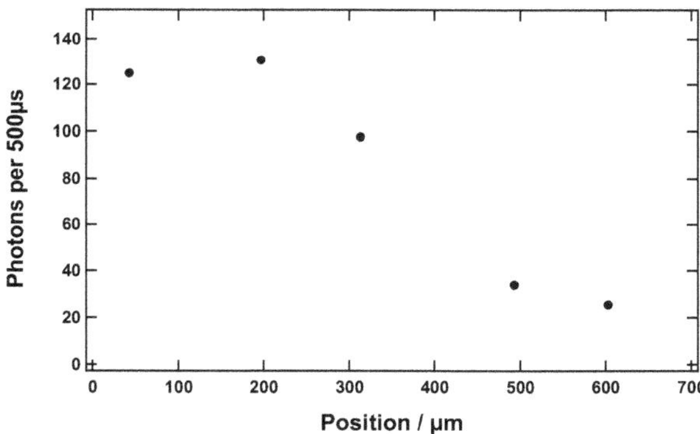

Figure 2: Average detected photons per $500\,\mathrm{\mu s}$ from fluorescence of fluorescein at various positions across the channel between the y-junction and the herringbone structure (in µm) during a 2 s shot. Fluorescein was mixed with diluted HCl (pH$\sim$2).

Fig. 3 shows the result of the GFP denatuartion experiment described in 2.5. The number of detected photons ($500\,\mathrm{\mu s}$ bin-time) for six consecutive shots (A-F) with a mixing ratio of 1 to 1 is shown. The observation time after each shot was 150 s. After an initial peak at the time of mixing (A: 50 s, B: 200 s, C: 350 s, D: 500 s, E: 650 s, F: 800 s) the signal decays, showing a double exponential process. The corresponding rate constants k_1 and k_2 determined by double exponential curve fitting are shown in Table 1. The waveform of shots A-D are quite similar even though the absolute values differ from shot to shot. Shots E and F are significantly different to the previous four. This fits to the difference in rate k_2 in Table 1.

Problems arose by fluorescein sticking to the channel walls

even after intensive washing with ethanol and water, producing a high background fluorescence level which decayed due to photo-bleaching at the point of observation (focal spot) within a few minutes. However, the influence of this contamination on the measurements due to slight movement of the mixer chip during the shots, slightly shifting the point of observation is neglectable.

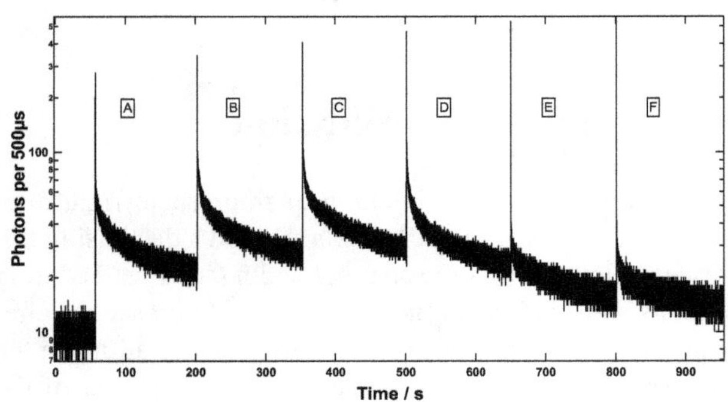

Figure 3: The recorded data of six consecutive shots (A-F) are shown. GFP (0.66 µM in 50 mM TRIS, pH 6.5) was mixed with SDS (0.67% in 50 mM TRIS, pH 6.5) in an 1 to 1 ratio (10 µL each per shot). Number of photons detected per 500 µs plotted against time (in seconds). The signal shows a double exponential decay.

Table 1: determined rate constants (corresponding to shots A-F in Fig. 3)

shot	k_1 (s^{-1})	k_2 (s^{-1})
A	$0.25 \pm 4 \cdot 10^{-3}$	$0.022 \pm 2 \cdot 10^{-4}$
B	$0.30 \pm 3 \cdot 10^{-3}$	$0.020 \pm 1 \cdot 10^{-4}$
C	$0.32 \pm 3 \cdot 10^{-3}$	$0.017 \pm 1 \cdot 10^{-4}$
D	$0.30 \pm 3 \cdot 10^{-3}$	$0.021 \pm 2 \cdot 10^{-4}$
E	$0.33 \pm 9 \cdot 10^{-3}$	$0.013 \pm 3 \cdot 10^{-4}$
F	$0.34 \pm 8 \cdot 10^{-3}$	$0.012 \pm 3 \cdot 10^{-4}$

4 Conclusion

The results of the GFP denaturation show that it is possible to measure reaction processes in real-time with the presented apparatus. However, further work has to be done to ensure and proof reproducibility of the experiments. Stronger bondings as well as seals inside the connectors and the ports on the chip should be included to ensure safe flow and to enable the use of higher flow-rates to reduce the dead-time. An empiric determination of the dead-time (as described e.g. in [5]) has yet to be done to be able to produce valid scientific data.
The pH-quenching of fluorescein can be used to visualise the mixing when observed with a CCD camera and a non-confocal microscope [7].
After a few month the bond between the carrier plate and the lid of the mixer showed signs of corrosion possibly impairing the integrity of the mixer. For further work a new mixer chip should be acquired. Furthermore the use of a custom designed mixer and more durable materials (e.g. PEEK tubing, mixer from fused silica) may be an option and would spare the necessity of bonded connections and improve the reliability of the setup.

Acknowledgement

The work has been carried out at Institut für Physik, Universität zu Lübeck.
Special thanks are due to Dr. Young-Hwa Song and Manfred Mischok for their competent support.

5 References

[1] S. V. Kathuria, A. Chan, R. Graceffa, R. P. Nobrega, C. R. Matthews, T. C. Irving, B. Perot, and O. Bilsel, "*Advances in turbulent mixing techniques to study microsecond protein folding reactions*," Biopolymers, vol. 99, no. 11, SI, pp. 888–896, 2013.

[2] D. McQuarri, "*Stochastic approach to chemical kinetics*," Journal of Applied Probability, vol. 4, no. 3, pp. 413–&, 1967.

[3] R. Harvey, "*A Simple Stopped-Flow Photometer*," Analytical Biochemistry, vol. 29, no. 1, pp. 58–&, 1969.

[4] S. M. H. Khorassani, A. Ebrahimi, M. T. Maghsoodlou, M. Shahraki, and D. Price, "*Establishing a new conductance stopped-flow apparatus to investigate the initial fast step of reaction between 1,1,1-trichloro-3-methyl-3-phospholene and methanol under a dry inert atmosphere*," Analyst, vol. 136, no. 8, pp. 1713–1721, 2011.

[5] P. Brissette, D. Ballou, and V. Massey, "*Determination of the dead time of a stopped-flow fluorometer*," Analytical Biochemistry, vol. 181, no. 2, pp. 234–238, 1989.

[6] L. Böswirth and S. Bschorer, *Technische Strömungslehre*. Wiesbaden, Germany: Vieweg+Teubner Verlag, 2012.

[7] Z. Majumdar, J. Sutin, and R. Clegg, "*Microfabricated continuous-flow, turbulent, microsecond mixer*," Review of Scientific Instruments, vol. 76, no. 12, 2005.

[8] O. Shimomura, F. Johnson, and Y. Saiga, "*Extraction, purification and properties of aequorin, a bioluminescent protein from luminous hydromedusan, aequorea*," Journal of Cellular and Comparative Physiology, vol. 59, no. 3, pp. 223–&, 1962.

[9] K. Alkaabi, A. Yafea, and S. Ashraf, "*Effect of pH on thermal- and chemical-induced denaturation of GFP*," Applied Biochemistry and Biotechnology, vol. 126, no. 2, pp. 149–156, 2005.

Fluorescence Properties and Cytotoxicity of Nanoparticle-based Ratiometric Fluorescent Thermometer on RPE Cells

S. Adler [1], G. Hüttmann [2] and Y. Miura [3]

[1] Medizinische Ingenieurwissenschaft, Universität zu Lübeck, stephanie.adler@miw.uni-luebeck.de

[2] Institue of Biomedical Optics, Universität zu Lübeck, huettmann@bmo.uni-luebeck.de

[3] Institute of Biomedical Optics and Department of Ophthalmology, Universität zu Lübeck, miura@bmo.uni-luebeck.de

Abstract

To overcome the difficulties of determination of the temperature-resolved biochemical responses of retinal pigment epithelial (RPE) cells during/following hyperthermia, it is desired to establish a method for temperature measurement at the cellular level. Recently introduced dual colour ratiometric nanothermometer (RNT) consist of the temperature-sensitive fluorescent dye Eu-TTA (λ_{ex} = 340 nm, λ_{em} = 614 nm) and the thermo-insensitive rhodamine 101 (λ_{ex} = 540 nm, λ_{em} = 596 nm). In this study, the temperature-dependent fluorescence spectra of RNT were measured using a spectrofluorometer, and then the effect of RNT on RPE cell viability was examined using a MTT assay. The measurement of the fluorescence spectra of RNT confirmed the temperature-sensitivity of Eu−TTA and the relatively stable fluorescence intensity of rhodamine 101, while fading phenomenon of Eu−TTA fluorescence is still to be solved. MTT assay results suggest that RNT can be cytotoxic in high concentrations, thus the concrete molecular concentration for non-cytotoxic use should be determined.

1 Introduction

Many diseases of the fundus of the eye, such as age-related macular degeneration (AMD) or diabetic retinopathy, are significantly related to the dysfunction of retinal pigment epithelial (RPE) cells [1], [2]. Since the RPE cells adhere and interact with the photoreceptor outer segments (POS) at their apical side, the disturbance or loss of the RPE function might lead to the loss of visual function. Therefore, the RPE serves as a critical therapeutic target. There are different laser-based therapeutic approaches targeting RPE cells, as for instance photocoagulation, selective retina treatment (SRT) and transpupillary thermotherapy (TTT). Some of them (e.g. photocoagulation and TTT) are applied for the purpose of the use of laser-induced thermal effects. Due to the high variety of individual tissue properties of the RPE and the choroid, as especially melanin contents, the temperature increase at the irradiated site varies with location. Therefore, control of the thermal dose at laser irradiation is almost impossible without dosimetry. Most recent development allows to control the thermal dose during irradiation [3], [4]. These possibilities motivated us to investigate temperature-dependent RPE cell biological responses towards the establishment of a new therapeutic strategy to induce sublethal RPE hyperthermia. Sublethal temperature increase-dependent biochemical responses of RPE cells are still not known very well. Previous reports suggested that the intracellular temperature increase could lead to valuable repercussions whereby cellular functionality could be improved [5]. However, since there are still only a few studies performed, temperature-dependent biochemical responses of RPE cells should be further elucidated in order to clarify the effects of sublethal RPE hyperthermia. To monitor the temperature-dependent cellular responses in detail, measuring the intracellular temperature has been desired. Most of the previous studies regarding RPE cell responses to hyperthermia have been conducted with a thermometer for the extracellular temperature measurement [5]. For the intracellular measurement, a molecular thermometry that could be performed in aqueous solutions and also in biological cellular environment is desired. Different approaches have been taken by different workgroups from single-emission fluorescent probes to ratiometric fluorescent ones [6]. Here, we used nanoparticle-based ratiometric fluorescent probes designed and synthesized by our collaborator, Madoka Suzuki, Ph.D. and his workgroup from the Waseda Bioscience Research Institute in Singapore [7]. These ratiometric nanoparticle are of great interest as it was reported that they spontaneously enter living HeLa cells via endocytosis and serve as a walking nanothermometer in cells [7], [8]. In this study, we examined first the fluorescence properties of the nanothermometer, which were kindly provided by M. Suzuki, Ph.D. with our laboratory setup. Then, towards the application in temperature measurement of our RPE cell cultures, the effect of the nanothermometer on RPE cell viability was investigated.

2 Material and Methods

2.1 Cell culture

To obtain a primary RPE cell culture, porcine RPE cells were isolated from freshly enucleated porcine eyes. The cells were cultured in Dulbeccos Modified Eagle Medium (DMEM), supplemented with 10 % porcine serum, 1.0 % antibiotics/antimycotics and 1.1 % sodium pyruvat (purchased from Sigma-Aldrich) at 37 °C and 5 % CO_2. One day after seeding, the cells were washed with phosphate buffer saline without calcium chloride and magnesium chloride (PBS^-) to remove non-adherent cells. When grown to confluence, the cultures were passaged by trypsinization using trypsin and ethylenediaminetetraacetic acid (EDTA) (0.05 g trypsin + 0.1 g EDTA / 100 ml PBS^-). This subculture process was repeated when the cells were grown to confluence again. The cell culture dishes of the second generation were used for experiments.

2.2 Fluorescent ratiometric nanothermometer (RNT)

The fluorescent RNT were kindly provided by a research group of Dr. Suzuki, Waseda University Singapore. In addition to the thermosensitive europium(III) thenoyltrifluoroacetonate (Eu-TTA: λ_{ex} = 340 nm, λ_{em} = 614 nm), the thermo-insensitive rhodamine 101 (λ_{ex} = 540 nm, λ_{em} = 596 nm) is also encapsulated in a hydrophobic poly(methylmethacrylate) (PMMA) core. This core is additionally coated with positively charged poly(allylamine) hydrochloride (PAH) to shield from interactions with the surroundings. An overview of the nanoparticle structure can be seen in Fig. 1. The mean diameter of the nanoparticle has been given as 140 $\pm$ 59.9 nm (mean $\pm$ standard derivation) [7]. The obtained nanoparticles were diluted in 1 ml of distilled water (stock solution). Since the dry weight of the solution had not been measured, the concentration (w/v) and the molar concentration of the nanoparticle solution could not be determined in this study.

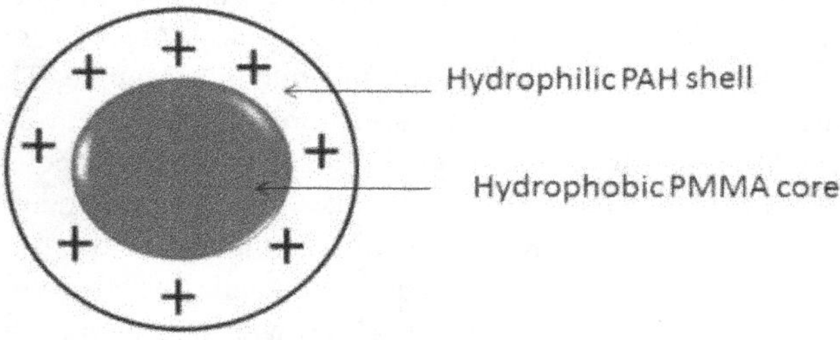

Figure 1: Overview of the nanoparticle structure. The core, encapsulating the fluorophores Eu-TTA and rhodamine 101, consists of hydrophobic poly(methylmethacrylate) (PMMA), the shell consists of positively charged poly(allylamine) hydrochloride (PAH).

2.2.1 Measurement of the temperature-dependent fluorescence spectra of RNT

To measure the temperature-dependent fluorescence spectra of RNT, including Eu-TTA and rhodamine 101, a tenfold dilution of the stock solution was made with PBS^-. Three wells of a 96-well-plate (Sarstedt, No. 82.1581) were filled with 100 μl of the diluted nanoparticle solution, and some wells were filled with 100 μl PBS^- to determine the background fluorescence. Fluorescence spectra at the excitation wavelengths of 340 nm with no cut-off for Eu-TTA and at 540 nm with a cut-off at 550 nm for rhodamine 101, were measured for the emission wavelength range of 570 nm to 650 nm (2 nm steps) with a spectrofluorometer (SpectraMax M4, Molecular Devices, USA) linked to its specific computer program (SoftMax® Pro, Molecular Devices). These measurements were performed at some temperatures in the range of 22.5 °C to 46 °C (22.5 °C, 30 °C, 38 °C, 46 °C). After the measurement was conducted in ascending order of temperature, the temperature of the device was cooled down to approximately 24 °C and the measurement was repeated, in order to examine if the change of temperature-dependent fluorescence intensity is reversible. The mean value of the background fluorescence was calculated and was subtracted from the mean fluorescence intensity of the samples. The ratio of the fluorescence intensities between those at the excitation with 340 nm (Eu-TTA) and with 540 nm (rhodamine 101) was calculated at each temperature setting.

2.2.2 MTT assay: determination of the effect of RNT on RPE cell viability

The MTT (3-(4,5-dimethylthiazol-2-yl)-2,5-diphenyltetrazoliumbromide)-assay was conducted according to the protocol developed by Mosmann [9]. Porcine RPE cells were seeded on some wells of a 96-well-plate (5000 cells in 100 μl medium per well). When the cells were grown to confluence, the culture medium was replaced with a dilution of RNT in culture medium (10-, 100-, 1000- or 10000-fold dilution of the stock solution). For each dilution, four wells were provided to calculate their mean value afterwards. Additionally, the cells in four wells were not exposed to RNT to assign this mean value as the non-treated control. The cells were then incubated for 48 h at 37 °C in the 5 % CO_2 incubator. After incubation, 20 μl of MTT solution (5 mg/ml) were added to each well with RPE cells, followed by the short rotation on the plate shaker at 150 rpm for 5 min, and the next incubation at 37 °C in the 5 % CO_2 incubator for 3 h. In the next step, the cell culture supernatant was removed and replaced by 100 μl dimethylsulfoxid (DMSO). Another rotation was carried out at 150 rpm for 5 min to stir it thoroughly with the cells. This is followed by the measurement of the light absorption at 570 nm with the spectrophotometer (SpectraMax M4, Molecular Devices, USA). The intensity of the absorption value indicates the amount of formazan, which was formed through the conversion of MTT by the function of a mitochondrial dehydrogenase. Therefore, the obtained value can be utilized as an indicator of the number of the vital cells.

3 Results and Discussion

3.1 Temperature-dependent fluorescence spectra

Fluorescence spectra of Eu-TTA and rhodamine 101 at different temperature settings are shown in Fig. 2 and 3, respectively. The measured data confirm the fluorescence maxima of Eu-TTA at 614 nm and rhodamine 101 at 596 nm for the given excitation wavelength. As can be seen in Fig. 2, the fluorescence intensity of Eu-TTA declines with increasing temperature (71.13 % decrease by ascending temperature from 22.5 °C to 46 °C, at λ_{ex} = 340 nm, λ_{em} = 614 nm). The fluorescence intensity of rhodamine 101 also showed slight decline (11.81 % decrease at λ_{ex} = 540 nm, λ_{em} = 596 nm) (cf. Fig. 3), which was smaller compared to the one of Eu−TTA. Fading phenomenon was observed with both dyes. After the temperature of the spectrofluorometer was cooled down to approximately 24 °C, their fluorescence intensity was not as high as the one measured beforehand at a similar temperature (Fig. 2 and 3, thin continuous lines). In Fig. 4, the ratio of the fluorescence intensities of Eu-TTA and rhodamine 101 was calculated for the corresponding wavelengths. The ratio declines for each wavelength with rising temperature. Since the influence of the fading phenomenon of Eu-TTA was apparent as shown above, the ratio could reach approximately only the half of the inital value after cooling of temperature down to 24 °C. For the repeatable and precise temperature measurement in the studies on cells, it is surely necessary to produce minimal fading fluorescent RNT.

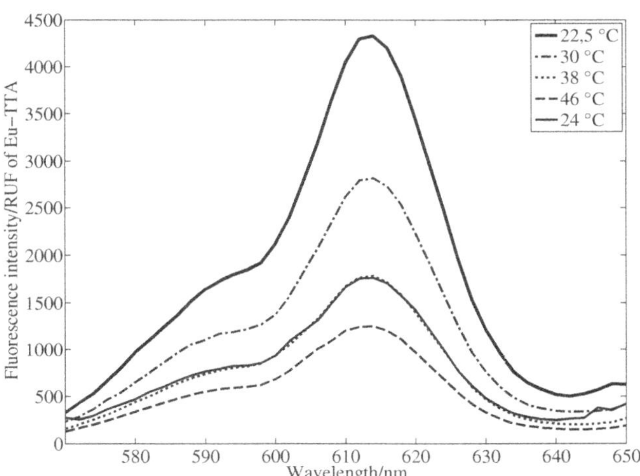

Figure 2: Temperature-dependent fluorescence spectrum of Eu-TTA for the emission wavelength range of 570 nm to 650 nm (λ_{ex} = 340 nm). In the measurements with ascending temperature, the fluorescence intensity decreases with increasing temperature. However, as seen with the thin continuous line (24 °C), which describes the spectrum after the temperature was cooled down, fading phenomenon was confirmed as the fluorescence intensity was not as high as before.

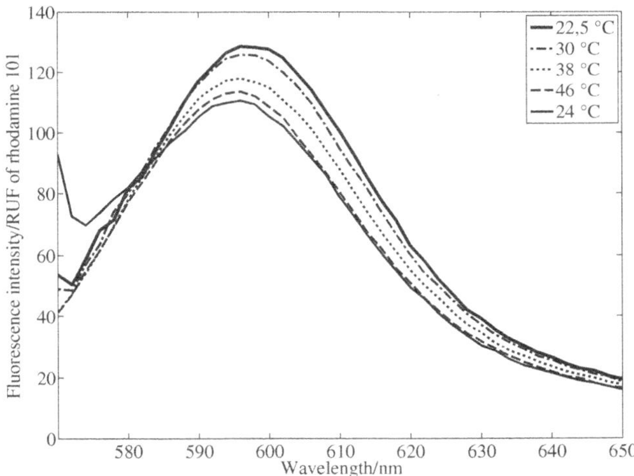

Figure 3: Temperature-dependent fluorescence spectrum of rhodamine 101 for the emission wavelength range of 570 nm to 650 nm (λ_{ex} = 540 nm). The thin continuous line (24 °C) describes the spectrum after the temperature was cooled down.

3.2 MTT assay

As can be seen in Fig. 5, higher concentration of RNT (small dilution rate) decreased the light absorption values in the assay, indicating the decrease of RPE cell viability. The light absorption values were scaled as the relative value to the non-treated control group in percent. To determine if there is a significant variation within the different groups of RNT dilution and to include the whole sample in the analysis, a one-factorial analysis of variance (ANOVA) was conducted. The p-value of the ANOVA indicates that there are significant differences (p = 6.5E-16). Afterwards, a post-hoc two-tail t-test was conducted on the data to determine which groups are significantly different. The significance needs to be adjusted to avoid a cumulation of errors. The adjustment was carried out by a bonferroni correction, where the significance value was divided by the number of comparisons. The results yield that all dilutions tested in this study lead to a significant decrease in cell viability, where the higher dilution rate (1000- and 10000-fold dilution) showed significantly less toxicity than the low dilution rate (100- and 10-fold dilution). These results suggest that RNT may be cytotoxic. However, the toxic effect seems to be concentration-dependent, and therefore, in order to confirm the possibility of their usage on RPE cells in experimental research, we need to investigate further to find the safe dilution rate as well as the determination of the molar concentration corresponding to it.

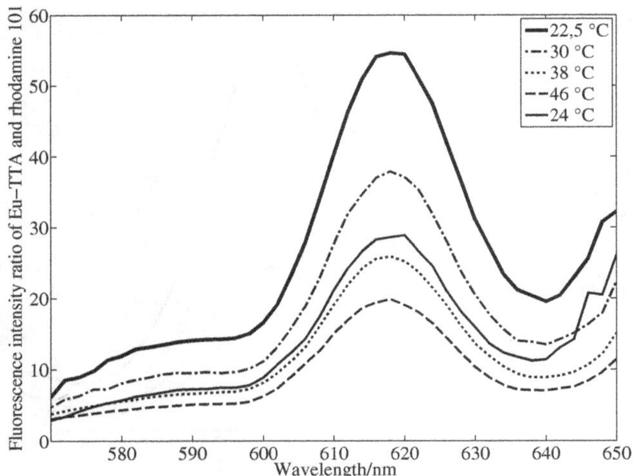

Figure 4: Ratio of the fluorescence intensities of Eu-TTA and rhodamine 101 dependent on wavelength and temperature. The thin continuous line labels the spectrum which has been measured after the temperature of the spectrofluorometer was cooled down back to 24 °C.

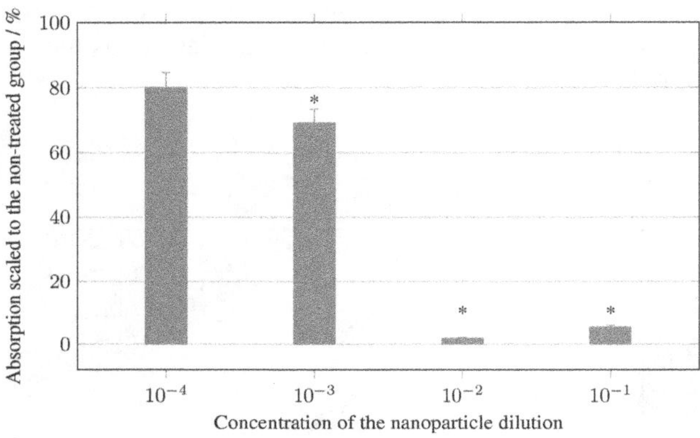

Figure 5: Non-treated group is assigned 100 %. The RNT dilution treated groups are scaled dependent on their absorption value. * indicates a significant difference between the p-values of the non-treated group and the treated groups.

4 Conclusion

The ratio of the fluorescence intensities of the RNT that we examined is temperature-dependent, although it is reversible only to some extent due to the fading phenomenon. Those fading problem needs to be solved in the future RNT development. RNT showed a concentration-dependent cytotoxic effect on RPE cell culture. For experimental research, the toxicity of RNT on RPE cells needs to be further investigated.

Acknowledgement

This work has been carried out at the Institute of Biomedical Optics of the Universität zu Lübeck. Special thanks go to M. Suzuki, Ph.D. from the Waseda Bioscience Research Institute in Singapore for providing the RNT.

5 References

[1] J. Ambati, J. P. Atkinson, and B. D. Gelfand, “Immunology of age-related macular degeneration,” *Nature reviews. Immunology*, vol. 13, pp. 438–51, June 2013.

[2] I. S. Samuels, B. A. Bell, A. J. Pereira, J. E. Saxon, and N. S. Peachey, “Early retinal pigment epithelium dysfunction is concomitant with hyperglycemia in mouse models of Type 1 and Type 2 diabetes,” *Journal of Neurophysiology*, Nov. 2014.

[3] R. Brinkmann, S. Koinzer, K. Schlott, L. Ptaszynski, M. Bever, A. Baade, S. Luft, Y. Miura, J. Roider, and R. Birngruber, “Real-time temperature determination during retinal photocoagulation on patients,” *Journal of biomedical optics*, vol. 17, p. 061219, June 2012.

[4] S. Koinzer, K. Schlott, L. Ptaszynski, M. Bever, S. Kleemann, M. Saeger, A. Baade, A. Caliebe, Y. Miura, R. Birngruber, R. Brinkmann, and J. Roider, “Temperature-controlled retinal photocoagulation–a step toward automated laser treatment,” *Investigative ophthalmology & visual science*, vol. 53, pp. 3605–14, June 2012.

[5] H. Iwami, J. Pruessner, K. Shiraki, and R. Brinkmann, “Protective effect of a laser-induced sub-lethal temperature rise on RPE cells from oxidative stress,” *Experimental Eye Research*, vol. 124, pp. 37 – 47, 2014.

[6] C.-Y. Chen and C.-T. Chen, “A PNIPAM-based fluorescent nanothermometer with ratiometric readout,” *Chemical communications (Cambridge, England)*, vol. 47, pp. 994–6, Jan. 2011.

[7] Y. Takei, S. Arai, A. Murata, M. Takabayashi, K. Oyama, and S. Ishiwata, “ARTICLE A Nanoparticle-Based Ratiometric and Self-Calibrated Fluorescent Thermometer for Single Living Cells,” *ACS Nano*, vol. 8, no. 1, pp. 198–206, 2014.

[8] K. Oyama, M. Takabayashi, Y. Takei, S. Arai, S. Takeoka, S. Ishiwata, and M. Suzuki, “Walking nanothermometers: spatiotemporal temperature measurement of transported acidic organelles in single living cells,” *Lab on a chip*, vol. 12, pp. 1591–3, May 2012.

[9] T. Mosmann, “Rapid colorimetric assay for cellular growth and survival: Application to proliferation and cytotoxicity assays,” *Journal of Immunological Methods*, vol. 65, pp. 55–63, Dec. 1983.

Comparative Study of the Gamma-Spectrometers Berthold LB2040's and Berthold LB2045's Performance based on the Half-life Determination of the Radioactive Isotope Ba-137m

C. Treig [1], J. Schorch [2], E. König[1] and C. Schmidt [2]

[1] Medizinische Ingenieurwissenschaft, Universität zu Lübeck, {christoph.treig, enno.koenig }@miw.uni-luebeck.de

[2] Isotopenlabor der Sektion Naturwissenschaft, Universität zu Lübeck, {schorch, christian.schmidt}@isolab.uni-luebeck.de

Abstract

The gamma spectrometer Berthold LB2040 was acquired in 1983 by the Universität zu Lübeck to perform laboratory experiments for teaching purposes. The intended use was to determine the half-life of Ba-137m. After 31 years of service and due to a rising number of outtakes, the Berthold LB2045 was acquired. As part of the acquisition in 2014, it should be checked, whether it can deliver the same performance concerning LB2040's tasks. Focus of this work is a comparison between both devices, with regarding to functionality, the influence of different acceleration voltages and the general performance by determining the half-life of Ba-137m. The result is, that the Berthold LB2045 can handle all requirements. It can even provide a broad range of additional capabilities for the future.

1 Introduction

Since 1983 the Isotopenlabor der Sektion Naturwissenschaft of the Universität zu Lübeck has used the nuclear radiation measuring device Berthold LB2040 for teaching purposes, especially in the context of the radiation safety course. In 2014 the Berthold LB2040 was replaced by the new gamma spectrometer Berthold LB2045. Both devices are capable of detecting gamma-photons,[1] which occur at nuclear decay. Thereby, they allow the identification of different types of nuclides as well as the determination of the half-life in radioactive samples.

In the Isotopenlabor der Sektion Naturwissenschaft at the Universität zu Lübeck these devices are mainly used by students calculating the half-life of Ba-137m, the daughter nuclide of Cs-137. In this context, the devices shall be compared in order to determine the technical differences. In detail, the researches include the energy properties, the functionality and the effect of different acceleration voltages on the current counting rate.

2 Material and Methods

In the following subsections the basics as well as the experimental setup and the device properties are described.

2.1 Basics

An isotope generator by Eckert & Ziegler Nuclitec GmbH® is used for the tests. It contains up to 370 kBq Cs-137[2] with a half-life of 30.02 years. Cs-137 as long-lived parent nuclide decays by emission of beta radiation into the stable isotope Ba-137.

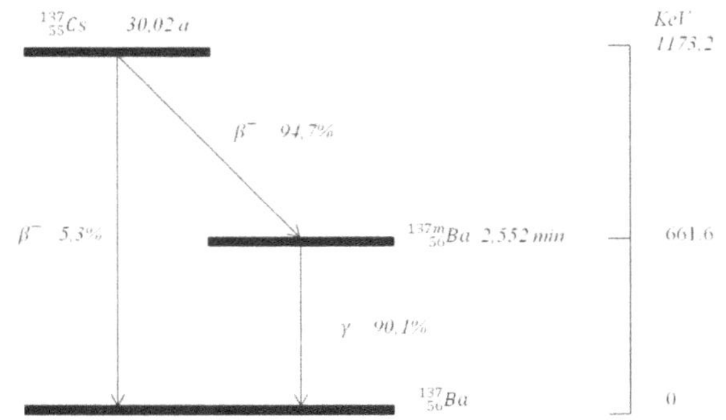

Figure 1: Term diagram of Cs-137 decay [1]

As shown in Figure 1, Cs-137 decays directly with a 5.3 % probability into the stable energy state of Ba-137. In 94.7 % of cases, the conversion takes place via the metastable, excited energy state of the daughter nuclide Ba-137m. In contrast to Cs-137, Ba-137m has a very short half-life of only 2.552 min. Ba-137m decays into the stable state of Ba-137 with a 90.1% probability by emission of gamma radiation.

[1] Detection of alpha and beta radiation is not possible.

[2] Date of acquisition: 10/02/2012

The energy of this transition is 661.66 keV.
In the remaining 9.9 % cases, there is internal conversion of the Ba-137m following characteristic energy lines, including the prominent K_α at 32.194 keV.
Within the generator Cs-137 and Ba-137m exist in a secular equilibrium, which develops if the half-life of the parent nuclide is long compared to that of the daughter. In the state of equilibrium, the activity of the daughter equals the parent's [2]. To dissolve the Barium, a saline eluting solution is used. After elution, the re-establishment of equilibrium or the decay of Ba-137m can be measured with both devices.

A. Berthold SZ50U - Scintillation Detector
In the scintillator, the detection material is arranged in a lattice. The ionizing radiation transfers energy on the lattice's electrons (see Figure 2) [5]. When this energy is released, small light flashes are generated. For preventing further ionization due to the released electrons, an energy buffer in form of a donated atom is added in the lattice. The light flash releases electrons in the photocathode of the photomultiplier (see Figure 3). High voltage allows to accelerate the electrons towards the anode thereby releasing further electrons in an avalanche effect, that can be detected as a current impulse at the anode [5]. Its magnitude depends on the energy of the incoming radiation. The most commonly used scintillator material is doped sodium iodide (NaI), as it is used in the Berthold SZ50U [6].

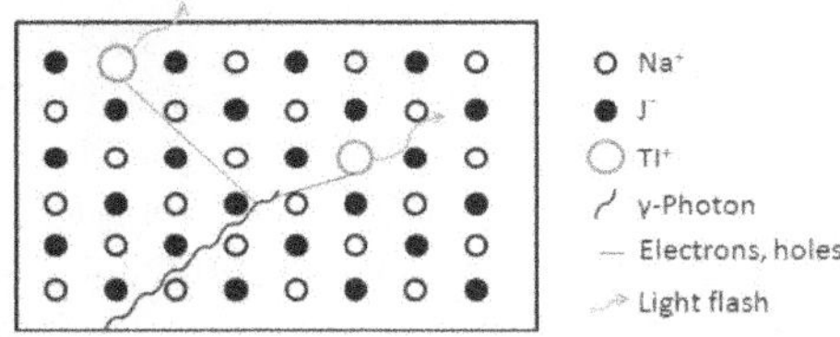

Figure 2: Generation of a light flash in a doped NaI - crystal

The iodide provides a high gamma-ray absorption. It also supplies a great light output and has an excellent energy resolution for a scintillation detector [2, 6].

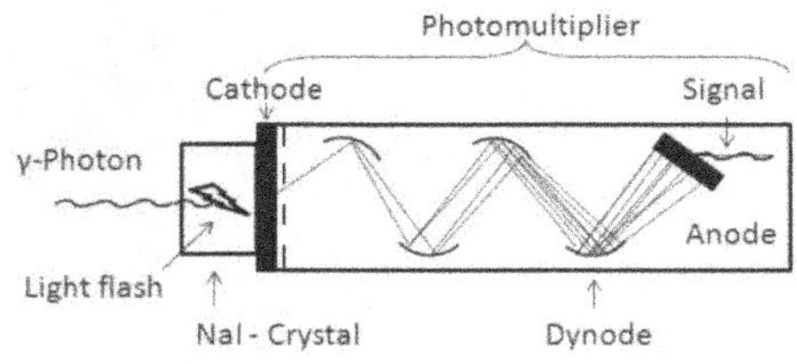

Figure 3: Principle of a NaI - detector [5]

However, there are some major disadvantages. It is brittle and sensitive to thermal gradients as well as to thermal shock. Moreover, it is hygroscopic and must be encapsulated at all times [2, 6].
During the measurement, the detector is placed in a lead shielding to reduce background radiation at all times. The shielding is 160 mm in diameter and has a material thickness of 35 mm.

B. Berthold LB2040
The Berthold LB2040 measuring system consists of a high voltage unit, a pulse amplifier, a one channel discriminator, a digital counter and a rate meter.
The device compares the magnitude of the radiation's voltage pulse U_γ with two threshold voltages U_1 (Baseline) and U_2. If $U_1 \leq U_\gamma \leq U_2$, the pulses will be counted.
For measuring purposes, the Berthold LB2040 has to be connected to the Berthold SZ50U scintillation detector.

C. Berthold LB2045
The Berthold LB2045 is a modern gamma spectroscopy system used for the application in laboratories, nuclear medicine or for studying environmental samples.
The LB2045 is a modular built system consisting of a central processing unit and a graphical touch screen. Like the Berthold LB2040, it has to be connected to the SZ50U scintillation detector for measuring purposes. For measurement data acquisition, the system utilises a multi channel analyzer, which is capable of recording 2048 energy channels simultaneously. It provides different energy ranges (0-256 keV, 0-1024 keV and 0-2048 keV) as well as a nuclide library, an automatic energy calibration, a half-time correction and a background measurement.

2.2 Experiment Setup

At the beginning of the measurement, various presettings on the Berthold LB2040 are applied. At first, it is important to identify the operating voltage in which the detector is in the plateau. The plateau is the voltage range, where no further electrons are dissolved out of the dynode by the applied high voltage. Therefore, the LB2040 and the SZ50U are connected and the Cs-137 radiation source is placed in front of the detector. Now the voltage, beginning with 250 V, is increased gradually by 50 V up to 1100 V (the upper limit is 1250 V).

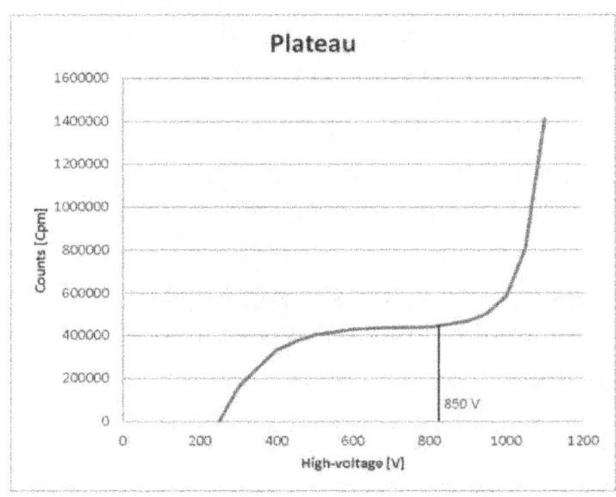

Figure 4: Voltage characteristics of the LB2040

Based on the determined curve (figure 4: Plateau), the operating voltage is set to 850 V for all following tests.
To get correct results, it is important to know the background radiation. Therefore, the Cs-137 is removed and the decays in the whole energy range are counted with 10

repetitions (see Table 1). After that an average, which will be subtracted from the received data, is calculated.

Table 1: Background radiation

Measurement	1	2	3	4	5	6	7	8	9	10	Average
Background radiation	310	260	270	240	350	340	260	250	370	220	± 287

Finally, the Cs-137 spectrum is recorded to find the characteristic energy peaks, so that the data can be used as reference for comparison during later tests. The energy range is 100 mV. The baseline U_1 starts at 0 mV and will be increased significantly up to 600 mV.

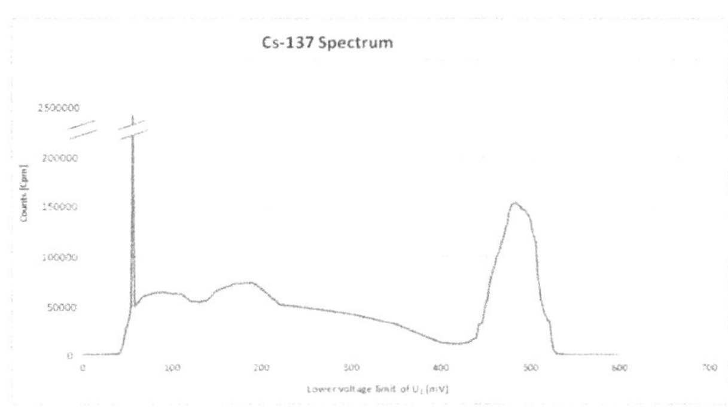

Figure 5: Energy spectrum of the Cs-137 determined with the LB2040 features two peaks.

Figure 5 shows two distinct energy peaks: The first one at about U_1 = 56 mV with approximately 2,500,000 counts per minute (cpm) and the second one at about U_1 = 484 mV with approximately 155,000 cpm. The first peak is equivalent to the characteristic 32.194 keV energy line and the second one to the 661.66 keV energy line of the Cs-137 spectrum. The peak position depends on the applied high voltage. For the following half-life measurements, the energy peak at 661.66 keV will be used.

The LB2045 is equipped with a built-in automatic energy calibration using a Cs-137 source.

2.3 Elution of Ba-137 and Half-life Calculation

For eluting Ba-137, a solution of 0.04 % HCl and 0.9 % NaCl is pressed through the generator with a syringe. The eluate is collected in a small vessel and quickly placed in front of the detector. The LB2040 is set to the previously determined voltage settings. To receive enough values, measurement intervals of 12 s over 15 min are chosen for both devices. For the LB2040, a short break of 8 s is necessary to manually record the data. On the contrary, the LB2045 transmits the data automatically to a PC. Therefore it is able to perform two more measurements per minute. The received data is plotted semi-logarithmic over time. To determine the half-life, the slope m of the straight line is calculated by

$$m = \frac{ln(\frac{Y_2}{Y_1})}{X_2 - X_1}, \tag{1}$$

and the half-life itself by the equation

$$T_{\frac{1}{2}} = \frac{ln(2)}{m}. \tag{2}$$

X represents a certain point of time and Y the corresponding count rate.

3 Results and Discussion

A. Precision of Half-life Determination

The activity plotted semi-logarithmic over time yielded to a declining straight line for each device, which is shown in Figure 6.

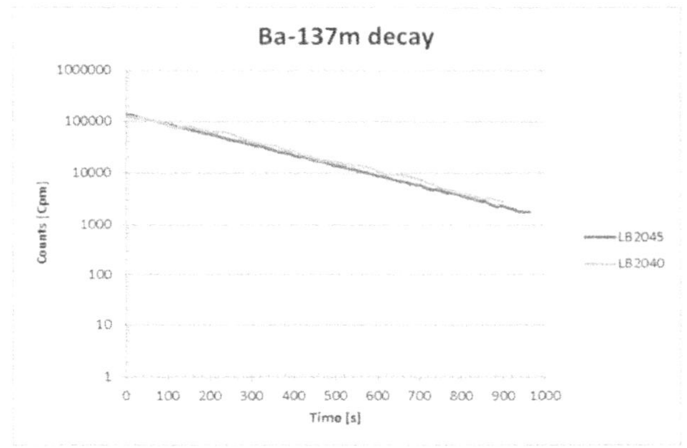

Figure 6: Semi-logarithmic plot of the decays over time

According to (1) and (2), the calculated half-life of Ba-137m was $T_{\frac{1}{2}}$ = 2.65 min for the Berthold LB2040 and $T_{\frac{1}{2}}$ = 2.52 min for the Berthold LB2045. Therefore, the error for the LB2040 to the given literature value of 2.552 min were 3.84 % and for the LB2045 1.19 %.

B. Acceleration Voltage

The acceleration voltage's influence could only be analysed at the LB2040. At the LB2045, it is an inherent part of the automatic calibration, so that it could not be changed manually.

Experiments of this kind were not possible with the new device. Apart from this fact, the LB2040 was not capable of holding the high voltage at a constant level over a long period. The reason for this was probably a defective contact. So it is hardly suitable for longer experiments in the future.

C. Energy Properties

The LB2040 offers 1000 different base-line voltage settings to choose. The smallest energy resolution is 2 mV, but there is no direct correlation with the gamma-photon's energy in keV. As shown in section 2.2, an additional measurement and recalculation is necessary. The LB2045, on the contrary, directly shows the gamma-photons energy in keV. The lowest possible energy resolution is 5 keV.

The main advantage of the LB2045 was its ability to measure and separate all energy lines at once and to show them in a spectrum. The LB2040, on the other hand, uses a one channel discriminator, which detects only one certain energy interval at the same time. For a full spectrum, a sampling of all baselines (energy lines) has to be done.

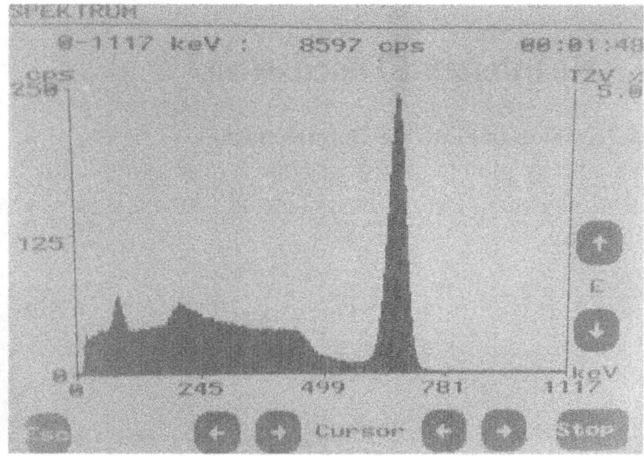

Figure 7: Cs-137 spectrum recorded with the LB2045

Figure 7 shows the measured spectrum with both specific Cs-137 peaks. Compared to LB2040's spectrum, the prominent 32.194 keV peak was less intense. The unexpected high intensity of this peak, observed with the LB2040, was probably caused by electronic disturbances due to the age of the device.

D. Functionality

There are generations between these two devices - the LB2040 is, after all, more than 30 years old. It works completely analogue except for a digital counter. Before each measurement, the plateau and the spectrum have to be determined. After that, every measurement is started manually. It is not possible to run automatic routines like at the LB2045 for repeating sequences for example. Due to the manual operating observational errors cannot be excluded.

The LB2045 is much more user friendly, because there is an automatic calibration, which takes only a few seconds. Settings for several nuclides can be selected, including different energy ranges and measurement sequences. Nevertheless, these measurement sequences have some disadvantages. If the measurement time is very long, the device produces an average over all occurred decays. This circumstance is problematic, especially when the measurement time is much longer than the half-life. At very short measurements the statistical error is quite big, because the acceleration voltage is switched on before each single measurement and needs some time to adjust.

4 Conclusion

Although, based on the results, both devices were capable of handling all assigned tasks, the LB2045 was definitely superior to the LB2040 regarding functionality, usability and performance. It could be used by persons without any specific knowledge. The handling was simple and the results were delivered in a quick and uncomplicated manner. Its use for teaching purposes is absolutely recommended. For the future, there are lots of different additional options with the LB2045, e.g. nuclide analyses[3], radioimmunoassays, or analyses of environmental samples [4][4].

On the contrary, the LB2040 required many presettings and -knowledge leading to a much longer measurement process in general. Furthermore, due to the device's high age, there were some electronic failures, which led to errors making it frequently necessary to repeat single measurements. This, in particular, strongly questions its reliability in the future.

Acknowledgement

The work has been carried out at the Isotopenlabor der Sektion Naturwissenschaft, Universität zu Lübeck.
Special thanks go to Prof. Dr. C. Schmidt, Dr. J. C. Schorch and E. König, who were always available to answer my questions.

5 References

[1] E. Brown and R. B. Firestone, *Table of Radioactive Isotopes*. John Wiley & Sons, England, 1986.

[2] Gordon R. Gilmore, *Practical Gamma-ray Spectrometry*. John Wiley & Sons, England, 2008.

[3] Berthold Technologies GmbH & Co. KG, *Operating Manual - Kernstrahlungsmessgerät LB2040*. Deutschland, 1983.

[4] Berthold Technologies GmbH & Co. KG, *Operating Manual - Gammaspektrometer LB2045*. Deutschland, 2014.

[5] Bildungsserver Baden - Württemberg, *Szintigraphie mit der Gammakamera*. Available: http://www.schule-bw.de/unterricht/faecher/nwt/unterrichtseinheiten/einheiten/medizin/arbeitsblaetter/31gammakamera_ab.pdf [last accessed on 09.02.2015].

[6] Konll F. Glenn, *Radiation Detection and Measurement*. John Wiley & Sons, England, 2000.

[3] By comparing spectra with literature values.

[4] E.g. waste water, rock samples and soil samples.

Re-setup of a Nitrogen Cooled Ge-Detector in Combination with a Canberra Multi Channel Analyzer for Determination of Terrestrial Radiation Sources

E. König[1] , J. Schorch [2], C. Treig [1] and C. Schmidt [2]

[1] Medizinische Ingenieurwissenschaft, Universität zu Lübeck, {enno.koenig, christoph.treig}@miw.uni-luebeck.de

[2] Isotopenlabor der Sektion Naturwissenschaft, Universität zu Lübeck, {schorch, christian.schmidt}@isolab.uni-luebeck.de

Abstract

The gamma spectrometer, a combination of the Canberra® multi channel analyzer DeskTop-InSpector and an Ortec® high-purity germanium detector, is used by the Isotopenlabor der Sektion Naturwissenschaft of the Universität zu Lübeck since 2001 for determining radioactive nuclides in samples. For the upcoming tasks, it has to be updated. To test the system's functionality, some terrestrial samples are analyzed with a new developed identification sequence. The results show, that the system could be updated successfully. Several radionuclides are found in the samples, proving the device's operational capability for the future.

1 Introduction

The Isotopenlabor der Sektion Naturwissenschaft of the Universität zu Lübeck uses the multi channel analyzer Canberra® - DeskTop-InSpector in combination with a Ortec® - high-purity germanium detector for gamma spectroscopy, especially in the context of the radiation safety course. In 2014 Microsoft® terminated its service for Windows XP. Therefore the detector's operating software shall be reinstalled on a Windows 7 operating system, checked for the corresponding compatibility, calibrated and finally tested on terrestrial radiation sources. Furthermore, for automatic nuclide identification, the existing nuclide library shall be modified and a new analyzing sequence be created. The aim is to determine radionuclides in different samples.

2 Material and Methods

For optimal measurement conditions, it is important to know the devices' functional principles. Setup and test execution depend on it.

2.1 Germanium Detector

For the detection of γ-radiation NaI- or germanium detectors are usually used.

In solid structures the precisely determined energy levels of atoms are broadened into energy bands. Between these bands are energy regions, which are forbidden to electrons. The energy difference between the two upper-most (valence band and conduction band) is called band-gap. For electrons to migrate through the material (current), they must gain sufficient energy to jump from the valence band across the band-gap into the conduction band. In semiconductors, like germanium, the band-gap is about 0.67 eV, so that most electrons are in the lower valence band and only a few in the upper. This provides a limited degree of conductivity, which depends on the current temperature - the higher the temperature, the higher the probability that an electron will be promoted to the conduction band. This resulting background current interferes with the actual measurement of γ-radiation and can be reduced by cooling.

Germanium is four valent and in a crystal lattice, surrounded by four other germanium atoms, each contributing electrons to the bounding between them. For improving its conductivity, it can be doped. On the one hand, a three valent atom, which produces a positive charged hole, can be inserted in the lattice (p-type germanium)[1]. On the other hand, it is possible to insert a five valent atom, which contributes an additional electron (n-type germanium)[2].

As shown in Figure 1, in a germanium detector the two types are combined and connected to a voltage source.

Due to the electric field, the positive-charged holes migrate to the negative side and the electrons to the corresponding positive side. The result is a region around the physical junction without charge carriers - the depletion region [1, 2]. Its size depends on the applied bias voltage and works practically as an insulator. However, if γ-photons of radioactive decay are absorbed in this region, they produce charge carriers due to ionization. The applied voltage pulls them through the whole depletion region leading to a measurable

[1] e.g. gallium or boron

[2] e.g. gallium or phosphor

current, which is proportional to the γ-photon's energy.

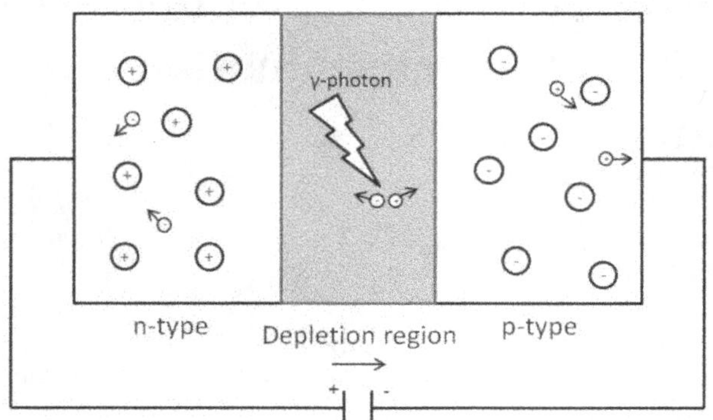

Figure 1: Basic construction of a germanium detector

The detector's main advantage towards gas detectors or scintillation detectors (e.g NaI - see paper C. Treig) is the much higher number of created charge carriers due to the low ionization energy. The statistical spread of the current's pulse height is consequently smaller leading to a much higher energy resolution. Furthermore, the transport of the charge carriers in semiconductors is much faster than the one of the ions in a gas detector [2].

The Ortec® - high-purity germanium detector is suitable for the energy range between 40 keV and 10 MeV [3].

2.2 Multi Channel Analyzer

The multi channel analyzer device Canberra® - DeskTop-InSpector is attached directly to the germanium detector. It basically sorts the generated pulses by height into different channels. Each channel number corresponds to a certain energy interval and an increasing channel number corresponds to the increasing γ-energy [2].

In the current constellation, the DeskTop-InSpector is set to 8192 channels covering a energy range from 0 to 2317 keV.

The device also provides the high voltage up to 4500 V, which creates the band-gap in the germanium detector [3].

2.3 Setup

As shown in Figure 2, the detector and samples are placed inside a heavy, 110 mm lead, a 3 mm copper and a 10 mm acrylic glass shielding to reduce all kinds of radiation to protect the operator from the radiation source inside the shielding as well as to reduce the impact of background radiation.

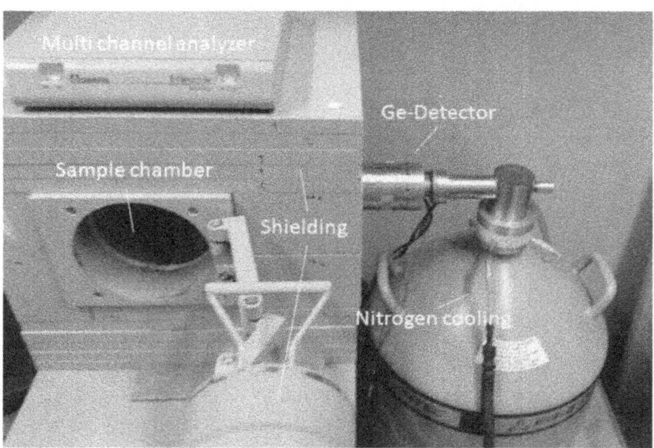

Figure 2: Detector system with shielding, multi channel analyzer and attached nitrogen cooling

The whole detector system is connected to an usual personal computer via a RS232-port. To operate the configuration, the corresponding detector software Genie-2000 is installed on a Windows 7 system. The software was originally designed for a Windows 95 and later updated for Windows XP system. There is actually a Canberra® Windows 7 support, but it is too expensive.

Two different Genie-2000 packages are installed, the basic spectroscopy software and the tool for automatic γ-analyzes. It provides, with the help of the integrated library, a full nuclide identification of a sample. For this, an automatic sequence is developed, which analyzes the recorded spectrum. The following steps are part of the sequence [5]:

- Peak search,
- peak area calculation,
- efficiency correction and
- nuclide identification with interference correction.

The peak search determines the location of the recorded peaks corresponding to a preset sensitivity. The peaks are fitted to a resembling Gauss-function.

In the next step, the area beneath this function and its boundaries are calculated. This yields the number of recorded photons within the peak.

The following efficiency correction is necessary, because photons with different energies are not detected with the same probability.

Finally, the peaks are assigned to the most likely nuclides comparing the energy lines with the library entries. The interference correction checks, if the activity of each energy line matches the probability of this certain decay. In this way, interfering peaks of two different nuclides are separated and reassigned.

Naturally, the identification only provides correct results, if the nuclide specific entries of the energy lines are recorded precisely and the instrument is calibrated correctly. Wrong or inaccurate values have to be edited first.

2.4 Test Execution

Before the measurement of terrestrial samples, the system has to be calibrated regarding to voltage, energy and activity.

A. Applied high voltage
To determine the best possible voltage (see 2.1), the activity of different nuclides is measured. The measurement time was set to 15 minutes and the voltage was increased each time by 500 V.

Table 1: Activity measurement of different nuclides under different voltages

		Counts [1/s]	
Voltage [V]	Co-57 (122 keV)	Ba-133 (356 keV)	Cs-137 (662 keV)
500	3.02	5.65	2.88
1000	5.21	9.34	15.2
1500	6.6	12.7	21.3
2000	7.93	14.3	24.3
2500	8.82	15.4	24.8
3000	9.31	16.1	26.2
3500	9.61	16.2	26.4
4000	9.71	16.5	26.7

Table 1 shows, that the voltage increase over 3000 V did not improve the number of detected decays significantly. To avoid unnecessary strain on the detector, the voltage was set to this particular value.

B. Energy Calibration
For the energy calibration, a Cs-137[3] and a Co-60[4] source are used. With the help of these lines, a three-point calibration is run. This ensures, that the detected unknown nuclide's energy lines match the real ones.

C. Activity Calibration
For the activity calibration, a corresponding solution is used. It consists of different nuclides with known start activities A_0 and known γ-emission rates G. These two values must be calculated at this juncture

$$A = A_0 * e^{\frac{-ln(2)*t}{T_{\frac{1}{2}}}} \tag{1}$$

with the half-time $T_{\frac{1}{2}}$ and t, the days past since the manufacturing date. The same equation applies for the γ-emission rate (A is changed into G). The quotient of G and A yields the decay probability p

$$p = \frac{G}{A}. \tag{2}$$

The quotient of the actual measured counts Z and G is the detection efficiency W of the detector

$$W = \frac{Z}{G}. \tag{3}$$

[3]Main γ-energy at 661.67 keV
[4]Main γ-energies at 1173.24 keV and 1332.5 keV

With these values, the activity of a measured sample can be calculated

$$A = \frac{Z}{p * W}. \tag{4}$$

D. Measurement of Terrestrial Radiation Sources
At last, the automatic nudclide identification is tested on different samples. Primarily, to prove the device's functionality, but also to determine the radiation sources, which are part of the present environment.
List of the examined samples:

- Lignite,
- volcanic rocks,
- uranium rocks,
- uranium pearls,
- a gas mantle,
- dolomitic lime and
- milk powder.

The measurement time was set to 6 h for the U-samples, the volcanic rocks and for the gas mantle due to the expected high activity. For the other three, it was set to 24 h.

3 Results and Discussion

The installation of the detector software Genie-2000 on a Windows 7 system was successful, although some packages, using a MS-DOS or Windows 98 environment, could not be integrated. However, these were not essential for the practical use. Due to the Windows 7 extended support, which continues until 2020, the important safety updates are guaranteed for the future.

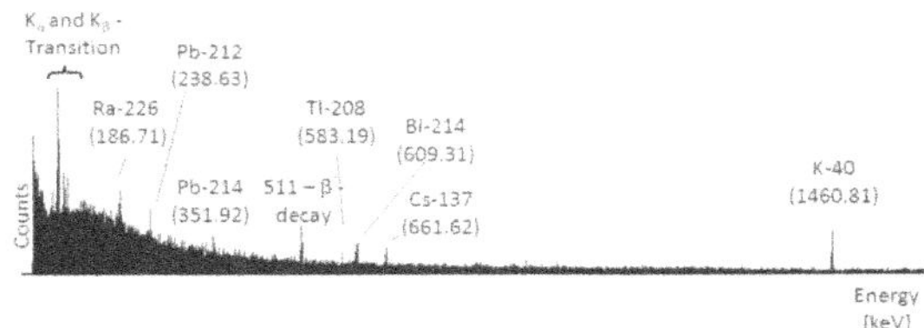

Figure 3: The lead shielding's background spectrum

The background spectrum (see Figure 4) was generated, because of the impurity of the lead shielding. Products of the Th-232 and the U-238 decay chains could be found. Furthermore, the radioactive nuclides led to a K_α and K_β - transition due to ionization (around 74 keV and 88 keV) measurement of the shielding material. Therefore this spectrum had to be subtracted from all following.

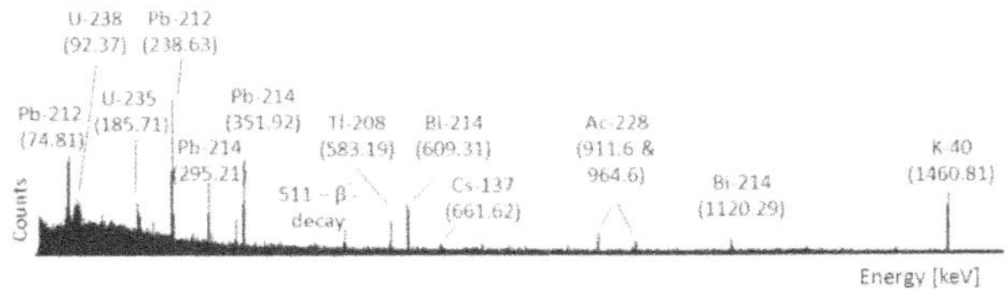

Figure 4: Volcanic rocks spectrum

Figure 4 shows exemplary the spectrum of the volcanic rocks (Figure 3 and 4 are not in scale). The prominent lines are marked. After subtracting the background, the automatic nuclide identification sequence found the following nuclides in different samples:

Table 2: List of nuclides found in the examined samples

Background	Milk powder	Lignite	U-pearls
K-40	K-40	K-40	K-40
Cs-137	Ga-67	Cs-137	Zr-97
Tl-208	Cs-137	–	Th-231
Pb-212	–	–	Pa-234m
Pb-214	–	–	Th-234
Bi-214	–	–	U-235
Ra-226	–	–	Am-243
Np-237	–	–	–
Am-243	–	–	–

Table 3: List of nuclides found in the examined samples

U-rocks	Volcanic rocks	Dolomitic lime	Gas mantle
Ti-44	K-40	Ga-67	Be-7
Co-57	Tl-208	Cs-137	K-40
Kr-87	Bi-212	Tl-208	Ti-44
Zr-97	Pb-212	Bi-211	Mn-54
I-126	Bi-214	Pb-212	Rb-89
Xe-133	Pb-214	Bi-212	Sb-122
Bi-211	Ra-224	Pb-214	Xe-133m
Bi-214	Ac-228	Ra-224	Ce-141
Pb-214	Th-231	Th-231	Eu-155
Ra-226	U-235	Np-237	Tl-208
Ac-227	Np-237	Am-243	Bi-211
Th-227	U-238	–	Bi-212
Pa-231	Am-243	–	Pb-212
Th-231	–	–	Ra-224
Pa-234m	–	–	Ac-228
Th-234	–	–	Th-231
U-235	–	–	Th-232
Np-237	–	–	Pa-234
U-238	–	–	U-238
Am-243	–	–	Am-243

The results in Table 2 and 3 show, that radioactive nuclides were detected in each sample. Most of them were part of the three natural decay chains of U-238, 235 and Th-232 [4]. With this knowledge in mind, it was possible to determine some additional nuclides, whose peaks were not detected by the peak analyze due to its missing accuracy[5] [4]. Additional some nuclides could be excluded, which were not likely to occur in the sample. Their γ-energies often laid in the lower energy range, where backscattering and X-ray fluorescence interfered with the actual spectrum leading to false higher peaks. Especially Am-243[6], detected in almost each analyzes, was unlikely to be present due to the fact that a quadruple neutron capture of Pu-239 is necessary for its generation [4].

Particularly noteworthy was the difference between the U-pearls and the rocks. Many of the U-238's decay chains products were missing in the pearls. The reason was, that they had been cleaned up during the manufacturing process. Only the products until Pa-234m could have build up so far. K-40 was detected in almost every sample, because it is a wide-spread primordial nuclide.

The Cs-137, as a fission product of U-235, was descended most likely from the 1986 nuclear plant accident in Chernobyl, Ukraine.

[5] e.g. Bi-211 and Th-227 (U-235 chain) and Ra-226 (U-238 chain) at the volcanic rocks

[6] main γ-energies at 43.53 keV and 74.66 keV

4 Conclusion

The software installation on a Windows 7 system succeeded without significant problems. The installed software packages works stable and suffice, especially for the radiation safety-course's requirements. This guarantees the device's full functionality in every aspect for the future.

The developed nuclide identification sequence provides an easy and fast way to get a first brief overview of the radionuclides contained in unknown samples. However, with some additional knowledge and experience it can be improved. Furthermore, the quality of the identification depends on the lexical scope and accuracy of the edited library.

The examinations of the samples yielded, that no terrestrial sample is free of radioactive materials.

Acknowledgment

The work has been carried out at the Isotopenlabor der Sektion Naturwissenschaft of the Universität zu Lübeck.
Special thanks go to Prof. Dr. C. Schmidt, Dr. J. C. Schorch and C. Treig, who never got tired of answering my questions.

5 References

[1] Knoll F. Glenn, *Radiation Detection and Measurement*. John Wiley & Sons, England, 2000.

[2] Gordon R. Gilmore, *Practical Gamma-ray Spectrometry*. John Wiley & Sons, England, 2008.

[3] PerkinElmer instruments, *Operator's Manual - Solid-State Photon Detector*. Oak Ridge TN , U.S.A., 2001.

[4] E. Brown and R. B. Firestone, *Table of Radioactive Isotopes*. John Wiley & Sons, England, 1986.

[5] Canberra Eurisys GmbH, *Genie-2000 - Benutzerhandbuch-*. Germany, 2004.

4
Biomedical Engineering

Dispensation of a bead suspension into small vessels

N. Blimke [1], E. Hoffmann [2], R. Rahmanzadeh [3] and L. Richter [2]
[1] Medizinische Ingenieurwissenschaft, Universität zu Lübeck, blimke@miw.uni-luebeck.de
[2] Development Analysis Techniques, EUROIMMUN AG, Lübeck, Germany, {e.hoffmann, l.richter}@euroimmun.de
[3] Institute of Biomedical Optics, Universität zu Lübeck, rahmanzadeh@bmo.uni-luebeck.de

Abstract

Particle-based automated laboratory is a relatively new advanced method for in-vitro diagnostics. For this purpose magnetic beads labeled with certain antigens are used for automated immunoassay devices. Here, we present an experimental setup for a reproducible filling procedure of a bead suspension into small vessels. First, an agitation system is used to keep the suspension homogeneous. To avoid sedimentation of the bead suspension, homogeneity is an essential requirement of this process. Afterwards, to fill the suspension into small vessels a reservoir connected with a peristaltic pump is mandatory. In this work, an appropriate bead reservoir was designed. The evaluation shows, that an agitator is more suitable than a standard mixing device for small volumes. For avoiding sedimentation of the beads inside the reservoir more turbulences have to be generated. However, new specifications are necessary for a bead reservoir to fill each small vessel by an automated liquid handling system.

1 Introduction

Automated laboratory machines are getting more and more popular for in-vitro diagnostics due to the high throughput and high quality of the analyses and reproducibility of the results [1]. The degree of automation of these machines ranges from semi-automated washing units or measurement devices to liquid handling systems [2] and to fully automated analyzers, performing complete sample processing as well as measurement and evaluation [1].
Currently, the application of magnetic beads for automated immunoassay devices is a well-established method [3]. The size of magnetic beads that we used is adjustable from 1 µm to 3 µm. The beads consist of several nanometer-sized iron particles that are wrapped with a layer of polymers. Even though beads are not magnetic or ferromagnetic, they behave in a magnetic field similar to iron filings.
For human antibody analysis, the beads are coated with certain antigens, e.g. VlsE (variable major protein-like sequence, expressed) or Borr. sucmo (Borrelia sucmo) [3].
For a novel fully automated analyzer, currently under development at EUROIMMUN, magnetic beads are employed as single test filled in small vessels. The challenge by using beads, is the rapid sedimentation. To avoid sedimentation a continuously maintained homogeneous bead suspension is a prerequisite. Thus, the amount of beads filled in the vessels must be highly reproducible.
The focus of this work is the dispensation with a reproducible amount of bead suspension into small vessels. For this purpose, the development of a bead mixing unit is necessary. Additionally, the construction of a bead reservoir is required.

2 Material and Methods

In this section, the two main parts for filling operation are presented: The experimental setup of a bead mixing unit and the design of a bead reservoir. Each part is analyzed with appropriate experiments. We will start, however, with a brief description of the general setup.

2.1 General setup

2.1.1 Hardware components

To maintain the homogeneity of the reprocessed bead suspension, a suitable method must be found. This is done by a mechanical agitator, which adequately mixes the bead suspension comparable to a roller shaker. As illustrated in Fig. 1, an one-liter-bottle with a wide bottleneck is used for the experiments. A peristaltic pump (323Du/MC304, Watson Marlow, MA USA) is applied, so that the bead suspension flows from the bottle to the reservoir and back again. The filling of each small vessels can then be done with an automated liquid handling system [2].

2.1.2 Quantifikation of beads

For counting the beads in suspension, Fluorescent-activated cell sorting (FACS) as a laser-based measurement method is used. Since beads in our application are not fluorescent, only the cell counting functionality of FACS is declared. Inside the FACS device (CyFlow Space, Sysmex Partec GmbH, Görlitz, Germany), particles pass a flow cuvette and are irradiated by a laser spot. This light is scattered by the particles and detected with photomultipliers.

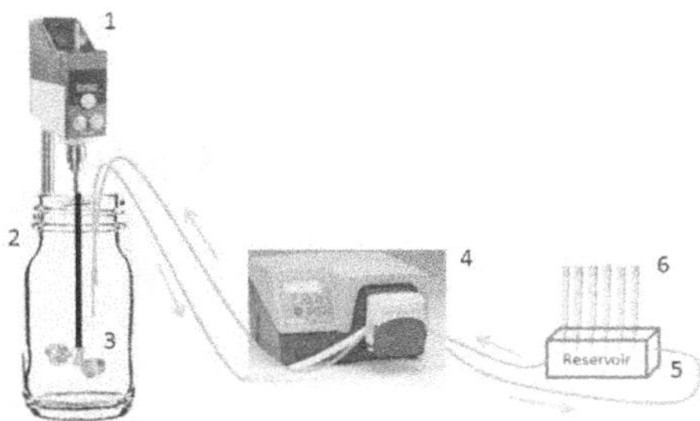

Figure 1: Experimental setup. The bead suspension inside an one-liter-bottle (2) is pumped by a peristaltic pump (4) through a reservoir (5) and afterwards back to the bottle. A precise amount of the suspension is pipetted with an automated liquid handling system (6). The homogeneity of the suspension is maintained by an agitator (1) and stirrer (3).

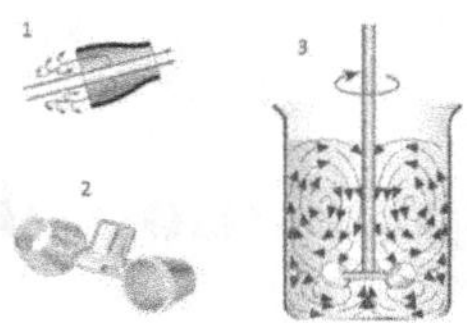

Figure 2: Turbulent equity ratio of swirling (3) are produced by the turbine-like design (1) of the dual impeller stirrer (2) from ViscoJet.

The forward scattered light (FSC) is used for determination of the cell size and the sideward scattered light (SSC) is applied for the detection of granularity and structure of cells [4]. The flow cytometry can differentiate between single beads and clusters. However, the amount of beads forming a specific cluster, can not be determined.

2.2 Bead mixing unit

2.2.1 Requirements

To mix a solution by a stirrer, certain requirements are mandatory. It is essential that no foam formation occurs while mixing. Due to foam, beads might sediment. Thus, the bead suspension will loose its homogeneity. Furthermore, a low dead volume is particularly important, in terms of wasting any bead suspension which might be not mixed. To achieve an equal distribution in the small vessels, the most important requirement is the avoidance of sedimentation.

2.2.2 Experimental evaluation

For evaluation the stirrer VISCO JET dual impeller d = 60 mm (VISCO JET Agitation Systems, Waldshut-Tiengen, Germany) and the agitator RZR2041 (Heidolph instruments, Schwabach, Germany) are used, which offers up to 2000 rpm for the stirrer. Fig. 2 shows the concept of the stirrer by VISCO JET which consists of a turbine-like design. In the following experiment, homogeneity produced by the stirrer is compared to the homogeneity produced by a roller shaker (RS-TR 5, Phoenix Instrument GmbH, Garbsen, Germany), which is a standard for smaller volumes. Secondly, the influence of foam to the bead sedimentation is evaluated.

2.2.2.1 Homogeneity

First, it must be shown if the stirrer and the roller shaker, which was used as reference, provide equal results. Thus, a homogeneity check must be verified. For this test MyONE beads labeled with Borr. sucmo were utilized in a concentration of 0,4 µg/ml. The bead suspension was diluted with blot wash buffer in a ratio of 1:167. The total volume contained approximately 400 ml. The bead suspension was mixed by a roller shaker for 15 min. Afterwards, 4 ml were taken as a reference sample. During the entire test, the reference sample was mixed by the roller shaker. The remaining amount of bead dilution was mixed in an one-liter-bottle with the agitator at a speed range of 302 - 313 rpm. Now, 3x 100 µl were taken from the stirrer beads as well as from the reference sample every 15 min. This was performed for 130 min. Each of the 100 µl samples was filled with 900 µl of sheath buffer and the amount of beads was measured with the FACS as described in Section 2.1.2. This way, homogeneity was evaluated over time.

2.2.2.2 Influence of foam formation

First, we have evaluated if the beads settle in foam during the continuos mixing process. Thus, the bead concentration would probably decrease over time. The agitator was therefore set to 1000 rpm, so that foam formation was occured in the bead suspension.
For this experiment, the same approach of the previous attempts was used. For pre-treatment the bead suspension was mixed by the stirrer at 300 rpm for 40 min. To compare the results, 3x 100 µl were taken every 5 min from the surface of the solution. Afterwards the same dilution (100 µl of the bead suspension with 900 µl of sheath buffer) was used for the FACS measurement. After 20 min the rotation speed was increased to 1000 rpm. The range of removal remained constant.
As a continuative experiment, we repeated the above described test but for a longer period of time. In this case, the bead suspension was mixed by the roller shaker for 85 min. Subsequently, the suspension was mixed at 300 rpm for 20 min by the agitator and afterwards at 1000 rpm. The measurement time was performed for 4 h 15 min.

2.3 Bead reservoir

2.3.1 Requirements

To avoid sedimentation of the beads, certain requirements are mandatory for a bead reservoir. The two main components are the rounding of all edges as well as the prevention of undercuts. Undercuts are zones, that will practically not be mixed. Here, the probability for bead sedimentation is extremly high. To connect the peristaltic pump with the reservoir, tubes are essential. Indeed, undercuts produced by the tube connectors are inevitably. Furthermore, a purification of the reservoir must be possible for reutilization. To minimize evaporation, the surface must be rather small but loarge enough for access.

2.3.2 Design

As a first concept a reservoir with six individual wells is designed. For later processing the external dimensions of the reservoir corresponds to an usual SBS (ANSI-Standard on the recommandation of Society for Biomolecular Screening [5]) format. For constructing flexible tubes of the peristaltic pump, tube connectors suitable for inside diameter (ID) 2.54 mm/2.79 mm are constructed. All wells have in common, that an overflow is used to maintain a constant liquid level as well as a subsidence of a hole, which used for aspiration. As illustrated in Fig. 3 the variable parameters are width of the wells (w), designs of the inlet and outlet (x), differential length (y) and kind (z) of the aspiration hole.

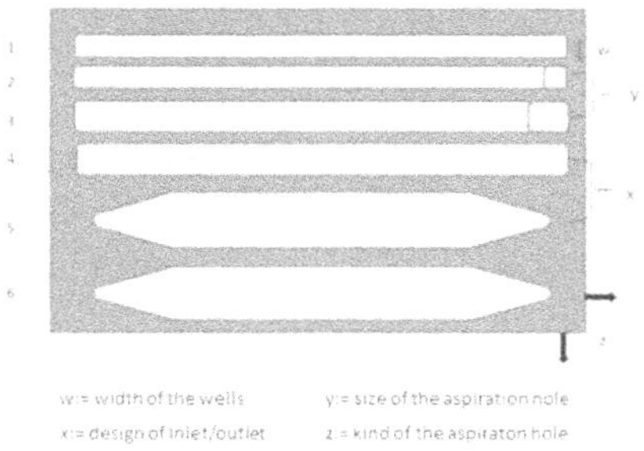

Figure 3: Schematic design of the bead reservoir with individual wells and parameters.

In Table 1 six wells with their individual parameters are listed. The reservoir is produced with an Objet Connex 3D Printer (Stratasys, Eden Prairie, MN USA). To design a fine-detail and stable model the object is printed by the transparent material VeroClear-RGD810 [6].

Table 1: Individual parameter of the wells

Parameter		1	2	3	4	5	6
width (w)	2 mm	x	x				
	3 mm			x	x		
	6mm					x	x
inlet/ outlet (x)	parallel	x	x	x	x		
	conic					x	x
length of the aspiration hole (y)	1.65 mm				x	x	
	4.65 mm	x	x	x			
kind of the aspiration hole (z)	lateral	x		x	x	x	
	bottom-up		x				x

In Fig. 4 the constructed bead reservoir with the individual parameters is illustrated. All descripted requirements are implemented.

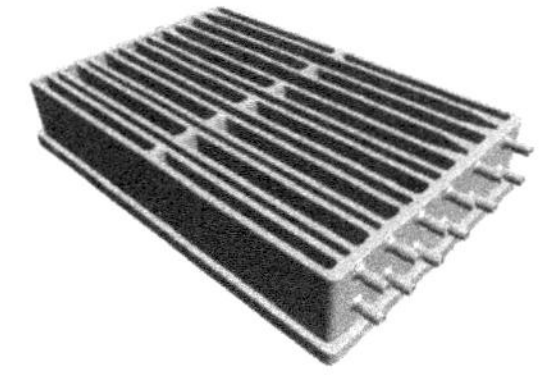

(a) General view

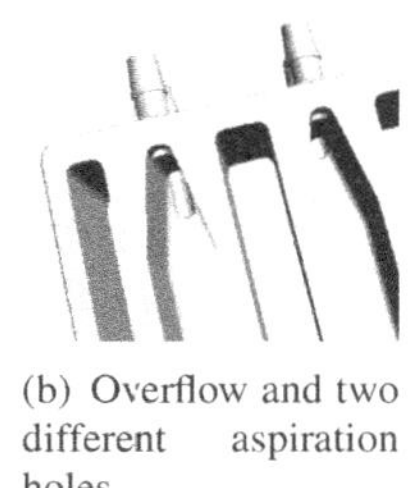

(b) Overflow and two different aspiration holes

Figure 4: Design of the bead reservoir.

2.3.3 Experimental evaluation

To check the functionality of the bead reservoir for potential sedimentation places, well 1 and well 6 were filled alternately with distilled water and red dye. Thus, the peristaltic pump was connected with the bead reservoir, so that the liquid circulated. The rotation speed of the peristaltic pump was set to 60 rpm. In addition to sedimenation places flow conditions are analyzed. Potential sedimentations of dye molecules could be easily recognized. Thus, new insights and requirements can be gained to design an improved reservoir.

3 Results and Discussion

In this section, we present the results of the tests of the bead mixing unit as well as the experimental test of our bead reservoir.

3.1 Bead mixing unit

3.1.1 Homogeneity

As illustrated in Fig. 5 the homogeneity between a roller shaker used as reference and an agitator is approximately equal. Thus, the bead suspension is sufficiently mixed by the agitator at 300 rpm. A minimal outlier exists after 30 min. But there is also a high standard deviation at this particular time. However, clusters are not disrupted by stirring, because the amount of clusters as well as the amount of single beads does not increase.

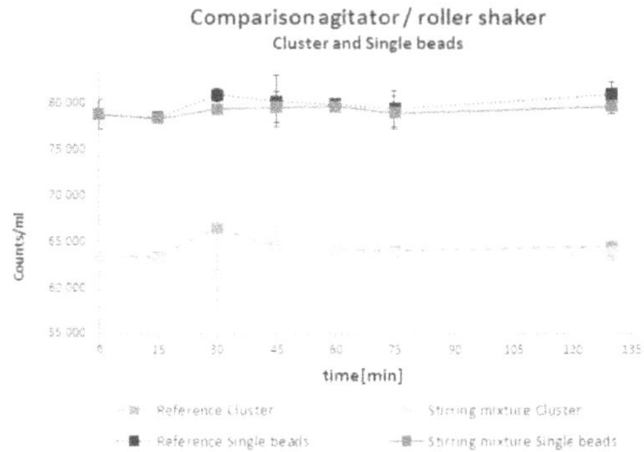

Figure 5: Comparison of homogeneity by the stirrer (300 rpm) and the roller shaker.

3.1.2 Influence of foam formation

To analyze the influence of foam formation, the rotation speed was increased to 1000 rpm after 20 min. The line graph (Fig. 6) shows the increased amount of single beads. As we have shown in later tests clusters are be produced by wash buffer over time. We analyse primarily the temporal process of single beads and clusters. Thus, the amount of beads per milliliter varies at starting time. In addition, the count of clusters in the bead suspension increases slightly. This means that clusters are broken up to smaller clusters and single beads. Initially, it was assumed that a large amount of beads would settle in foam, and the amount of beads decreases at a high number of rotations. As illustrated in Fig. 6, we showed the opposite with our experiment. To confirm the results, the test was repeated over a longer period.

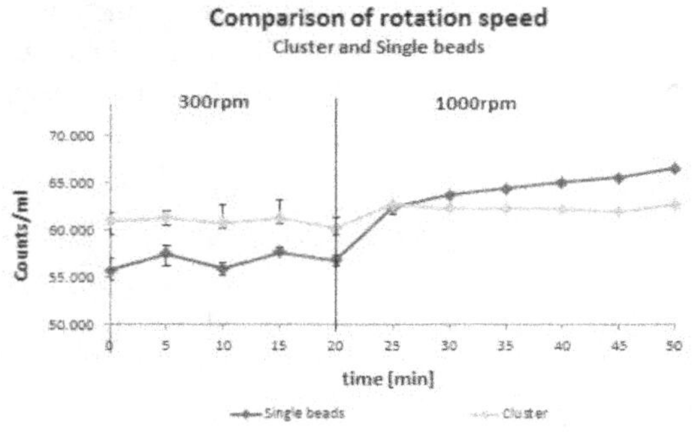

Figure 6: Comparison of Clusters/Single beads at 300 rpm and 1000 rpm.

As illustrated in Fig. 7 the results were confirmed: There is an increase of single beads in suspension. The amount of clusters also increases. Our assumption of cluster disaggregation is intensified. According to this, we assume clusters are broken up to smaller clusters and single beads. However, the amount of beads remained constant after 195 min. The homogeneity the reference sample is constant during the entire process.

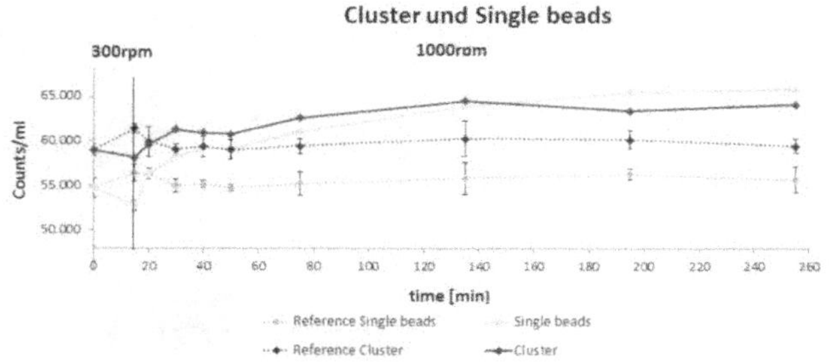

Figure 7: Comparison of Clusters/Single beads at 1000 rpm.

3.2 Experimental evaluation of the bead reservoir

Sedimentations of red dye molecules are visible at the aspiration hole as well as at the side walls. By the second aspiration hole, the dye solution flows directly against the wall between the two aspiration holes. The local sedimentations would be probably identical if the red dye would be replaced with the bead suspension. Due to conical in-/ and outlet the flow condition in well 6 is most suitable. In the wells 1 to 4 undercuts are predominant. However, the flow conditions in all wells are still insufficient due to the narrow width of the wells.

4 Conclusion & Outlook

We have shown that the agitation system is a suitable method for homogenous mixing of a bead suspension. Our result suggests, that clusters are broken up in case the rotation speed is high enough. To produce a minimal foam formation as well as a cluster disaggregation, the rotation speed must be adapted accordingly.
Furthermore, the constructed reservoir must be adapted to avoid sedimentation of the bead suspension. The wells are to narrow for producing a turbulent flow. Thus, the individual wells of the reservoir have to be enlarged to a major reservoir. Other requirements are a major radius of the roundings as well as a conic hole of the in-/ and outlet.
Thus, we could prove a number of factors that manipulate the loading of a bead suspension in small vessels with a reproducible amount. As a next step, we plan to integrate the designed bead reservoir in combination with the presented mixing unit into an EUROLabLiquidHandler for an automated filling of the bead suspension into small vessels.

Acknowledgement

The work has been carried out at EUROIMMUN AG.

5 References

[1] David Wild, Rhys John, Chris Sheehan, Steve Binder and Jianwen He, *The Immunoassay Handbook: Theory and applications of ligand binding, ELISA and related techniques.* Elsevier, UK, Fourth Edition 2013.

[2] EUROIMMUN AG, *EUROLabLiquidHandler - Intelligent pipetting*, product description, Lübeck, 11/2012.

[3] DYNAL, *Surface-activated Dynabeads*, A wide product portfolio for flexible molecular separations, 2010.

[4] Partec, *CyFlow space Instrument Operating Manual.* Münster, Rev. 004, 2007.

[5] American National Standards Institute, *for Microplates - Footprint Dimensions*, Society for Laboratory Automation and Screening, ANSI/SLAS 1-2004.

[6] Stratasys, *PolyJet Materials Data Sheet*, Eden Prairie, MN USA, 05-2014.

Simulation of torque acting on the joints of an exoskeleton for stroke rehabilitation

G. Männel [1], A. Gabrecht [2] P. Weiss [2] and E. Maehle [2]

[1] Medizinische Ingenieurwissenschaft, Universität zu Lübeck, maennel@miw.uni-luebeck.de
[2] Institute of Computer Engineering, Universität zu Lübeck, {gabrecht,weiss,maehle}@iti.uni-luebeck.de

Abstract

This paper describes the development of a MATLAB simulation to calculate the acting toques at the joints of an exoskeleton used in post stroke rehabilitation. The simulation uses object-oriented programming to create a finger model, basically consisting of three joints and their associated guiding points of the tendon used for actuation. The simulation is used to examine the trajectory of the acting torque. It was found that the torque at the joints can decrease down to 37.6 % while closing the hand. It was possible to reduce the decrease at one joint to 0.9 % by constructing an arch over the joint. Also the simulation is used to examine the influence of one's joint orientation on the acting torque at another joint. It was found that the angles of the metacarpophalangeal joint (MCP) and proximal interphalangeal joint (PIP) have an influence on the torque at the respective other one.

1 Introduction

Stroke is the leading cause of acquired disabilities worldwide [1]. In 60 % of the cases stroke patients suffer an impairment of the hand for a longer time period, whereas only 5 to 20 % of all patients recover full functionality [2]. Impairments of the hand functions causes problems in activities of daily living, such as opening a bottle or using a computer.
Stroke rehabilitation is based on the concept of neuronal plasticity, the capability of lifelong cerebral reconfiguration, which is a long term process. This leads to long and expensive therapies. In combination with demographic changes in the western civilization, socio-economic problems arise. Today 2 to 5 % of healthcare costs in western civilization goes directly toward stroke treatment and rehabilitation [3]. In Germany the costs for first time ischemic stroke is estimated to sum up to 108 billion Euro over 20 years from 2010 till 2030. An estimation of the WHO states that the absolute number of stroke patients in the EU and the EFTA-states will grow about 36 % over 25 years. Predicting that the number will rise from 1.1 million patients in the year 2000 to 1.5 million in 2025 [3].
The basis of motor learning is repetitive, task-specific training [4], which makes it suitable for robots assisting the therapist. Although studies did not yet show a significant improvement in activities of daily living, the functionality and the strength of the impaired limb may improve through robot assisted therapy [5]. In addition to the supportive part in traditional therapy, robotic rehabilitation holds the opportunity of additional exercise in home environment independent from therapist and clinics. Therefore, those systems have to be inexpensive, transportable, and easy to use.

The approach of the **m·ReS**-project is to develop a **m**odular **Re**habilitation **S**ystem using different robotic devices for specific training tasks and hand functions instead of an all in one device. So the complexity of the single modules can be reduced, lowering the production cost and achieving more custom training possibilities. The system's module for pinch and grasp training is an exoskeleton dorsally mounted to the patient's hand [6]. To use exoskeletons in post stroke rehabilitation, it is important to prevent misalignment between the motion axis of the device and the anatomic joints of the user [7] [8], otherwise causing soreness, stiffness, or even pain for the patient. In order to avoid the usage of adaptation mechanisms, a parameterized computer-aided-design (CAD) model was created. Using these parameters to control the dimensions of the exoskeleton allows us to fit the model to the user's hand. By applying rapid prototyping techniques, such as 3D-printing, it seems possible to produce customized rehabilitation devices with a minimum joint misalignment [9].
It is furthermore possible to reduce the price by using fewer actuators then independent movable degrees of freedom (DOF). In the examined exoskeleton only one actuator for each finger is used. The achieved force is conveyed with Bowden cables to the exoskeleton. The tendon runs from the back of the hand over guiding points to the finger tips. The acting torque $\vec{M}$ at one joint is given by

$$\vec{M} = \vec{F} \times \vec{r}. \tag{1}$$

Assuming the joint is placed in the origin, then $\vec{r}$ is representing the last tendon guiding point in front of the joint. The direction of $\vec{F}$ is given by the difference from $\vec{r}$ and the vector of the next guiding point. It's length is given by the applied force of the actuator. A rotation in the joint leads to

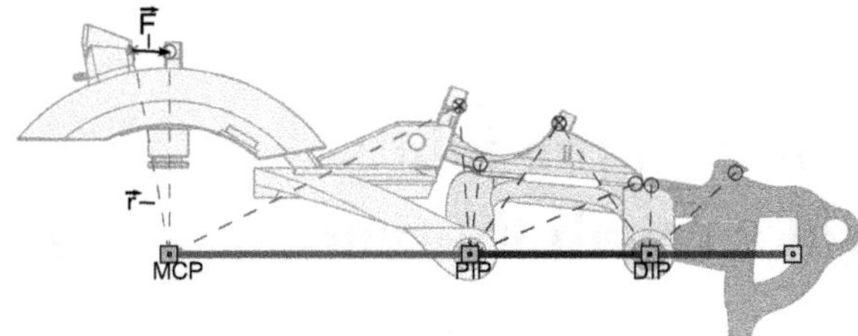

Figure 1: Visualization of the simulated finger model laid over the 2D-projected CAD-Model of the index finger. The bold lines represent the finger links and the bright squares the joints of the exoskeleton. The dashed lines represent the association of points with a joint, by connecting them. A circle at the end stands for a fix relation to the joint, so it moves in space when the joint is rotated. An X at the end indicates that the point is fix in space for the respective joint. If an X is in a circle the same point is associated twice to different joints. So when a rotation in the joint takes place, the point moves in space but keeps it relation to the other joint, because the joint rotates also around the other joint. The associated points in this image also represent the approximated position of the potential guiding points. On the MCP is $\vec{r}$ and $\vec{F}$ from (1) are marked.

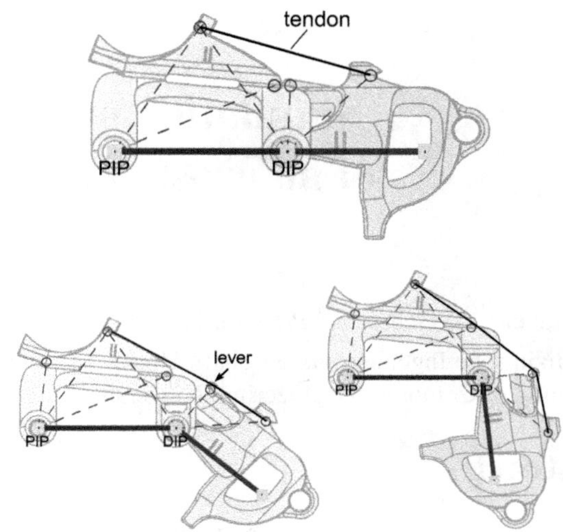

Figure 2: Illustration of the switch between guiding points at the distal interphalangeal joint (DIP) of an index finger. In the top the joint is fully extended enabling direct convey between the two initial guiding points. This direct transmission is disturbed as the lever, keeping the tendon away from the users skin, interferes as new contact point (bottom left). On the bottom right it can be seen that at about 90 degrees joint angle another guiding point takes the place of the initial one left of the joint.

a change of the relation between the guiding points, causing a change in the acting torque. This dependency on the joints angles makes it hard to control the acting torque by only applying a single force. The Vectors $\vec{r}$ and $\vec{F}$ are also marked on the metacarpophalangeal joint (MCP) in fig. 1.
This paper presents the preparation of the next prototype iteration and the base for a new controlling algorithm. A simulation implemented in MATLAB is used to calculate the acting torques at each joint. It takes into account that the guiding points can change depending on the joint angles. Based on these results it is examined how the orientation of one joint influences the torques acting on the other joints. Furthermore additional guiding points were simulated to determine their effect on the acting torque.

2 Material and Methods

The simulation was developed in MathWorks MATLAB version 2010b. Additionally the robotic toolbox version 9.9 by Peter Corke [10] was used. Using object-orientation for each joint and the finger allowed to parameterize the finger model in the simulation in a similar fashion as the CAD-Model, using the same Excel-Spreadsheet as data basis.
Each object of the class *joint* holds the information about its position in space when the finger is fully extended, its Denavit-Hartenberg (D-H) parameters, and the limits in which it is possible to flex the joint. Also it is possible to associate points to the joint and save their relative position to it. Furthermore each object has the functionality to create the D-H parameters for the finger link's end point and for rotation around the joint.
To create an object of the class *finger* three *joints* are needed. Each object sets the three links in relation to each other, so it holds the information of every joint position and its associated points. The class also provides the functionality to set any joint to a desired angle within its limits and plot the finger. Fig. 1 shows thereby the MATLAB-plot from the simulation on top of a 2D-projected CAD-Model of the index finger using the same parameters.
By using the model it is possible to calculate the torque over each joint at any joint angle. First the initial guiding points, when the joint is completely extended, were determined. This is necessary for taking into account that the guiding points can vary depending on the configuration of all joints. Depending on the joints angle the guiding point can change, because another contact point moves into the direct connection between the former points deflecting the tendon. This circumstance is illustrated by fig. 2, displaying the possible guiding point of the distal interphalangeal joint (DIP) and the joint rotation angle where the change takes place. The exact position of the guiding points is thereby changing all the time, considering having a surface instead of a point. The simulation just considers an approximation of all points capable of becoming a guiding point and calculates the corresponding flip angle. Knowing the points between which the tendon is tensioned at each joint angle allows us to apply (1).

2.1 Examination of the torque trajectory

Using the simulation, the trajectory of the torque for each joint as a function of its angle is evaluated. The model used for creating the trajectory is based on the measured parameters of a 31 year old male's right hand index finger. The hand was not impaired by stroke. Further information about the measurement of the parameters is given in [9]. The exoskeleton model used for this part is shown in fig. 1. The other joints are fully flexed, in order to minimize the influ-

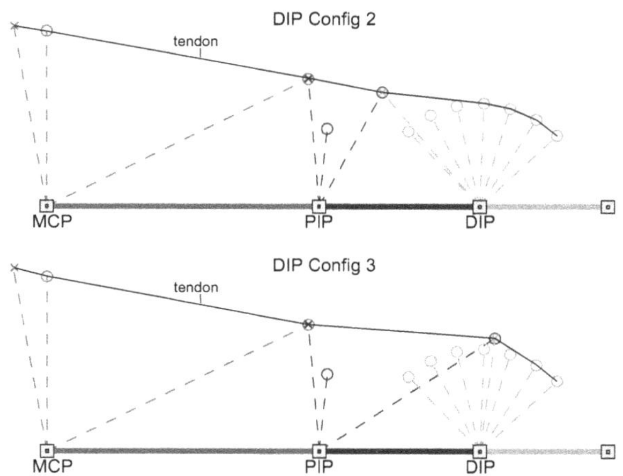

Figure 3: The alternatively examined guiding points configuration at the DIP. In configuration 2 (top) an arch expanding over the DIP is created. In configuration 3 (bottom) the guiding point, centrically placed over the PIP-DIP-Link in configuration 1 and 2, is moved directly over the arch.

ence of the other joints on the acting torque.
Furthermore new guiding point configurations are examined exemplary for the DIP. In the second examined configuration an arch, extending over the joint, was created by associating multiple points to the joint. The opening angle of the arch is 90 degrees. Additionally in a third configuration the guiding point in front of the joint was moved further in distal direction. Both alternative configurations are shown in fig. 3.

2.2 Influence of the joint configuration on the acting torque at a single joint

In order to examine the influence of the joint configuration on the acting torque at another joint, the torque trajectory for each joint configuration is created. The joint configurations are in the common physiological range of motion (ROM) discretised by half degree steps. The simulation results create a data space of three dimensions. Each dimension represents the angle of one joint. The value at each data point is the acting torque at the examined joint, in relation to its maximum. The data is used to interpret the acting torque as function of the respective other joints.

3 Results and Discussion

The plot of the torque acting on each joint while the other joints are flexed is shown in fig. 4. On all three joints the torque decreases while flexing the finger. The decrease of torque at the proximal interphalangeal joint (PIP) is 62.4 %, which is the highest decrease among the examined joints. But also the decrease of 57.1 % at the DIP is problematic, especially considering that the ROM is 20 degrees smaller. At the metacarpophalangeal joint (MCP) the decrease is only 34.0 %. This is caused by relatively small offset between the guiding points.

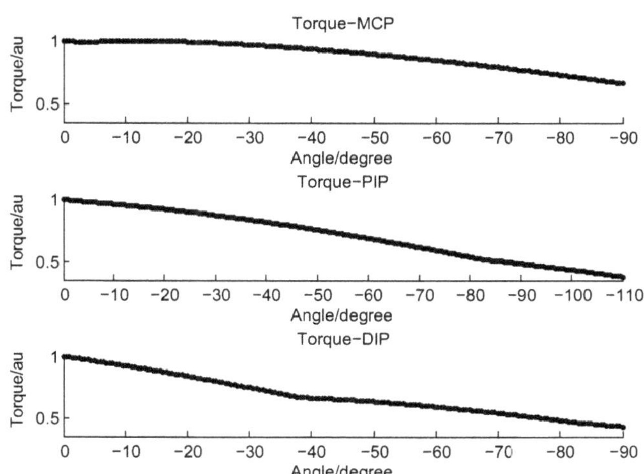

Figure 4: Plots of relative results from the simulation of the torque at each joint, while the other joints are completely flexed.

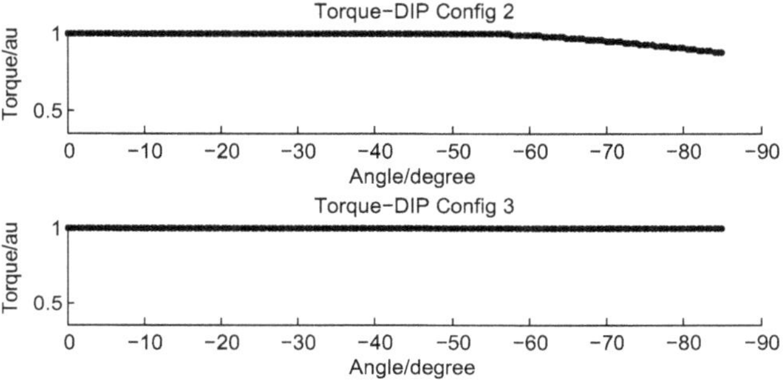

Figure 5: Plot of simulated relative torques at the DIP with the other joints completely flexed, using alternative guiding point configurations presented in fig. 3.

Furthermore it can be seen that a change of guiding points flattens the curvature of the decreasing plot. Is is best visible in fig. 1 on the DIP at about -38 degrees flexion, where the incline of the torque trajectory clearly changes. By placing extra guiding points on an arch the torque decrease can be reduced rapidly. As seen in fig. 5 the additional contact points on the arch structure flattens the curvature in the beginning of the flexion and delays the decrease. So the total decrease was reduced to 12.8 %. Placing the guiding points closer together in configuration 3 reduces the decrease to only 0.9 % generating an almost constant torque.
The analysis of the joint independence delivered only a small influence of the joint configurations to the acting torque at one joint. It can be said that torque acting on the DIP is completely independent from the configuration of the other joints and also the angle of the DIP has no influence on the other joints.
The MCP and the PIP have a small influence on each other. As seen in fig. 6 the torque decreases if the joint is moved. If either one is flexed over 3.5 degrees the trajectory is a flat line indicating no influence. The cause of the influence is the tendon bypassing all guiding points on the link between MCP and PIP. The maximal decrease of the torque is with 0.53 % slightly higher on the PIP as the decrease of maxi-

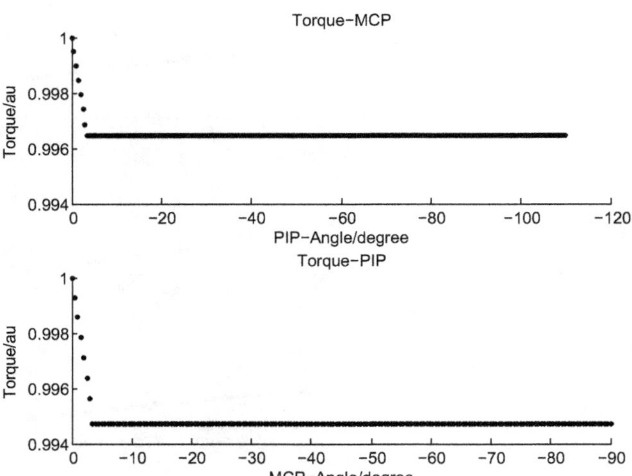

Figure 6: On the top the torque acting on the MCP is plotted as function the PIP's angle. The MCP is thereby fully extended. On the bottom the torque acting on the PIP is plotted as function of the MCP's angle, with the PIP fully extended.

mal 0.36 % at the MCP. This can be explained with relative difference of the lever length caused, by the joints location.

4 Conclusion

In this work we presented a MATLAB simulation in order to predict the acting torques on the joints of an exoskeleton used in post stroke rehabilitation. The model is object-oriented designed using the same parameters as the CAD-model. This makes it easy to alter the model and adapt it to other exoskeletons as well.

The simulation was used to examine torque trajectory for each joint. The discovered decreases of the torque closing the finger are unwanted and lead to testing different guiding point configurations. Concluding that creating an arch construct over the joints guiding the tendon flattens the torque curvature. Also a short distance between the contact points is of advantage.

Furthermore the independence of the joints was analysed. A small influence of the MCP and PIP was found, when both joints are nearly extended. Since the joints are influencing each other problems to control the applied force can arise. The simulation can help to prevent those shortfalls in next prototype iterations.

The next step is an evaluation of the simulation's accuracy and using the simulation for quantitative predictions of the applied torque at each joint. So the simulation can be used as base for controlling the force applied by the actuators. Also the found solution for minimizing the torque decrease are incorporated into the next prototype iteration.

Acknowledgement

The work has been carried out at the Institute of Computer Engineering, Universität zu Lübeck.

5 References

[1] S. C. Johnston, S. Mendis and C. D. Mathers, *Global variation in stroke burden and mortality: estimates from monitoring, surveillance, and modelling*. The Lancet Neurology, vol. 8, no.4, pp. 345–354, 2009.

[2] G. Kwakkel, B. J. Kollen, J. van der Grond and A. J. H. Prevo, *Probability of regaining dexterity in the flaccid upper Limb Impact of severity of paresis and time since onset in acute stroke*. Stroke vol. 34, pp. 2181–2186, 2003.

[3] P. U. Heuschmann, O. Busse, M. Wagner, M. Endres, A. Villinger, J. Röther, P. L. Kolominsky-Rabas, P. L. and K. Berger, *Schlaganfallhäufigkeit and Versorgung von Schlaganfallpatienten in Deutschland*. Akt Neurol, vol. 37, pp. 333–340, 2010

[4] H. Woldag and H. Hummelsheim, *Evidence-based physiotherapeutic concepts for improving arm and hand function in stroke patients*. Journal of Neurology, vol. 249, no.5, pp. 518–528, 2002.

[5] J. Mehrholz, A. Haedrich, T. Platz, J. Kugler and M. Pohl, *Electromechanical and robot-assisted arm training for improving generic activities of daily living, arm function, and arm muscle strength after stroke*. Cochrane Database Syst Rev, vol. 6, 2012.

[6] P. Weiss, L. Heyer, T. F. Münte, M. Heldmann, A. Schweikard, E. Maehle, *Towards a Parameterizable Exoskeleton for Training of Hand Function After Stroke*. in: Rehabilitation Robotics (ICORR), 2013 IEEE International Conference on, 2013.

[7] A. Schiele, *Ergonomics of exoskeletons: Objective performance metrics* in: EuroHaptics conference, 2009 and Symposium on Haptic Interfaces for Virtual Environment and Teleoperator Systems. World Haptics 2009. Third Joint, pp 103–108, IEEE, 2009.

[8] A. Chiri, M. Cempini, S. M. M. De Rossi, T. Lenzi, F.Giovacchini, N. Vitiello, M. C. Carrozza, *On the design of ergonomic wearable robotic devices for motion assistance and rehabilitation*. in: Engineering in Medicine and Biology Society (EMBC), 2012 Annual International Conference of the IEEE, pp. 6124–6127, IEEE, 2012.

[9] P. Weiss, G. Männel, T. Münte, A. Schweikard and E. Maehle, *Parametrization of an Exoskeleton for Robotic Stroke Rehabilitation*. in: Replace, Repair, Restore, Relieve–Bridging Clinical and Engineering Solutions in Neurorehabilitation, pp. 833–843, Springer, 2014.

[10] P. I. Corke, *Robotics, Vision & Control: Fundamental Algorithms in Matlab*. Springer, 2011

Determination of Measurement Characteristics of a Sensor for Blood Leakage in Hemodialysis

D. Prox [1], and A. Röse [2]
[1] Medizinische Ingenieurwissenschaft, Universität zu Lübeck, prox@miw.uni-luebeck.de
[2] Fresenius Medical Care Deutschland GmbH, Bad Homburg, andreas.roese@fmc-ag.com

Abstract

Blood leak detectors are an important protective system in hemodialysis. They protect the patients from an extracorporeal blood loss to the dialysate. Blood leaks appear in case of a rupture in the semi-permeable membrane of the dialyzer. The detectors must be able to detect very low amounts of blood in the dialysate. This requires an exact calibration of the detectors after production and a reliability review of the sensitivity to blood. Currently, the calibration is performed using diluted bovine blood. This work investigates several confounding factors for calibration. For that purpose, the output voltages of blood leak detectors of a pre-series production were measured at different conditions, such as flow rate, used blood stabilizer and degree of hemolysis. It was demonstrated that the optical properties of the blood mixture had changed during the day. A blood-free calibration might be a better approach to perform the calibration.

1 Introduction

The hemodialysis is the only treatment option for chronical kidney failure besides kidney transplantation. About two million patients rely on hemodialysis worldwide. In hemodialysis, the blood is cleaned in an extracorporeal circuit (illustrated in Fig. 1). The most fundamental component of the hemodialysis is the dialyzer which serves as a synthetic kidney. The dialyzer consists of about 10 000 hollow fibers with semi-permeable membranes. The blood of the patient flows inside this fibers and the dialysate flows outside of the fibers. A concentration gradient between blood and dialysate induces a diffusion of low-molecular substances (e. g. uraemic toxins, water) from blood to dialysate [1], [2].

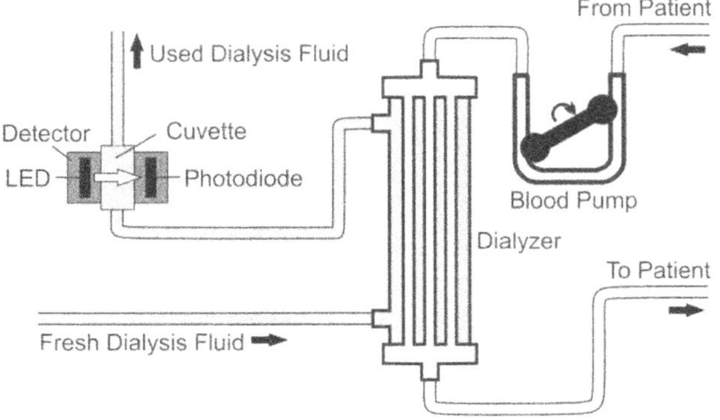

Figure 1: Simplified schematic representation of an extracorporeal blood circuit with blood pump, dialyzer and blood leak detector

Blood leaks are a possibly appearing complication in hemodialysis. A blood loss to the dialysis fluid can be induced by a rupture in the semi-permeable membrane of the dialyzer. Blood leaks can cause a hazardous blood loss for the dialysis patient and a contamination of the hydraulic part of the hemodialysis machine. The International Electrotechnical Commission (IEC) demands a protective system to protect the patient from a hazardous blood leak. The norm of the IEC defines a non-hazardous blood leak as a blood loos of 0.35 ml/min with a hematocrit of 32 % [3]. Therefore, a blood loss over this limit has to be detected by a blood leak detector.

At present, a new blood leak detector (BLD) for hemodialysis is developed at the company Fresenius Medical Care. The new blood leak detector is intended as successor to the existing detector for mounting in new dialysis machines and as replacement for malfunctioned detectors in existing dialysis machines. Fig. 2 shows the BLD. The optical transmission of light is used for the detection of blood. During the transmission of light through a liquid, the light gets absorbed and scattered. However, the absorption dominates at a high dilution. The extinction of light can be approximately described by the Beer-Lambert law

$$E_\lambda = \lg\left(\frac{I_0}{I_1}\right) = \epsilon_\lambda * c * d \qquad (1)$$

where E_λ represents the wavelength-dependent extinction, I_0 the intensity of the incoming radiation into the cuvette, I_1 the intensity of the emerging radiation from the cuvette, ϵ_λ the wavelength-dependent spectral absorption coefficient, c the concentration of blood and d the path length. The detection of blood in a fluid is based on the different transmission of light at different wavelengths. The spectrum of blood with a high oxygen content has e. g. several absorp-

tion maxima at 415 nm, 545 nm and 578 nm [4].
The BLD consists of a custom-made two-color LED, which emits light of the green and red wavelength range. This allows the detection of effects that affect the same change of extinction on both wavelengths (e. g. a calcification of the cuvette). Besides, the BLD consists of two photodiodes. One photodiode receives the light which has passed the cuvette. Additional, a second photodiode receives the light which has passed a reference light path. Thereby, the deterioration of the LED can be compensate [5]. The BLD can distinguish between minor and massive blood leaks. Therefore, the BLD has two output voltages, a blood leak channel U_{bll} and a dimness channel U_{dim}. The output voltage U_{bll} represents the ratio between the transmission of light of both emitted wavelengths. In contrast, the output voltage U_{bll} describes the transmission of light at only one wavelength. A minor blood leak is signalized to the dialysis machine by the output voltage U_{bll}, whereas the output voltage U_{dim} represents a massive blood leak [6]. In case of a blood leak, the dialysis treatment is stopped immediately by the machine.

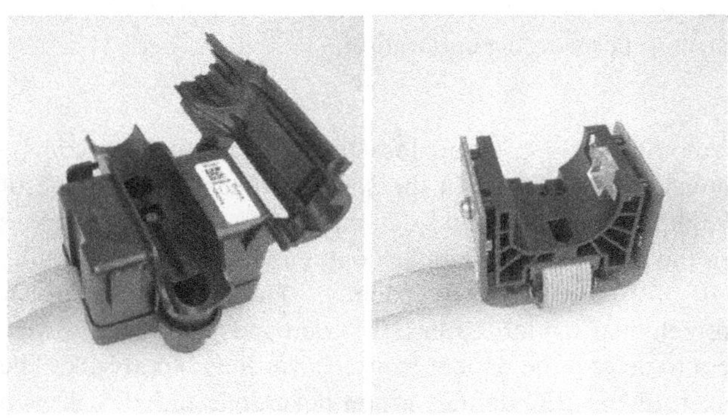

Figure 2: New Blood Leak Detector with cover (left) and without cover (right).

Before mounting the BLD into the dialysis machines, the BLD have to be calibrated. Following, the currently performed calibration process is described. The calibration is executed with a test fluid which contains small amounts of bovine blood. First of all, the hematocrit of each blood sample is determined, in order that the required blood volume for the test fluid can be calculated. Afterwards, a blood mixture with a concentration of 1 ml blood (with a hematocrit of 25 %) per 1 000 ml dialysate has to be prepared daily which gets pumped in a closed circuit during the calibration. The calibration process of the detectors occurs basically in two steps. In the first step, the detectors are calibrated on a cuvette filled with a hemofiltration fluid. In the second step, the detectors are placed on the cuvette, in which the diluted blood flows. Then the detectors are tested for their ability to detect blood in the liquid. Detectors that pass the test can be built into dialysis machines. Detectors that do not pass the test will be rejected and repaired if possible. The blood used for calibration is purchased externally and is obtained from living donor animals. Blood is a natural product whose quality subjects to fluctuations. Additionally, the optical properties of blood are influenced by other parameters, e. g. flow rate or degree of hemolysis [4]. For a reliable calibration it is obligated that all detectors are calibrated and tested under the same constant conditions. Consequently, it is necessary to investigate several influences on the output voltages of the BLD.

2 Material and Methods

For the experiments, 15 detectors of a pre-series production of the BLD were used. For each experiment, a separate closed circuit consisting of sterile 'LifeLine Beta' blood hose systems of the company Fresenius Medical Care was established (illustrated in Fig. 3). The blood which was stabilized with Acid-Citrate-Dextrose (ACD) or heparin has been mixed with a 9 % aqueous solution of NaCl, with reverse osmosis water (RO water) or with a hemofiltration solution in a laboratory bottle according to the mixing ratio used in calibration of the BLD. A magnetic stirrer which was operated at 200 revolutions per minute was used for mixing of the diluted blood. The circuit was designed so that the blood mixture flows from the laboratory bottle through an external line roller pump, through a cylindrical transparent cuvette and afterwards back to the laboratory bottle. The laboratory bottle was sealed by parafilm.

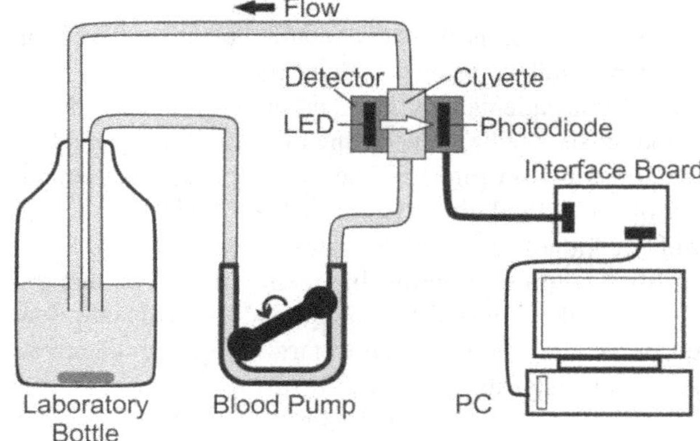

Figure 3: Schematic representation of the measuring setup

The detectors were connected in a random order on an interface board which has been specially prepared for the development of the BLD. With the interface board all input and output voltages of the detector can be measured. In addition, the debug output of the detector can be readout with a connected PC. A running-in of approximately five minutes before starting the measurement make sure that there are not any electronic drifts and the output voltage of the detectors are stabilized. Afterwards, the detectors were fixed by a clamp on a cuvette filled with RO water. After stabilization of the output voltage the voltages U_{bll} and U_{dim} are saved by a LabView program. In the next step, the detectors were fixed on the cuvette filled with diluted blood (showed in Fig. 4) and the output voltages are measured. The calculated difference between the two output voltages is the so called measured effect of the blood mixture.

To investigate the influence of the flow rate of the blood mixture to the output voltages a circuit was constructed as described above and the external blood pump was operated with six different revolutions (20 min^{-1}, 30 min^{-1}, 40 min^{-1}, 50 min^{-1}, 60 min^{-1}).

In a second experiment, the influence of the solvent of the blood mixture was examined. For that purpose, two identical circuits were build. In the first circuit, the blood was mixed with a NaCl solution. In the second circuit, the blood was mixed with a hemofiltration solution ('multiBic') of the company Fresenius Medical Care.

To determine the temporal change of the optical properties of the diluted blood two circuits were assembled in the same way described above. The first circuit was filled with ACD-stabilized whole blood, whereas the second circuit was filled with heparinized whole blood. These measurements were performed with all detectors one, four and six hours after preparing of the blood mixture. This temporal investigation was repeated with hemolyzed blood. For that purpose, the ACD-stabilized blood and the heparinized blood was mixed with RO water. The RO water induced the lysis of the erythrocytes, the so-called hemolysis.

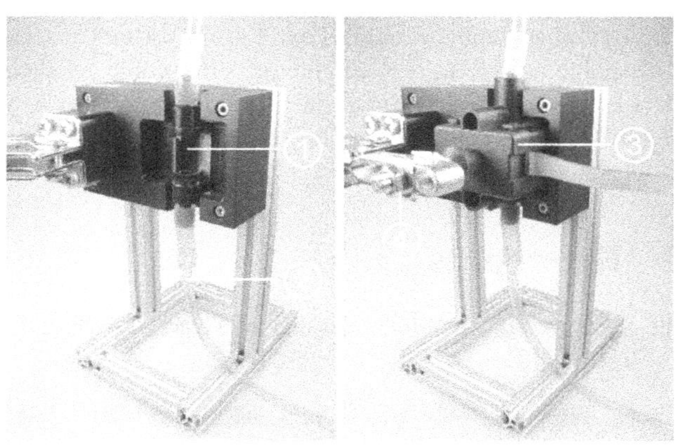

Figure 4: Measuring stand with a cylindrical transparent cuvette (1) and blood hose system (2). The diluted blood flows from the bottom to the top of the cuvette (left). The blood leak detector (3) is fixed by a clamp (4) to the cuvette (right).

3 Results and Discussion

The results of the measurements in each case with 15 detectors are visualized as box plots in the following diagrams. The ends of the whiskers represent the minimum and maximum of all of the data.

The determined measured effects ΔU_{bll} and ΔU_{dim} at different flow rates are visualized in Fig. 5. A significant difference of the output voltages U_{bll} and U_{dim} could not be determined on the investigated flow rates. The overall mean value was -3.357 V for the measured effect ΔU_{bll} and -0.693 V for the measured effect ΔU_{dim}. This signifies that the used blood concentration is too marginal so that a different flow rate does not affect the output voltages of the BLD. Flow fluctuations are therefore uncomplicated for the calibration of the BLD.

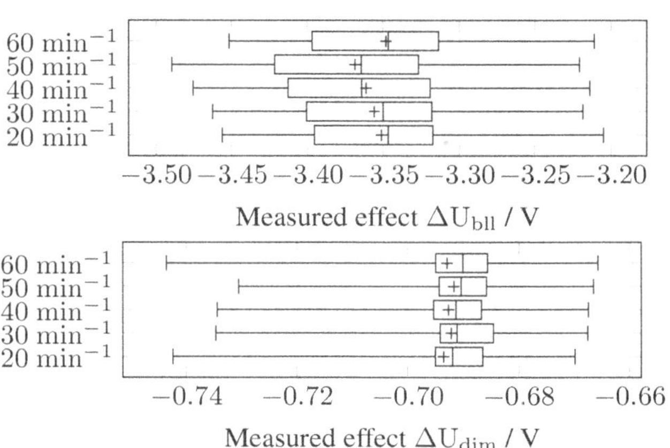

Figure 5: Measured effect at different flow rates (20 min^{-1}, 30 min^{-1}, 40 min^{-1}, 50 min^{-1}, 60 min^{-1}).

Fig. 6 shows the measured effects of the whole blood diluted in NaCl solution and in the hemofiltration solution 'multiBic'. As well, there was no significant difference of the output voltage U_{bll} at different solutions determined. The choice of solution has no effect on the blood, so that the wavelength-dependent absorption is not affected. However, it was ascertained that the output voltages U_{dim} showed a significant difference. The mean value difference of the measured effect ΔU_{dim} between the NaCl solution and the hemofiltration solution was 0.060 V. This difference is caused by the different refraction indexes of the blood-free solutions. The determined voltage difference is not relevant for calibration, because the calibration process takes the transmission of the blood-free solution into account.

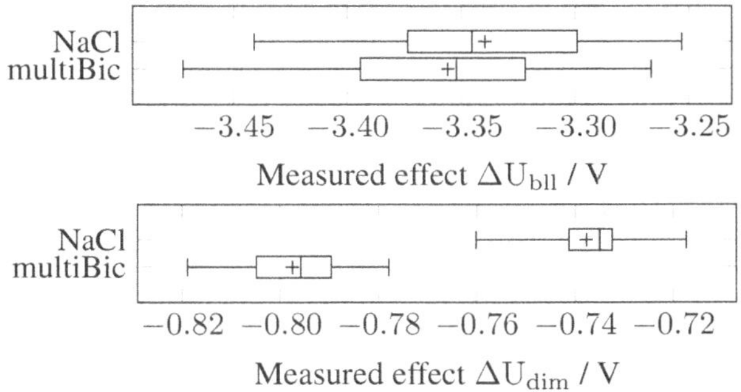

Figure 6: Measured effect at different chosen solutions. 'NaCl' represents the diluted blood in a 9 % aqueous solution of NaCl. The abbreviation 'multiBic' represents the diluted blood in the hemofiltration solution 'multiBic' of the company Fresenius Medical Care.

The results of the temporal investigation with whole blood are visualized in Fig. 7. Thus, it appears that the measured effect ΔU_{bll} decreased over the course of the day. The average measured effect ΔU_{bll} decreased by 0.169 V for the ACD-stabilized whole blood and by 0.157 V for the heparinized whole blood. In contrast, the measured effect

ΔU_{dim} had not changed significantly.

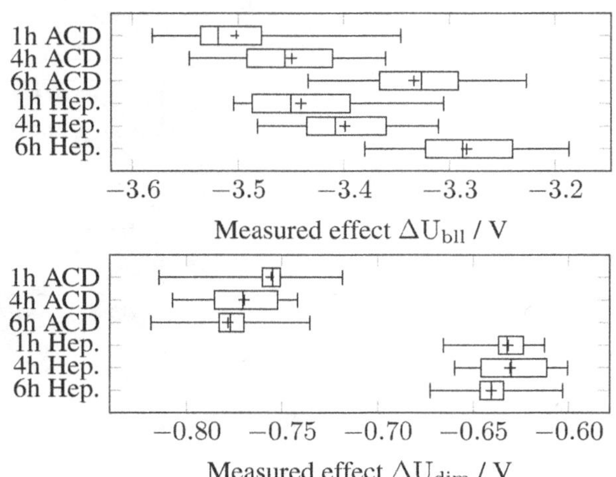

Figure 7: Measured effect at different times (1 h, 4 h, 6 h) after the preparation of the whole blood mixture. 'ACD' represents the ACD-stabilized whole blood and 'Hep.' represents the heparinized whole blood.

Also a temporal change of the output voltages could be measured in the blood mixture with hemolyzed blood (visualized in Fig. 8). The average measured effect ΔU_{bll} decreased by 0.146 V for the hemolyzed blood with ACD-stabilizer and by 0.228 V for the hemolyzed blood with heparin. In contrast, the measured effect ΔU_{dim} increased during the day by 0.054 V on the hemolyzed blood with ACD-stabilizer and by 0.098 V on the hemolyzed blood with heparin. After the preparation of the blood mixture, the output voltages significantly distinguished. This difference is minimized during the course of the day.

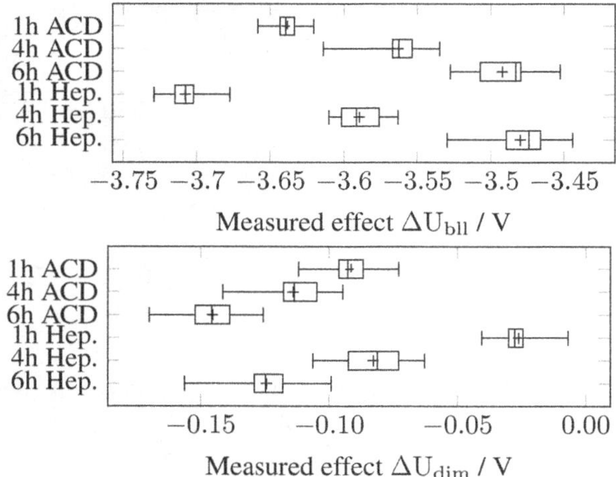

Figure 8: Measured effect at different times (1 h, 4 h, 6 h) after the preparation of the hemolyzed blood mixture. 'ACD' represents the hemolyzed blood with ACD-stabilizer and 'Hep.' represents the hemolyzed blood with heparin.

By comparing the measurements, it appears that the measured effect ΔU_{bll} at hemolyzed blood was greater than the negative measured effect ΔU_{bll} of the whole blood. This confirms that the absorption coefficient of hemolyzed blood in the red wavelength range is greater than the absorption coefficient of the whole blood. In contrast, the measured effect ΔU_{dim} of the hemolyzed blood was less than of the whole blood. This different is based on the low dispersion coefficient of hemolyzed blood compared with the dispersion coefficient of whole blood.

4 Conclusion

The laboratory scaled experiments reveals that fluctuations of the flow rate and the choice of the solution for preparing the blood mixture are uncomplicated for the calibration of blood leak detectors. However, it has been demonstrated that the optical properties of the diluted blood are changed during the day. This requires a continuous monitoring of the optical parameters of the blood mixture during the calibration process. In the future the technical feasibility of a blood-free calibration has to be investigated.

Acknowledgement

The work has been carried out at Fresenius Medical Care Deutschland GmbH, Bad Homburg. Fresenius Medical Care is a provider of products and services for patients with kidney failure. Thanks goes to the entire BLD team for their support.

5 References

[1] S. Geberth and R. Nowack, *Praxis der Dialyse.* Springer, Berlin/Heidelberg, 2014.

[2] R. Nowack, R. Birck and T. Weinreich, *Dialyse und Nephrologie für Fachpersonal.* Springer, Berlin/Heidelberg, 2009.

[3] International Electrotechnical Commission, *Medical electrical equipment-Part 2-16: Particular requirements for basic safety and essential performance of haemodialysis, haemodiafiltration and haemofiltration equipment*, Geneva, 2012.

[4] M. Friebel, *Bestimmung optischer Eigenschaften von humanem Vollblut in Abhängigkeit von verschiedenen physiologischen und biochemischen Zustandsparametern.* Laser- und Medizin-Technologie Berlin, Berlin, 2007.

[5] A. Röse, *Component Design Document (CCD). Neuer Blutleckdetektor NBD: Messverfahren und Schnittstelle zu 2008, 4008, 5008.* Fresenius Medical Care Deutschland GmbH, Bad Homburg, 2014.

[6] A. Gagel, *System Design Document (SSD): Softwarebeschreibung des Blutleckdetektors.* Fresenius Medical Care Deutschland GmbH, Bad Homburg, 2012.

Checking the usability of a valve system to control a pressure controlled valve from a breathing machine

R. Holzhause [1], B. Adametz[2] and S. Franke[2]
[1] Medizinische Ingenieurwissenschaft, Universität zu Lübeck, holzhaus@informatik.uni-luebeck.de
[2] Weinmann Geräte für Medizin, Hamburg-Eidelstedt, {b.adametz, s.franke}@weinmann.de

Abstract

Breathing machines are used to treat sleep apnea. To compensate the respiratory interruptions as good as possible it is important to know when inserting a breathing drop-out and how the ventilation must be set. Depending on the breathing therapy pressure, flow and gas composition have to be measured. With the usually used fix expiration leak the measurement is inaccurate and a correction of the deviation is necessary.
With an integrated valve system it is possible to measure exactly and to optimize the ventilation. Therefore, a pressure controlled valve on the respiratory mask, controlled with a direct operated proportional piezo valve and a fix leak, was tested. A usability test is made, to ensure that the valve system works accurate and to identify which parts should be adjusted for trouble-free function.

1 Introduction

A breathing machine is a device which helps people to breath when they are unable to get enough air on their own. This symptom means that the person has a sleep apnea, a breathing arrest that mostly occurs during sleep.
There are two different types of sleep apnea, the central sleep apnea and the obstructive sleep apnea. The central sleep apnea is a rare form of it. It is caused by damage to the central nervous system and is characterized by a missing respiratory impulse.

The obstructive sleep apnea is the most common. It is often caused by strong relaxation of annular muscles to the upper respiratory tract in the sleep. Thus, the throat is no longer able to resist the vacuum that is created while breathing. It follows that the respiration collapses as a consequence disability.
Apnea leads to sleep disorders and lack of oxygen in the blood which can lead to other failures of important vital functions within a very short time [1], [2].
Ventilation therapy can be used to treat sleep apnea. For obstructive sleep apnea the throat space is splint with a continuous positive pressure. Central sleep apnea is treated with a traditional resuscitation. Then inspiration and expiration is completely taken over by the ventilator. This is why it is important to have a reliable and accurate breathing machine.
In the ventilation therapy for obstructive sleep apnea there are often fix leak systems for the expiration. Here, the flow losses are compensated during the inspiration with more pressure. Pressure and flow on the patient have to be calculated and are not as accurate as a direct flow and pressure measurement. With a pressure controlled expiration valve on the patients' mask a more accurate ventilation is achievable.

A breathing machine can be connected with an one-tube system or a two-tube system. Both systems may have a pressure controlled expiration valve.

The advantage of such valves is the controlled regulation, because it allows to define exactly when the valve should be opened or closed. Additionally, in combination with a two-tube system, a pressure controlled valve controls that the exhaled air does not flow back into the blower. The exact pressure and flow as well as the exact gas composition can be measured continuously [4]. There are different options to realize the exact pressure at the pressure controlled valve:

- One 2/2 ways valve with a fix leak
- Two 2/2 ways valves with a fix leak
- One 3/3 ways valve

The pressure can be generated with high precision by an electric piezo valve. These valves are the better alternative to conventional magnetic valves.

This usability test is to determine which piezo valve system, in combination with a fix leak, is suitable to regulate a pressure controlled valve for an optimized ventilation of a breathing machine. Therefore, a valve system with one 2/2 ways valve and a fix leak and two 2/2 ways valves with a fix leak are analysed.

2 Material and Methods

To test the usability of the valve system with the 2/2 ways valve in combination with the fix leak the knowledge of the operating principle of a proportional piezo valve is required.

2.1 Function of a piezo electric valve

Piezo electric valves are small and light, very durable, fast and energy-efficient. Furthermore, they have almost no self-heating because they do not need any energy to hold a steady state. In addition, the valves work in proportion and are very resistant. Also beneficial is that they are almost silent, which is very important for ventilation at night [3].

The piezo valve has an inlet port and an output port. It has also a ribbon cable with three connections and two holes in the housing to fix it on a flange. Inside the valve a piezoelectric ceramic is placed. The indirect piezoelectric effect is used by the valve. In response to an applied voltage the ceramic deforms. The piezo ceramic inside the valve is located on a passive conductive carrier which bends up due to the contracted ceramic.

Bending the material opens the valve and allows for regulating the flow. The contraction of the piezo ceramic is proportional to the applied voltage. If no voltage is applied the piezo valve is closed. The higher the applied voltage, the further the valve is opened and the flow of the medium increases.

To control the used valve properly, the additional pressure of $2,068\ bar$ has to be supplied. On one hand the pressure supply prevents the valve from functioning at too low pressure. On the other hand a lower voltage is necessary to open the valve with the supplied pressure. Therefore, the valve is capable of easy dosing of concentrations and allows stepless adjustment.

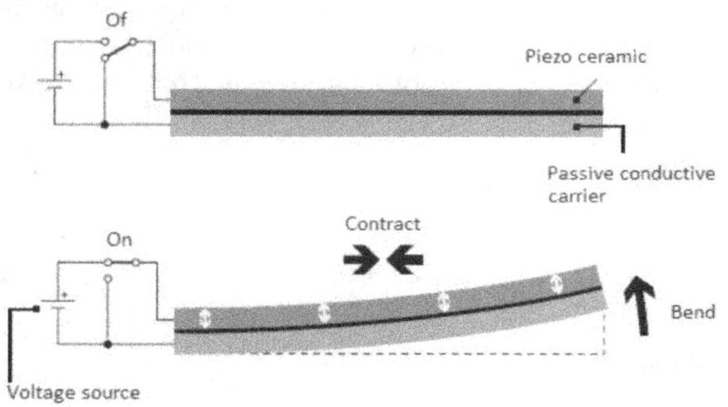

Figure 1: With applied voltage the ceramic deforms and bands the conductive carrier above.

The valve works in a voltage range from $0\ V$ till a maximum voltage and has a resistor to secure the system of the valve. Pin one from the ribbon cable must be connected to the control stage. Pin two and three must be connected to ground.

With a laboratory power supply which can generate $60\ V$ and a high-voltage amplifier, a maximal voltage can be generated like the data-sheet in Fig. 2 shows.

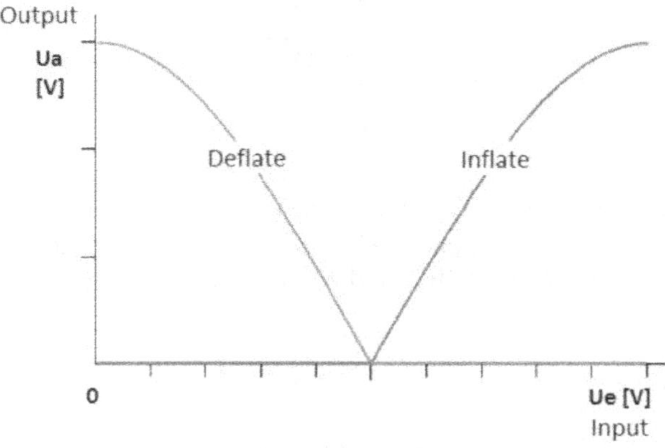

Figure 2: The figure shows that the venting in and out are zero until an applied voltage.

2.2 Function of a pressure controlled valve

The pressure controlled valve from GaleMed, Taiwan is shown in Fig. 3 a) and b). It consists of two cones with a cross-section of $22\ mm$ on the right and left side and one of $15\ mm$ in the middle. The $22\ mm$ cone on the right side can be connected to a mask. In Fig. 3 b) is shown that the expiration flow puts out through the right cone into the valve and lifts the membrane (2) against the control pressure. The control pressure comes through the tube (1) and is spreading on the upper side of the membrane. Then the expiration flow circulates through the valve into the left tube, connected to a breathing machine.

The diameter of the membrane is $31.7\ mm$, it equates to a face of $790\ mm^2$, and the valve seat inner diameter is $16.3\ mm$ what equates to an area of $208\ mm^2$. Because of the bigger face for the control pressure the expiration pressure can be higher then the control pressure without opening the patient valve [5], [6].

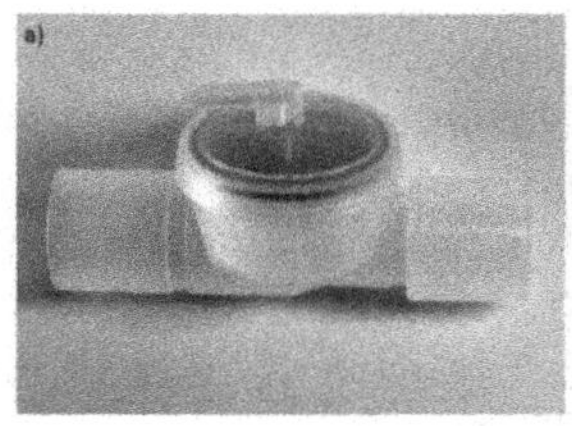

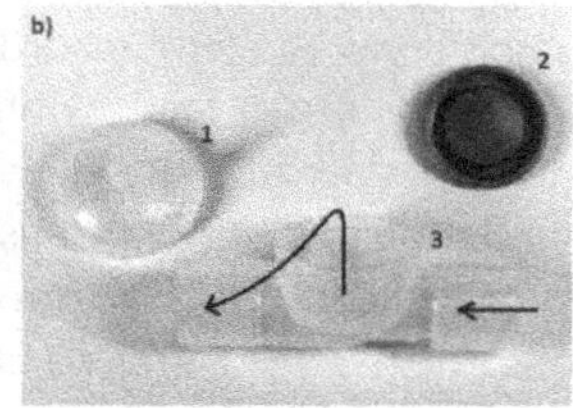

Figure 3: Photograph from a patient valve from GaleMed, Taiwan. In photograph a) the valve is complete. In photograph b) it is shown in component parts with the direction of the flow from the right to the left site if the valve is open. 1) is the cap with the tube for the control pressure, 2) is the membrane to close the pressure controlled valve 3).

2.3 Usability tests

To check the usability of a piezo valve in combination with a fix leak to control the pressure controlled valve usability tests are necessary.
The first test is shown in Fig. 5. Here, the functionality of the piezo valve is checked. The valve must close and open as shown in data sheet in Fig. (2).
The second test is verifying if the control pressure is high enough to close the pressure controlled valve on the patient mask (see Fig. 6). The control pressure is generated from the piezo valve in combination with a fix leak.
The last test is illustrated in Fig. 7. It is checked if the combination of two piezo valves and one fix leak increases the efficiency by verifying if the resulting control pressure increases in comparison to a single piezo valve.

For all tests, a flange is necessary guarantee a lossless transition of gas. The flange is a connection block between the inputs and outputs of a valve and the associated tube connections. It is typically made of aluminium and has holes inside for the lead of the gas.
For this experiment the flange is constructed in Pro Engineer (short: *proE*[1]) on the base of the mechanical drawing of the valve (see Fig. 4). Based on this drawing the flange was milled.
After the mechanical and electrical connection of the valve, the breathing machine has to be connected with a tube system and a pressure controlled valve (see Fig. 5).

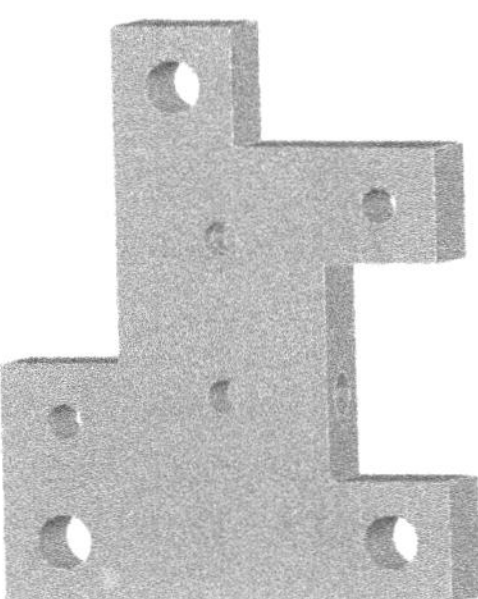

Figure 4: 3D-construction of a flange.

The following tests are only to check the usability of the piezo valve to control the pressure controlled valve. Therefore the set-up is simple and the pressure controlled valve is used like an inspiration valve.

2.4 Test 1

In the first test (see Fig. 5) it is analysed if the valve opens and closes correctly. The breathing machine with a constant pressure of 20 hPa is started while the manometer (PF 300) measures the pressure after the outlet from the valve. Then the laboratory power supply and a high-voltage amplifier are started. The change of the voltage can be controlled by the laboratory power supply. According to the opening status of the piezo valve the flow increases. As soon as the piezo valve opens, the control pressure is expected to be the same as the adjusted pressure on the breathing machine.

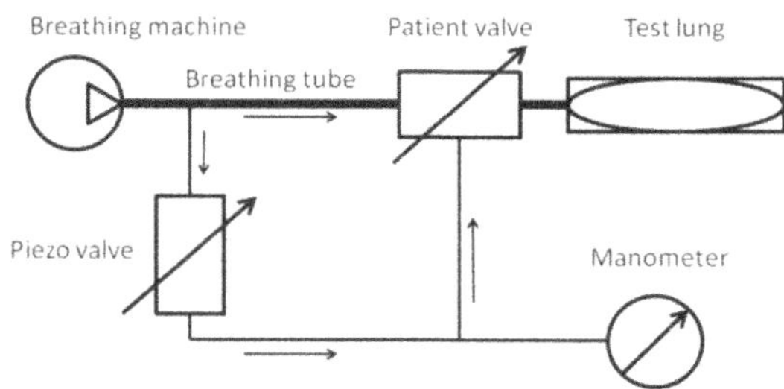

Figure 5: Connection set-up.

2.5 Test 2

For the second test (see Fig. 6) the fix leak is included and the maximal resulting pressure on the pressure controlled valve is measured with the manometer. Therefore, a constant pressure of 20 hPa is applied. As long as the piezo valve is closed, no control pressure is applied to the pressure controlled valve. The patient valve is opened and the flow can stream into the test lung. When the piezo valve is opened the flow should not steam into the test lung, because the control pressure should close the patient valve. For this reason it is necessary that the pressure is high enough to close the pressure controlled valve completely.

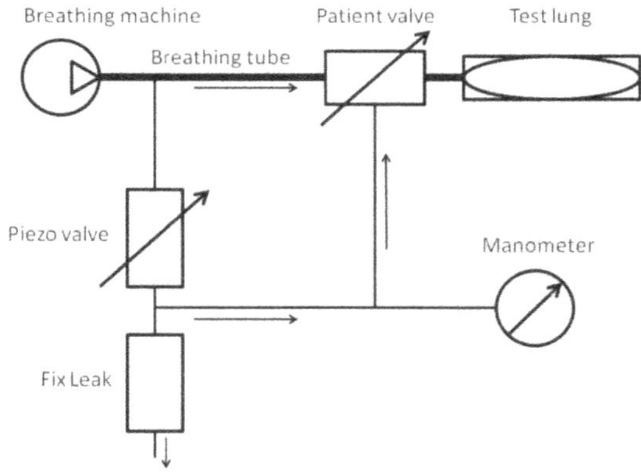

Figure 6: Connection set-up.

2.6 Test 3

For the third test (see Fig. 7) two piezo valves in parallel and one fix leak are connected by flexible thin tubes. The rest of the set-up remains the same. Because of the two piezo valves connected in parallel the lateral cut is bigger and the control pressure should increase.

[1] proE is a construction tool

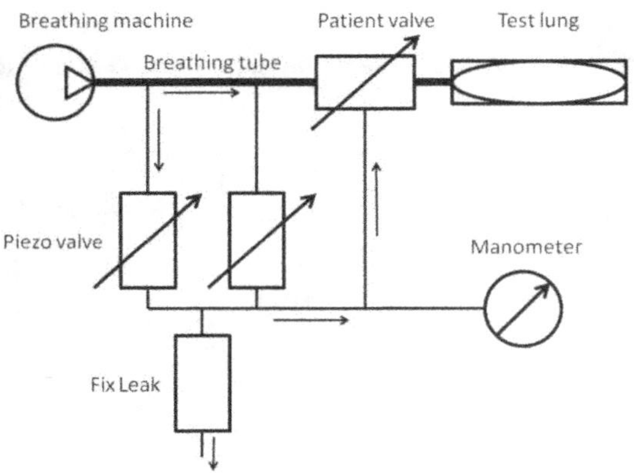

Figure 7: Connection set-up.

3 Results and Discussion

During the preparation phase it turned out that the piezo valve is lined to a working pressure of 2.068 bar which corresponds to 2068 hPa. Because of the much lower applied pressure of 20 hPa generated from the breathing machine, the valve could not open. So it was necessary to open the valve first with a pressure of 2068 hPa. That was realized with a compressed air pump. But if the piezo valve should be integrated in a breathing machine, it must be adapted to the used pressure range. Such valves are available but for the usability tests it was not necessary.

The first test was positive, the piezo valve opened and closed and the flow increased and decreased proportional to the applied voltage. Also the maximum control pressure of the 2/2 way piezo valve reached only 18.5 hPa. These results did not correspond with the theory that the control pressure should be the same like the applied pressure from the breathing machine. One probable reason is the set-up which can have leaks. Another reason could be the resistance of the thin tube which connects the piezo valve with the manometer. This can be concluded due to the observed interrelation that the longer the thin tubes were, the lower the measured control pressure was. However, further investigation is worthwhile as the causes of the errors can be fixed.

The second test provided a maximum pressure of 12.78 hPa. Because of the fix leak (0.8 mm cross section) in the combined valve system, the measured control pressure was much lower then in first test. Nevertheless the control pressure was high enough to close the pressure controlled valve. Anyway, for save breath control it is necessary to optimize the system to increase the control pressure.

In the last test two piezo valves were connected with the fix leak. As a result the cross section increased by 1.6 mm. Because of that the measured control pressure is with 18.89 hPa higher then in test two. The control pressure is close to the applied pressure. So it can be concluded that one has a good control of the pressure controlled valve.

4 Conclusion

The usability test showed that the valve system consisting of two 2/2 way valves and a leak is a good basis to control a pressure controlled valve. But there are different problems which have to be solved before the system can be installed. For instance the length of the thin elastic tubes have to be as short as possible and the connections should be checked for leakages. The whole valve system should be checked with a set-up, which uses the pressure controlled valve as an expiration valve. First with CPAP[2] and second with BIPAP[3]. Furthermore it has to be checked if a smaller valve system like only one 3/3 way valve can be used. A next step is to test one of the valve systems integrated into a breathing machine and with a two-tube system.

Acknowledgement

The work has been carried out at Weinmann Geräte für Medizin, Hamburg, Germany. I would also like to thank Prof. Dr. Hübner from the Institute of Physics, Universität zu Lübeck, Germany.

5 References

[1] H. Hein and D. Kirsten, *Schlafapnoe und Heimbeatmung*. Dustri, Münschen/Deisenhofen, 1997.

[2] F. Ritter and M. Döring, *Kurven und Loops in der Beatmung*. Lübeck, Dräger Medical GmbH, 2011.

[3] F. Festo, *Piezoventile in Medizintechnik und Laborautomatisierung*. Deutschland, Festo AG & Co. KG, Muster.

[4] J. Lingemann, *Nicht-invasive Beatmung BiPAP bei COPD und Lungenemphysem. Was ist notwendig, was ist medizinisch sinnvoll?*. Duisburg, COPD - Deutschland e.V., 04/2014.

[5] J. Kreuzer, *Project Work Thesis*. Hamburg-Harburg, Institut für Regelungstechnik, 12/2012.

[6] H. Wortelen, *Konstruktion eines Patientenventils*. Deutschland, Fachhochschule Oldenburg/Ostfriesland/Wilhelmshaven Standort Wilhelmshaven, 06/2005.

[2] Continuous positive airway pressure
[3] Biphasic positive airway pressure

5
Safety and Quality I

Investigation of the APICA ASC^{TM} access and closure device for the delivery of mitral valve therapies

M. Seiler [1], B. Cunniffe [2], C. O'Sullivan [2]
[1] Medizinische Ingenieurwissenschaft, Universität zu Lübeck, seiler@miw.uni-luebeck.de
[2] Apica Cardiovascular Ltd., Galway (Ireland), brendancunniffe@eircom.net, ciaranosull@gmail.com

Abstract

Mitral valve regurgitation is the second most frequent native valve disease, in Europe, behind aortic valve stenosis. In recent years the transcatheter aortic valve implantation (TAVI) has provided a new treatment opportunity for patients that present with high surgical risk. The ASC^{TM} device from Apica Cardiovascular Ltd. was able to advance those procedures with a device which reduces the bleeding, stabilize the delivery and closure the access site after the surgery. Since transcatheter devices for mitral valve replacement are in development, it is reasonable to review if the ASC^{TM} device is ready to be used for a mitral valve application. A comprehensive review of the mitral valve diseases and mitral valve transcatheter technologies with additional interviews concluded that the delivery system (in its current configuration) can be used in certain instances. Further testing must be carried out to give some indication of how the delivery system can be adapted.

1 Introduction

Mitral valve regurgitation (MR) is the second most common heart valve disease in western Europe and the USA, after aortic valve stenosis (AS) [1]. In a ranking according to the age, MR is the most common heart disease for patients with an age above 65. The increasing age of the patients with those heart valve diseases comes with an additional likelihood of co-morbidities and leads to an enhanced operation risk [2]. Most of the heart valve procedures are still conventional operations like an open heart sternotomy. Therefore the thorax of the patient will be opened and the cardiovascular system maintained by a heart-lung machine. Such procedures have minor risk for young and stable patients and still represent the preferred approach. For those older and bad conditioned patients would such a procedure represent a major risk [3].

For a lot of patients with an AS there are already alternative minimal-invasive operation methods, such as right lateral thoracotomy and transcatheter aortic valve implantation (TAVI), which were developed in the last few years. The number of TAVI procedures in Germany increased in the recent years from 528 (2008) to 9341 (2012) [2], most likely due to the increasing age of the patients and associated operative risk. In contrast to the conventional sternotomy, TAVI procedures be realized without a heart-lung machine. For a TAVI procedure the aortic valve is delivered in a folded/crimped configuration through a catheter into the heart. At target location, the new prosthetic valve is expanded inside the existing native valve. The calcified nature of the stenosed native valve allows the new implanted valve to gain good anchorage at the target location. TAVI procedures can be performed transfemoral, transapical or transaortical. Because of the antegrade approach through the apex of the left ventricle, the transapical access site is the 'easiest' access and many new devices are designed initially for that approach [4]. To improve the access, stabilization and closure on the transapical access site, Apica Cardiovascular developed a novel delivery and closure technology as illustrated in Fig. 1 (specified in chap. 2).

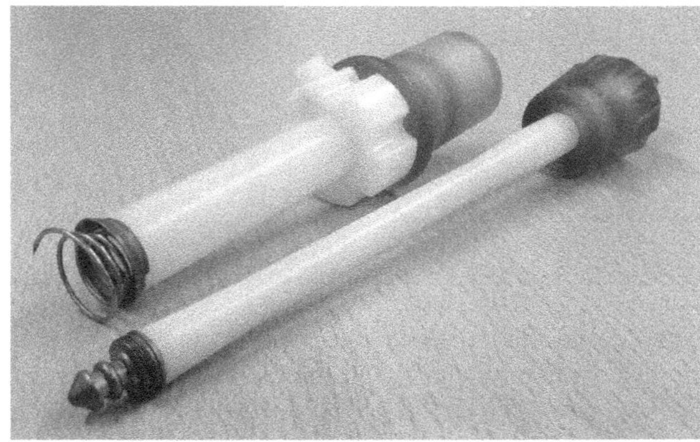

Figure 1: The access, stabilization and closure device of Apica Cardiovascular, Galway Ireland.

In contrast, devices for a transcatheter mitral valve replacement (TMVR) are still in preclinical development or early clinical testing [5]. As the mitral valve is located between the left atrium (LA) and left ventricle (LV), the transapical approach through the LV seems to be also a good opportunity for treatments of mitral valve diseases. Since the MR is a common valve disease in an older age group, which comes mostly with a higher operation risk, the ASC™ device from from Apica Cardiovascular should prove to be a valuable application system in the treatment of mitral valve diseases. It is therefore appropriate to analyse how the Apica Cardiovascular system could be used in the treatment of mitral valve diseases and if any mitral-valve-specific adaptations are necessary from the current commercially available system.

2 Material and Methods

The apical access, stabilization and closure device (ASC™, Apica Cardiovascular Galway, Ireland) is a transapical delivery and closure technology which supports the delivery of transcatheter heart valves for off-pump valve surgeries (so far on TAVI procedures). The system is basically built out of two primary components: a conical shaped titanium coil and a closure cap (each with its own individual delivery system) as shown in Fig. 1. The system is used in conjunction with the physician's choice of TAVI system and is compatible with all commercially available transapical TAVI systems at present. Through a small incision between the rips and with a minimal rip spreading, the introducer and sheath of the TAVI system is passed over the guide wire and passes through the myocardium in the normal way. The titanium coil of the ASC™ device is then torqued into the apical myocardium as shown in Fig. 2. In this way the entire apical access site of the heart has been stabilized and the physician is afforded secure control in a manner not possible with suture-mediated closure. Due to the conical

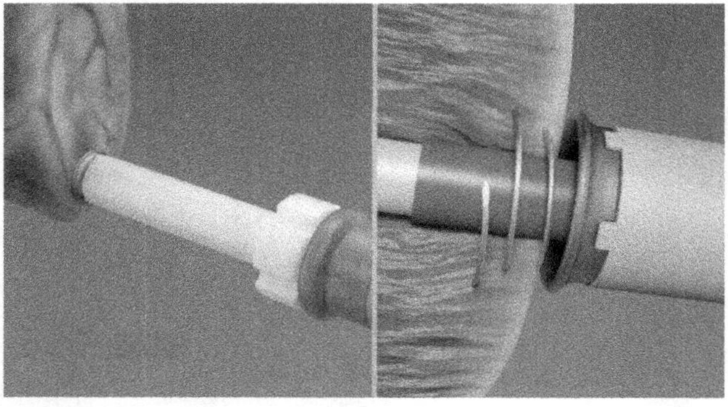

Figure 2: Insertion of the conical shaped titanium coil into the myocardium of the left ventricular apex (*Courtesy of Brendan Cunniffe, Apica Cardiovascular Ltd.*).

shape of the coil, the myocardium is mildly compressed against the valve delivery sheath, effecting haemostasis at the myocardial access site thereby preventing a peri-sheath bleeding during the procedure. The introducer is removed from within the TAVI sheath, leaving the sheath itself in place within the ASC™ device. The valve implantation then proceeds in the normal way. After the procedure, the guide wire and sheath of the delivery system can be removed. Two valves integrated into the titanium coil delivery device of the ASC™ device ensure that no blood loss occurs through the ASC™ device itself. One of the valves is adjustable in diameter in order to ensure that haemostasis is possible on a variety of diameters, e.g. form TAVI systems with outer diameter of 34 Fr down to guide wires with a diameter of 0.035 inch. Final closure of the access site is effected by torquing the closure cap into the titanium coil implant. Both Apica delivery systems are removed and the combination of titanium coil and closure cap is left as the final closure implant in the myocardium, leading to a rapid and complete closure of the access site.

So far the ASC™ system has only been used for TAVI procedures, where a transcatheter aortic valve is implanted into the old stenosed aortic valve. A thorough understanding of transapical TAVI procedures (as well as a detailed understanding of how the ASC™ system is used to improve those) is necessary before embarking on a study of how the adaptation of the system for a delivery of mitral valve therapies might proceed. A further literature review of the pathology of mitral valve diseases is necessary to allow an understanding of the disease states and the specific anatomy of the mitral valve. This will highlight any considerations specific to mitral valve disease which might have implications for the adaptation of the current delivery system and shall reveal key elements of the mitral valve therapies. Additional to that there will be a review of the current mitral valve repair and replacement devices that are commercially available or in development. This will allow an understanding of the therapies the adapted access, stabilization and closure device must be compatible with. Since the TMVR is a developing therapy to deal with mitral valve diseases, it is also valuable to conduct some interviews with surgeons specialized in minimal-invasive mitral valve surgeries. The interviews shall represent the personal experiences and opinions of the surgeons about possible left ventricular access points and their advantages and disadvantages, together with a comprehensive knowledge about the execution of mitral valve operations. With the assistance of a prepared questionnaire the surgeons are asked about the patient profile for mitral valve therapies, their comorbidities and the comparison to TAVI patient profiles. Furthermore it shall show which access sites the surgeons favour in the majority of their cases and if there are specific issues with those access sites which might be addressed through the use of a device such as the Apica ASC™ system.

3 Results and Discussion

The mitral valve is a lot more complex than the aortic valve. While the circular shaped aortic valve is located within the beginning of the aorta, a properly structured 'blood vessel', the mitral valve is located between the LA and LV without such a strong foundation supporting it. The mitral valve opens during the diastole and allows the blood flow from the LA to the LV and is an apparatus built out of different components (as you can see in Fig. 3: annulus, leaflets, chordae tendineae and papillary muscles) [6]. The annulus is a D-shaped dense connective tissue and gives attachment to the mitral valve between LA and LV. During systole the mitral valve annulus moves over 1 cm in the direction of the apex. This motion makes it additionally difficult to fixate an implantation into the valve. The mitral valve comprises of two leaflets attached to the annulus. The two leaflets are different in structure and shape and classed as anterior and posterior leaflets. The posterior leaflet has a narrow shape and extends over two-third of the annulus. The anterior leaflet however is much broader and comprises one-third of the annulus. The free ends of the leaflets are linked with the chordae tendineae, which are basically thin chords, through the papillary muscles to the LV wall [7].

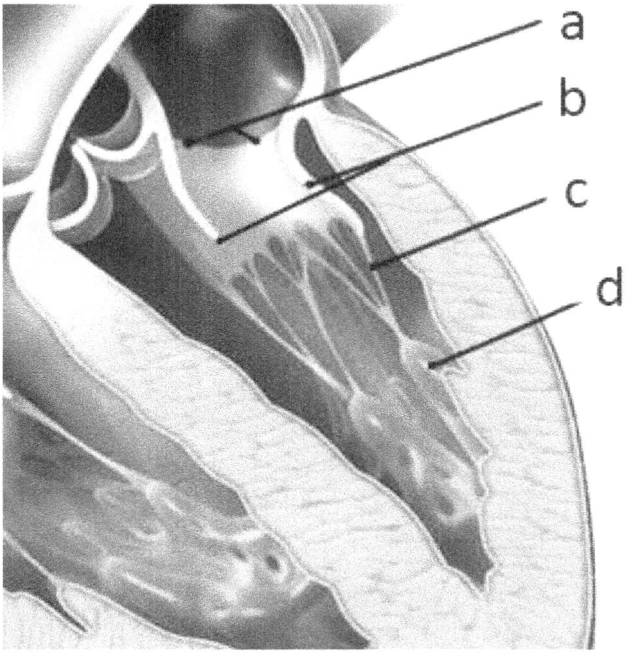

Figure 3: Components of the mitral valve apparatus with: a) mitral valve annulus, b) leaflets, c) chordae tendinae and d) papillary muscles. Adapted from: *http://www.apotheken-umschau.de/multimedia/231/198/257/65758421009.jpg*

The main types of mitral valve diseases are mitral valve stenosis and mitral valve regurgitation. With stenotic diseases the leaflets of the valve become thick or stiff and may fuse together. This leads to a narrowed valve area and reduces the blood flow from the LA to the LV. One of the primary causes for a mitral stenosis is a previous rheumatic fever in the patient, which has been treated through the administration of penicillin. In such situation, the stenosis is most typically treated with a simple percutaneous mitral balloon commissurotomy (PMBC) [8]. In contrast to this, mitral valve regurgitation is a significantly more complex disease due to the different components of the mitral valve and the fact that the leaflets are not capable to close completely for various reasons. Mitral regurgitation disease is typically split into acute and chronic disease. An acute regurgitation is often caused by a previous significant impact to the thorax or a strong myocardial infarction, where the chordae tendinae become detached and the leaflets can't close any more. The chronic regurgitation can further be categorized in a primary or secondary (also functional) regurgitation. At the primary regurgitation the problem are the components of the mitral valve itself. This may include stretched or detached chords (mitral-prolapse) where the leaflets bulge back into the atrium under pressure from the LV during systole as a result of insufficient tension in the chords, detached chords and/or poorly formed leaflets.

In the secondary/functional regurgitation the MV apparatus is morphologically normal. Instead a LV dysfunction is caused by another disease such as a related myocardial infarction or idiopathic myocardial disease. This results in a dilated LV that leads to a widened annulus or a papillary muscle displacement which, in turn, results in a leaflet tethering manifesting in a regurgitation through the MV. In most of the cases of a functional regurgitation the treatment is much less clear than for a primary disease since the regurgitation is just one resulting aspect of another primary disease. In contrast to the treatment of the aortic valve stenosis, (where the replacement is the standard treatment procedure), it is accepted that the optimal surgical treatment for a primary regurgitation is in most cases a repair of the valve [9]. However the surgical treatment for functional regurgitation is a bigger challenge and less clear. There are different percutaneous repair options like the MitraClip which connects the leaflets at its biggest gap and leads to two smaller openings in the mitral valve which can close again during the systole. Other options are, for example, percutaneous procedures to tighten the leaflets or replace them with synthetic chords and annuloplasty where a smaller ring is stitched to the annulus to tighten it up so that the mitral valve is able to close again in the systole [10]. Although the repair is currently the leading method, replacement is associated with potential advantages especially when facilitated by a transcatheter approach. Furthermore a transcatheter mitral valve replacement (TMVR) can be more reproducible and applied to the majority of the patients in particular patients with a serve mitral regurgitation that present with high surgical risk. Since the native mitral valve apparatus is such a complex structure, it can be expected that different approaches (represented by differences in form, size and fixation method) to its replacement are being developed. Currently there are a number of different TMVR devices already in preclinical and clinical development. Due to the size of the native MV and its inherent D-shaped annulus most of the developed TMVR devices are much larger than their commercially-available TAVI counterparts. All of the four first-in-human tested TMVR devices are designed for an transapical approach (CardiAQ valve *CardiAQ Valve Technologies*, Tiara valve *Neovasc Inc*, Tendyne valve *Tendyne Inc*, FORTIS TMV *Edwards Lifesciences Corp*) [5]. The question remains if these valve systems are compatible with the current ASC system. Since the TMVR devices are still in their respective development phases not all the details of those valves are published yet. However some of the companies have released the diameter of the delivery sheath they are using. So far it seems like the largest delivery systems come with a diameter of 32 Fr [5] ($1\,Fr \approx \frac{1}{3}\,mm$) .There are two different sizes of the ASC system. The 'L' size is compatible with therapeutic devices to 28 Fr in outer diameter whereas the 'XL' size is used up to 34 Fr. This means that the size of the delivery sheath for TMVR devices currently under development does not represent a challenge for the current iteration of the ASC system as the XL ASC device can be used without an adaptation of the geometry. However it is not yet clear (from the available published literature around the TMVR devices currently under development) which TMVR systems possess/require significant flexibility in their delivery sheaths. It must be assumed, that the placement of the TMVR devices must be straight in line with the mitral valve. The apical access point, as used so far used for TAVI procedures, is well aligned with the aortic valve but a distinct angulation must be effected to achieve a straight alignment to the mitral valve. Consideration must also be given to the changes in wall thickness that occur as a result of MV disease and what effects, if any, these have on the ability of the ASC system to torqued into the myocardium during delivery/positioning. The research and interviews with mitral valve surgeons that have been conducted as part of this paper has indicated those changes (i.e. LV wall thickness changes) do not represent any difficulties for the successful delivery/positioning of the ASC system since it is being more likely that the LV thickness will increase by the raised wall stress [11], thereby providing increased local myocardial structure into which the ASC system can engage. Furthermore the ability for ASC device to be re-accessible is a particularly attractive feature. A repaired mitral valve can be expected to last for 10 years or longer [12], after which a second/repeat operation may be necessary. The conjunction of closure cap and titanium coil potentially allows for a re-accessing of the same location to effect the second/repeat procedure.

4 Conclusion

Since we are trying to use the same apical access points for TMVR procedures as used currently in TAVI procedures it is necessary to know the limitations of that area and the particular challenges associated with such procedures. To get an antegrade access to the mitral valve with the same apical access, the ASC™ delivery system requires modification of the approach angle of approximately of 15-20° as compared to that for the aortic valve. Additional to that is the limited space between the ribs. To gain a further understanding of that space limitation and the challenges presented by the angulation issues bench testing will be carried out as part of this project. This testing will be performed on excised porcine hearts and will provide an understanding of how the myocardial tissue reacts under the additional stresses that result from the increased angulation. The results of this testing will be presented separately.

Acknowledgement

The work has been carried out at Apica Cardiovascular, part of Thoratec Corporation, Galway, Ireland.

5 References

[1] J. Seeburger, H. A. Katus, S. T. Pleger, U. Krumsdorf, F.-W. Mohr, and R. Bekeredjian, "Percutaneous and surgical treatments of mitral valve regurgitation," *Dtsch. Aerztebl; 108(48) 816-821*, 2011.

[2] *Deutscher Herzbericht 2013*. Deutsche Herzstiftung e.V., 2013.

[3] C. R. Smith *et al.*, "Transcatheter versus surgical aortic-valve replacement in high-risk patients," *N Engl J Med; 364:2187-2198*, 2011.

[4] T. Walther and J. Kempfert, "Transapical vs. transfemoral aortic valve implantation: Which approach for which patient, from a surgeons standpoint," *Annals of Cardiothoracic Surgery*, 2012.

[5] O. D. Backer *et al.*, "Percutaneous transcatheter mitral valve replacement: An overview of devices in preclinical and early clinical evaluation," *Circ Cardiovasc Interv. 7:400-409*, 2014.

[6] J. K. Perloff and W. C. Roberts, "The mitral apparatus: Functional anatomy of mitral regurgitation," *Circulation Journal ;46(2):227-39*, 1972.

[7] J. L. Zamorano, A. Gonzalez-Gomez, and P. Lancellotti, "Mitral valve anatomy: implications for transcatheter mitral valve interventions," *Euro Intervention ;10:106-111*, 2014.

[8] M. Al-Zaaibag, S. Al-Kasab, P. A. Ribeiro, and M. R. Al-Fagih, "Percutaneous double-balloon mitral valvotomy for rheumatic mitral valve stenosis," *The Lancet; 327: 757-761*, 86.

[9] E. C. for Practice Guidelines, "Guidelines on the management of valvular heart disease," *European Heart Journal 33:2451-2496*, 2012.

[10] P. T. L. Chiam and C. E. Ruiz, "Percutaneous transcatheter mitral valve repair - a classification of the technology," *JACC: Cardiovacular Interventrions; 4:1-13*, 2011.

[11] W. H. Gaasch and T. E. Meyer, "Left ventricular response to mitral regurgitation: Implications for management," *Circulation ;118:2298-2303*, 2008.

[12] C. Yankah, H. Siniawski, C. Detschades, J. Stein, and R. Hetzer, "Rheumatic mitral valve repair: 22-year clinical results.," *J Heart Valve Dis. ;20(3):257-64.*, 2011.

Technical Reequiping and Restructuring of Endoscopic Department at Demmin Hospital

Falk Mummert [1], Dipl.-Ing Christian Lehrkamp [2]
[1] Medizinische Ingenieurwissenschaft, Universität zu Lübeck, mummert@miw.uni-luebeck.de
[2] Kreiskrankenhaus Demmin, lehrkamp@kkh-demmin.de

Abstract

Due to the age of electronic data acquisition and data storage it is necessary to develop paths that integrate medical systems in the IT landscapes of hospitals. With the hiring of a new chief physician of internal medicine of the hospital Demmin new claims on the endoscopic instrumentation were made, to achieve a specific diagnosis and therapy. A switch from the previously guided device endoscopic inventory of the company Olympus to the manufacturer PENTAX medical had been completed by technical and economic aspects. The aim of this work is to plan an optimal workflow with the newly acquired technical components for the endoscopic treatment spectrum and to realize it. Different interface adapters from the examination declaration, the image capture to analysis and reporting, and archiving images are to be made with the involvement of a finding documentation system by the integration of endoscopy systems in the clinic structure .

1 Introduction

Endoscopy comes from the Greek language and means endon = within, inside and skopien = look. The task of endoscopes is to gain an insight into the interior of the body. This can be done in two ways. First, the endoscope can be introduced through natural orifices or percutaneously after surgical transection of the body surface. The endoscope can be regarded as an "extended mind" of the physician. By this technique, areas of the body can be achieved, that would not be seen without surgery. Meanwhile endoscopy systems are no longer just for endoscopic diagnosis, they are also used pre-, intra-, and postoperatively in visceral surgery [1]. The endoscope next to the image transmission still has other tasks, such as the introduction of probes and catheters, taking tissue samples or haemostasis by electrocoagulation. Endoscopy is associated with the medical technology, more than any other region in the clinical area [2]. This attachment to technology includes all units of an endoscopy system of mechanics, lighting to image acquisition, image processing and image storage. Endoscopy has become in almost all medical disciplines to the established standard. By realy simple beginnings with rigid endoscopes, highly complex medical systems have evolved. The image acquisition and image processing can be realized only by modern computer technology and data processing [1]. A finding report, for image documentation of endoscopic findings and endoscopic operations is required from a medical and forensic point of view according to defined criteria. That's the reason why endoscopy systems has to integrate in the hospital's IT [3],[4].

2 Material and Methods

In October 2014 new devices were procured for two fitted examination rooms of the endoscopic functional area in the district hospital Demmin. There was a change from the device manufacturer Olympus to the endoscopy components of the company PENTAX medical. On the one hand, this happened for economic reasons and on the other hand by the appointment of a new chief physician. This new chief physician has already substantial experience with the named endoscopy system. Furthermore, compared to Olympus the PENTAX medical video processors can use the i-scan image processing technology. A video processor EPK-i5000 and a video processor EPK-i7000, two mud pumps, two ITD endoscopy video cars, two 26 inch NDS Radiance monitors G2HB, a trolley uni-cart, a CO_2 insufflator, and various optics of the company PENTAX medical were bought. The following optics were purchased: two video gastroscopes type EC-2990i, a video gastroscope type EG29-i10, a video gastroscope type EC16-K10, two video colonoscope type EC-3890Fi2, a video colonoscope type EC38-i10F2, a video colonoscope type EC-3490TFi, a video-bronchoscope type EB-1975K and a video duodenoscope type ED34-i10T.
The table shows the technical data, diameter of insertion tube, diameter of distal end, diameter of instrument channel, the working lenght, the angle of view the angulation up and down and the angulation right and left, of three different endoscopes (a gastroscope, a colonoscope, a bronchoscope)[6] . The endoscopes are built according to the requirement of the investigation. The optics of PENTAX medical all have a high definition chip as well as a clean cap system. This is a removable cap at the distal end for

Table 1: technical data of some endoscopes

technical data	EG-2990i	EC-3890Fi2	EB-1975K
insertion tube Ø	9.8 mm	13.2 mm	6.4 mm
distal end Ø	10.8 mm	13.2 mm	6.3 mm
instrument channel Ø	2.8 mm	3.8 mm	2.8mm
working lenght	105 cm	150 cm	60 cm
angle of view	140 °	140 °	120 °
angulation up/down	210°/210°	180°/180°	180°/130°
angulation right/left	120°/120°	160°/160°	-/-

fast and secure mechanical cleaning of air and water channels. In addition, the endoscopes have an insertion tube with different flexibility gradation. Now, a short insight into the technical details of the newly acquired endoscopy units is given. The video processors support the ultra-modern endoscopic diagnosis. They combine illumination with an image quality in HD +. The i-scan imaging technology allows an assessment of surface structures with high precision. Using a 300 watt xenon light as source so the white light illumination supporting the orientation very fast. Even detection of small lesions are possible. Mucosal changes are easily recognizable by the HD image quality. The default i-scan profiles can be accessed at the touch of a button. In addition, both video processors provide an interface for an external USB mass storage. The video processor EPK-i7000 has a touch screen and a keyboard as a user interface and the other processor only a keyboard as a user interface [6].
The CO_2 insufflator from PENTAX medical has several options for health care. The device can be plugged directly into a container with sterile water and carbon dioxide or to the central supply. There is a central power supply to the endoscopy workstations of the hospital which provides both carbon dioxide and oxygen. The CO_2 insufflator is used, for example at a colonoscopy. As a result to supply carbon dioxide, the intestinal expands slightly and also narrow passages will meet with the endoscope. Carbon dioxide is absorbed rapidly compared to room air from the surrounding tissue, so that any complaints of the patient during the investigation and after the investigation are reduced. To get a better view of the gastrointestinal tract, its rinsed by warm water of the mud pump. Flushing is operated by a foot pedal. Water and carbon dioxide are each heated to body temperature, 37 degrees Celsius [6].
By the mobile endoscopy video car both endoscopy workplaces are autonomous and transportable. That means one endoscopic system can be driven in radiology station, for example by a ERCP (endoscopic retrograde cholangiography), and the other system remains in the endoscopy department. The video car makes it easy by its twin swivel castors and several shelves which can be loaded by a maximum of 50 kilogram. The endoscopy video car also features a rotating and tilting LCD display mount, and a height adjustable double-endoscope holder. The video car is electrically equipped with an isolation transformer (1600 volt amperes), a central on-off switch and an eight-fold power strip with a fuse and a POAG plug per socket. Electrical safety conforms to applicable standards and guidelines DIN EN 60742 (VDE 0551) and DIN EN 60601-1 (VDE 0750) [6] .

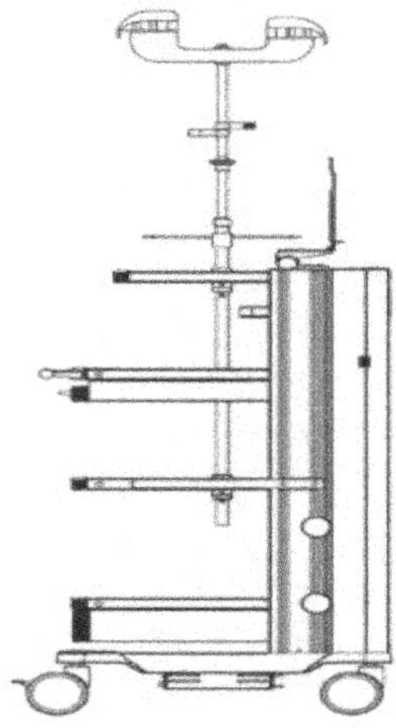

Figure 1: endoscopy video car for a mobile use of the endoscopic system

With the newly acquired tools, two endoscopy workstations wil be established.

2.1 Inventory of equipment

The endoscopic system with all its instruments had to be incorporated into the clinical area. For this, first an inventory was made and the equipment inventoried according to the Medical Devices Operator Ordiance (MPBetriebV). In this case, each newly acquired equipment is recognized in METOS and awarded new BMT numbers for each device. BMT stands for the Department of Biomedical Engineering. METOS is a programm for medical devices of the district hospital Demmin. Every medical device is listet in this programm whit an individuel BMT number and the clinical place. For the entire hospital staff it is possible to enter occurring disorders in METOS. The units of the endoscopy system pasted with the associated BMT numbers and the machines books were filed.

2.2 Imaging / Image transfer

For illuminating, endoscopes need a light transmission system. The light transmission by a flexible as well as rigid endoscopes happens by glass fiber bundle. The light is totally reflected at the interface between the mantle and the core of the individual fibers. Often, xenon or halogen lamps used as the light source. Filter and cooling fans prevent the equipment from overheating. The image transfer of rigid endoscopes is performed by lens systems. The image transfer of flexible endoscopes is performed by ordered glass fibers and a corresponding eyepiece. Meanwhile tiny television cameras are used as image sensor increases. The cameras are equipped by miniature CCD chips. This CCD sensors are sensitive electronic components that are based on the internal photoelectric effect. As a result, the resolution has improved and there are even HD systems on the market [1]. Only optics were purchased that use this type of image transmission. On this way they provide images in HD quality. Firmly on the endoscopy video car a video processor, a mud pump and a monitor installed. The following wiring diagram (Fig.2) shows the image capture and image transmission.

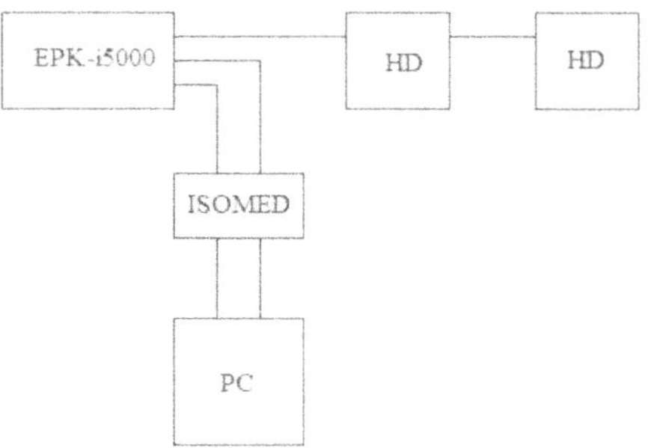

Figure 2: wiring diagram for the endoscopy workstation

The endoscope is connected to the video processor. The captured images will be sent to the monitor as a video signal. For both video processor and the monitor have a DVI interface. By this way the examiner see the images on the monitor in real time. The monitor is attached to the video car. For a better view for the examining or surgeon, a second monitor is required which is placed directly in his line of sight. The image transfer onto this monitor is done in one endoscopy room also by a DVI cable. At the other room the image transfer to the second monitor is wireless. This happens with an NDS ZeroWire, a video signal transmission system developed by NDS SURGICAL IMAGING. In video transmission over the ZeroWire receiver and transmitter modules, full HD video sources in real time can be transmitted with less than a frame latency. It is used for the ultra-wideband technology. The range is up to 10 meters. By a time-frequency coding system, several ZeroWire units might be operated without encountering the interfering channels [7]. But at this workstation its not used because two monitors are sufficient. In this way, no need for additional cables. So a trip hazard no longer exists and for mobile endoscopy systems the assembly and disassembly is easier. ZeroWire is compatible with the HDTV and HD video formats Medical and based on DVI video signal transmission level. Over those same DVI connection, the two monitors are connected to the transmitter and receiver. By the video processor in each case a video signal and a trigger signal for image acquisition are transferred through a video isolation amplifier to the PC system. It is used the video isolation amplifier of ISOMED. This has the function of the galvanic separation of the interfaces between two devices. In this case, one of the two devices meet the requirements of the Medical Devices Directive (MDD) and the other does not meet these requirements [5],[8].

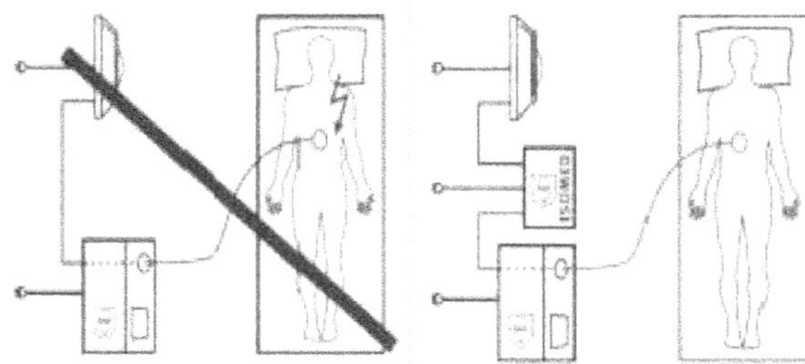

Figure 3: installation of ISOMED, on the left the incorrect use of ISOMED, on the right the correct use of ISOMED

The figure shows the correct use of ISOMED video isolation amplifier. Since the findings host is not meeting the requirements of the MDD, a use of ISOMED will be necessary at all.

On this way, medical devices, such as endoscopy devices can be connected to a monitor or PC-compatible image memory. The used isolation amplifier is capable of the type 4 channel BNC and is suitable for all kinds of video signal transmissions with 75 ohm input or output impedance. So there are four electrically isolated video channels with BNC connector for transmitting four composite signals. It is important to ensure that inputs and outputs are never connected simultaneously on the patient side. This ensures that there is no direct patient contact. The galvanic isolation from the input to the output side is performed by optical transmission. The ISOMED can be operated directly via mains plug by 230 V voltage. The appliance should be inspected at least annually in accordance by IEC 62353 / DIN VDE 0751 [8]. The video isolation amplifier is located together with the finding documentation system in the next room. The cable connection of isolation amplifier and video processor is provided by a small hole in the wall. Depending on the assignment of the function keys on the handset of the endoscope head, the triggered image signal can be transferred via the video isolation amplifier to the PC recording system. If an image is included, the default button pressed and the trigger output of the video processor take a signal pulse via the video isolaton amplifier to the graphics card of the finding computer. This captured the image, which is presented in real time and thus serves to image acquisition and processing in the findings and archiving process.

3 Results

For finding generation, on the respective computers of endoscopy anteroom a finding documentation of the client also newly purchased the finding documentation system

Viewpoint from the company GE are installed. These system is used for archiving of medical image data and provides the background for integration survey findings of a structured, implemented in the text and image. By the help of Viewpoint, the physician may be work quite intuitive by the program. All relevant items such as medication, indication, pathological content, diagnosis, complications, comments, biopsies or service entry can be queried. In this way, the finding can be write quickly and no important facts will remember. Before each examination, a requirement in the parent hospital information system (Orbis) of the hospital must be exist. This request is entered from the work list in the Viewpoint program. Without Indication of the patient's name, date of birth, name of the examining physician, name of the assistant staff and the endoscope that is used, the findings generation not released. After the required inputs, the acquired images are allocated to the patient. Viewpoint stores all already made inquiries. Therefore, findings of patients who investigated again are always available. To guarantee that no patients information are lost, at each workstation a 16 gigabyte USB stick is connected on the video processor. That also stores the images. The USB stick is also required if the endoscopic system is used mobile. Then there is no image capture cable by the video processor that added to the documentation computer. This may be, for example, in the case of an ERCP examination. It is already possible to store all video sequences via the external USB drive. This is currently being Viewpoint in the hospital Demmin royalty due not yet exist. The generated image data in the Viewpoint database stored its in .jpeg format. After the diagnosis is written and the images are stored in the Viewpoint server, the collected data on the USB flash are delated again. The finding, along with pictures, is copied to the hospital information system. Then it's available for the stations. In addition, printed the findings for external use and archived in electronic patient archive.

4 Conclusion

Endoscopy workstations are completed and meet the standards of the Medical Devices Directive (MDD). The chief physician is very pleased with the captured images. Since the integration of new endoscopy devices much more investigations were carried out as previously. As the program Viewpoint is not only suitable for reporting in endoscopy but also in sonography. So a concept for the standardized finding generation and archiving for ultrasound imaging is also planned and to develop.

Acknowledgement

The work has been carried out at the hospital Demmin.

5 References

[1] R. Kramme, *Medizintechnik.* 3.Auflage Springer, Berlin/Heidelberg , 2007.

[2] U. Bause, K. Forke, J. Matauschek, *Medizintechnik.* VEB Verlag Volk und Gesundheit, pp.119-120, Berlin, 1983.

[3] B. Lewerenz, *Bilddokumentation in der gastroenterologischen Endoskopie.* Available: http://edoc.ub.uni-muenchen.de/9702/1/LewerenzBjoern.pdf, 2009.

[4] T. Wittenberg,bP. Hastreiter, U. Hoppe, H. Handels, A. Horsch, H. P. Meinzer, *Bildverarbeitung für die Medizin 2003.* Springer, Berlin/Heidelberg,pp.191-192 ,2003.

[5] R. D. Boeckmann, H. Frankenberg, H. G. Will, *MPG and Co..* 4.Auflage TÜV Media, Köln, 2008.

[6] PENTAX medical Website, Available: www.pentaxmedical.de/Produktuebersicht.de , 2015.

[7] NDS SURGICAL IMAGING, Available: http://ndssi.com/data/uploads/pdf/Surgical/ZeroWire/nds-zerowire-sales-sheet.pdf , 2015.

[8] Manuel ISOMED video isolation amplifier, Ankrit, 2012.

Developing a procedure to test the compatibility of flexible endoscopes with an Endo-Thermo-Disinfector (ETD)

J. G. Grimm [1] and B. Ottens [2]
[1] Medizinische Ingenieurwissenschaft, Universität zu Lübeck, grimmj@informatik.uni-luebeck.de
[2] Olympus Winter & Ibe, Hamburg, benjamin.ottens@olympus-oste.eu

Abstract

The proper reprocessing of flexible endoscopes is essential for todays hygienic standards. When a new automated endoscopy reprocessor (AER) is developed, the user has to be informed which flexible endoscopes are compatible with the washer-disinfector. In this study, a test procedure was developed to test the compatibility of any flexible endoscope with a new AER. Therefore structures of flexible endoscopes and the components of an AER were investigated to understand, which functions of the AER are influenced by endoscopes. As result, a test procedure was developed, which can be used similar for all flexible endoscopes. Possible test results were discussed and solutions for non-compatible endoscopes were mentioned. The resulting data can be used to adjust analyzing algorithms of the AER and make modifications to eventually state the endoscope as compatible.

1 Introduction

Today endoscopes are used in nearly every section of a hospital, for example in gastrology, neurology, urology etc. [1], [2]. Flexible endoscopes are mostly designed to look into the natural body openings for diagnostics, biopsy and even therapy [1], [3]. After a flexible endoscope has been used, it has to be reprocessed sufficiently to prevent infections on other patients or hospital staff [4], [5]. Due to the structure and the surface material of flexible endoscopes, often sterilization is not possible, therefore cleaning and disinfection is used to reprocess endoscopes [5]. To standardize the reprocessing quality, various guidelines recommend using automatic endoscopy reprocessors [3], [6], [7]. In Germany medical equipment underlies certain guidelines for hygienics and safety [2]. For automatic reprocessing machines the most important guideline is the DIN EN 15883 [8] together with the recommendations of the Robert-Koch-Institut [7]. Due to constant modifications of guidelines and improvement in technologies, AERs are further developed. When a new AER is developed, not only the correct and safe functionality of the machine itself has to be tested, but also which endoscopes can be reprocessed correctly with the machine. To ensure that an endoscope is compatible with the machine a test procedure has to be developed. The procedure should be feasible for every flexible endoscope and documented the same way. For this study the different structures of flexible endoscopes were investigated and the different components and functions of an AER were analyzed to find out which units of the AER performe different according to the endoscope design and therefore have to be tested.

2 Material and Methods

The purpose of this study is to develop a test procedure which tests the compatibility of flexible endoscopes with a new endo-thermo-disinfector (ETD). The components and software of ETDs ensure not only a proper reprocessing but also prevent damaging the endoscope. The test procedure should only include those components which change the washing-disinfecting process depending on the design of the endoscope. In this section the structure of flexible endoscopes is described as well as the functionalities of an ETD.

2.1 Flexible Endoscopes Structure

The structure and design of flexible endoscopes can vary depending on the purpose, the imaging technology and the area of application [9]. Every flexible endoscope has either an ocular as eye piece or a *light guide plug* for video endoscopy, an *umbilical cord*, a *control piece* and the *insertion tube* [9]. Fig.1 shows an exemplary structure of the channel system of an endoscope. With the *light guide plug*, the endoscope is connected to the light source, the water supply and the air pump. New video endoscopes have a waterproof light guide connection, whereas older generations need a cap to prevent water damages during reprocessing [5], [9],[10].
The bending of the distal end of the endoscope can be adjusted with the *control piece*. The control piece additionally has a valve for suction, a for air/water control and a biopsy valve where instruments can be inserted. The part of the endoscope which enters the human body is called *insertion tube*. At the end of the insertion tube is the distal end which

can be bent from 90° to 210°. [5], [9]
The *channel system* can vary depending on the endoscope

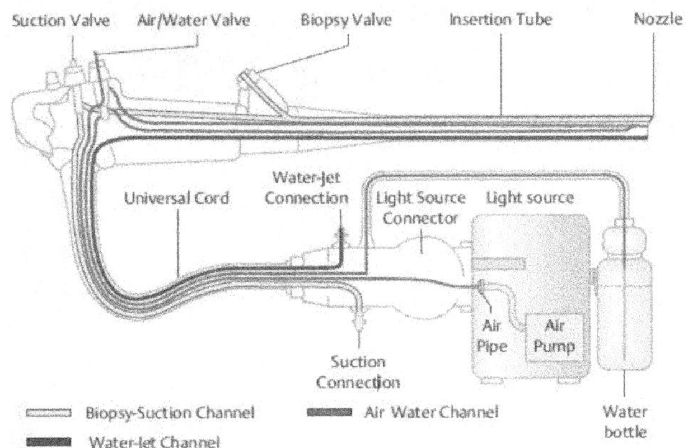

Figure 1: Structure of a flexible endoscope, adapted from [5]

type. There are differences in the number, the branches, the length, and the width of the channels. [3], [10]
Every flexible endoscope has a channel system which can contain different variations of suction- and biopsy channels, air-/water-system and auxiliary water channels or elevator channels. Instruments can be inserted through the biopsy channel which usually has the biggest diameter, the elevator channel on the contrary has the smallest diameter which can bend an instrument to the side, without bending the distal end. [3], [9]

2.2 Reprocessing of flexible endoscopes

Before the endoscope can be reprocessed, it has to be placed in the basket of the reprocessing machine. The basket has two holdings; one is for the control piece and the other one for the light guide plug. The fragile distal end of the endoscope can be fixed with an adjustable clamping piece. To rinse the endoscope channels, adapter hoses and channel separator have to be connected to each channel opening [4]. There are different adapters for different endoscopes, depending on the existing endoscope channels and the architecture of the endoscope. One adapter is for the leakage tester. After all adapter hoses are connected correctly to the endoscope, the basket with the endoscope inside can be put into the ETD and a reprocessing program can be started. A typical reprocessing program is shown in Fig.2. During the *pre-cleaning*, the outside of the endoscope and the endoscope channels are flushed with non-heated water to remove remaining residues after a manual cleaning. The *cleaning* removes all the soil with a detergent. A *rinsing* step removes all the chemicals used before. During *disinfection*, bacteria, mycrobacteria, fungi, yeasts, and viruses are inactivated to prevent contaminating the hospital staff and patients. The user can select either a long or a short *drying* program.[1], [4], [5], [7]
The ETD has different control devices to ensure a proper reprocessing. The devices depending on the endoscope are the *RFID* (radio-frequency identification), the *leakage tester* and the *flow control* [11].

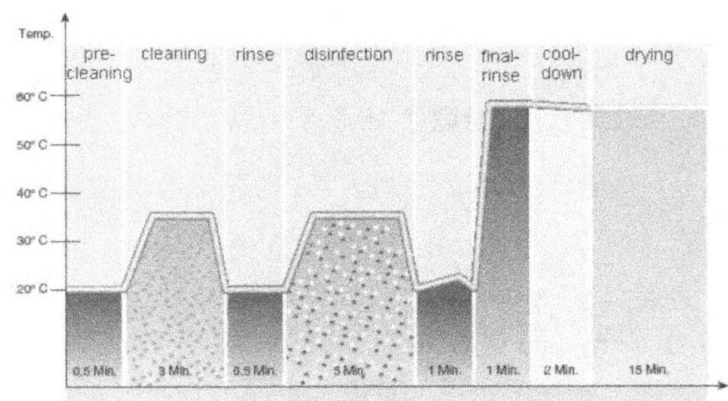

Figure 2: A typical reprocessing program, adapted and translated from [2].

Before the reprocessing starts, the ETD identifies the endoscope via RFID transponder on the endoscope, the endoscope depending reprocessing parameters are provided [2]. The ETD has a *leakage testing* device to detect leaks on the endoscope and ensures that no liquid enters the electronical and mechanical parts of the endoscope. A methode is used, where the sleeve of the endoscope is inflated and an over pressure is built up. If the endoscope has a leakage, the leakage tester detects a pressure decrease. The reprocessing program is aborted, if the pressure drops below a certain value in a defined time interval. During the reprocessing a permanent overpressure is held, to continuously detect leakages on the endoscope. [8]
The *flow control* ensures a permanent liquid flow through each channel of the endoscope. The sensors detect blockages in the endoscope and sends an alarm in case of an error. If an adapter or the channel separator is disconnected the ETD sends an alarm, as well, and the program is aborted. In those cases the user receives a message to control the channel connections or to manually brush the endoscope channels before restarting the reprocessing program. The flow values vary due to different channel diameters, layout and branches.[8]

3 Results and Discussion

Requirements have been defined for the test procedure. It is important that the test procedure can be performed with every endoscope type that is already on the market, every new endoscope and endoscope prototypes. Each test should be performed in the same order and documented the same way, to have comparable results. The order of the test procedure needs to be reasonable and no endoscope should be harmed during testing. Guidelines have to be followed such as the DIN EN 15883.

3.1 Test Procedure

In Fig.3 the individual steps of the test procedure are diagramed and will be specified in the following subsections.

Before the endoscope can be reprocessed, a set of param-

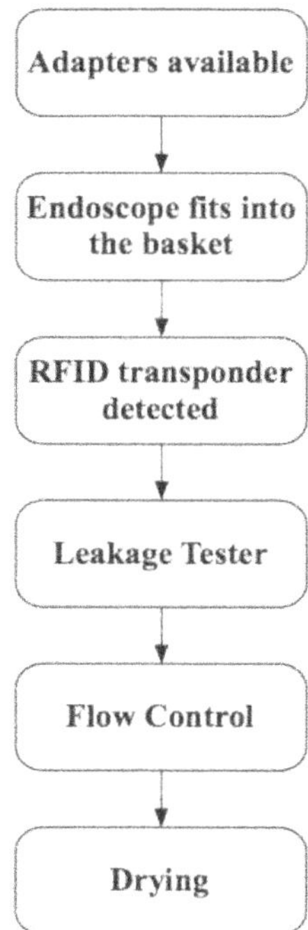

Figure 3: Diagram of the sequence of the components, the endoscope is tested with.

eters have to be chosen. The existing channels and the adapters define the parameter set. The parameters are chosen according to the channel designs and branches as well as the adapter ports. During reprocessing, the flow control and the leakage tester compare these reference parameters to the actual values. When all parameters are known, the test procedure can be started.

3.1.1 Mechanical compatibility

The first step is to check if an adapter is available for every channel of the endoscope to assure a correct reprocessing. If there is no adapter combination available, the test can be aborted and the following steps do not have to be performed.

The endoscope should be put into the basket and the light guide plug and the control piece should be put into the provided holders. The distal end shall be fixed with a clamping pice. It is important that the endoscope fits in those holdings to prevent it from moving during reprocessing and therefore prevent damages on the endoscope.

To identify the endoscope, every endoscope has to have either an built-in RFID transponder or an transponder which can be glued on the outside of the endoscope [2]. If the endoscope does not have an internal transponder or no suitable transponder is available which can be glued on, an external transponder which is attached to the basket in front of the reading device can be used. An external transponder also has to be used if the distance between the RFID transponder on the endoscope and the reading device is too far. When the endoscope type and the reprocessing parameters are known, a reprocessing program can be started.

3.1.2 Compatibility with the Leakage Tester

All parameters and values from the leakage tester unit measured during reprocessing have to be recorded for evaluation.

According to the DIN EN 15883 the leakage test has to be performed before the reprocessing and continuously during the reprocessing. A constant pressure is held on the endoscope; if the pressure drops under a specific value in a specific time, the reprocessing is aborted with an error message.

The endoscope tested does not have a leak, therefore the leakage tester should not abort the reprocessing program. However depending on the volume of the tested endoscope and due to changes in water temperature during reprocessing, the pressure could drop under the given limit and the reprocessing is aborted. If this is the case, the test is failed and can not be proceeded. The pressure data recorded during the leakage test will be evaluated and new parameters are chosen for this endoscope.

3.1.3 Compatibility with the Flow Control

All parameters and values from the flow control unit measured during reprocessing have to be recorded for evaluations.

The tested endoscope does not have any blockades in the channels per definition. If the reprocessing machine detects a blocked channel, the flow control parameters do not fit for the endoscope and the reprocessing program is aborted.

If the program is aborted, the test is failed and new parameters have to be evaluated.

In case of a successful reprocessing program, the endoscope has to be reprocessed a second time, but this time with adapters or the channel separator disconnected. The flow control data should be measured as well. The reprocessing program should be aborted by the flow control. If the reprocessing is not aborted, this part of the test is failed and new parameters have to be evaluated.

3.1.4 Drying according to DIN EN 15883

For a complete drying of the endoscope the DIN EN 15883 requires the following test after a reprocessing: A colored crepe paper has to be placed on a flat surface. Within 5 minutes after the reprocessing with a long drying program the endoscope has to be put on the crepe paper. The endoscope has to be kept horizontal at any times to keep residual water inside the endoscope channels. Any water dropping from the endoscope during unloading or dark spots, resulting from moisture have to be documented.

To test the dryness of the the channel, the endoscope has to be put in position being in a continuous fall from the light guide plug down to the distal end of the endoscope. The distal end should be place between 50 mm to 100 mm over a colored crepe paper. Every channel has to be discharged with 105 kPa to 120 kPa medical compressed air. The compressed air should be blown through every opening of the light guide plug and every opening of the control unit. Any residual humidity which can be seen as dark spots on the crepe paper, should be documented. If a complete drying is not possible, the endoscope has to be put in a special drying cabin. [8]

3.2 Result of the Test Procedure

When all tests are completed, the recorded data of the leakage tester unit and the flow control unit have to be evaluated even if the program was not aborted.
There are different results for a tested endoscope:

1. The reprocessing program was not aborted, the test procedure was smoothly conducted and the evaluated data was in the correct range:
   The endoscope can be classified as *compatible.*
   If every test was passed except for the drying, the user must be informed, that a complete drying is not possible.

2. The endoscope failed the test because of a wrong set of parameters or the evaluated data was not in the desired range:
   The parameters can be adjusted or a new set of parameters can be created for the endoscope. In this case the test has to be repeated with the new parameters.

3. The endoscope failed the test because the right adapters are not available or it does not fit in the basket:
   In this case the endoscope is classified as *not compatible* and it has to be evaluated if a redesign of the basket, the adapters or even the endoscope is economically reasonable.

4. The last choice is to classify the endoscope as *not compatible* and the endoscope cannot be reprocessed with the AER.

Endoscope which are tested as compatible can be added to the list of compatible endoscopes and can be reprocessed with the AER. The desired test result is, that every flexible endoscope which is commonly used in hospitals and medical practices is at last compatible with the new AER.

4 Conclusion

A test procedure was developed to test the compatibility of flexible endoscopes with a new AER. The structure of flexible endoscopes were investigated and then a new AER was analyzed. The test procedure was developed and different possible results were evaluated. Every endoscope has to pass the test procedure before labeled as compatible for the ETD machine.

Acknowledgement

The work has been carried out at Olympus Winter & Ibe, Hamburg. I want to thank Dr. rer. nat. K. Lüdtke-Buzug, my supervisor at the Universität zu Lübeck, Dr. S. Eschborn, B. Ottens, A. Weis and the entire ERS team for their guidance and support during my internship.

5 References

[1] K. M. Irion, M. Leonhard, *Endoskopie*. Medizintechnik (R. Kramme), Springer-Verlag, Berlin Heidelberg, pp. 379-401, 2011.

[2] Olympus Europa Media Center, *PDF Olympus informiert*, Volume 4|2013, Available: <http://www.olympus.de/medical/en/medical_systems/mediacentre/media_detail_75648.jsp>, last viewed 11.01.2015.

[3] C. Hilger, *Flexible Endoskope - Belastungsmerkmale und Beanspruchungsparameter*, Medizintechnik 123 Jg., Volume 5|2003, pp. 182-190.

[4] U. Beilenhoff, C. S. Neumann, J. F. Rey, H. Biering, R. Blum et al. *ESGE-ESGENA guideline: Cleaning an disifection in gastrointestinal endoscopy*, Endoscopy 2008, Volume 40, pp. 939-957.

[5] M. Jung and T. Ponchon, *Cleaning and Disinfection in Endoscopy*. Gastroenterological Endoscopy (M. Classen, G. N. J. Tytgat), Georg Thieme Verlag, Stuttgart, pp. 84-89, 2010.

[6] H. Feußner, A. Schneider, A. Meining, *Endoskopie, minimal-invasive Chirurgue und navigierte Systeme*. Medizintechnik - Life Science Engineering (E. Wintermantel, S.-W. Ha), Springer, pp. 1121-1161, 2009.

[7] *Anforderungen an Hygiene bei der Aufbereitung flexibler Endoskope und endoskopischen Zusatzinstrumentariums*, Robert Koch-Institut, Bundesgesundheitsblatt, Volume 42|2002, pp. 395-411, Springer-Verlag, 2002.

[8] International Organisation for Standardization. *DIN EN ISO 15883-4, Anforderungen und Prüfverfahren für Reinigungs-Desinfektionsgeräte mit chemischer Desinfektion für thermolabile Endoskope*, Deutsche Fassung, 2009.

[9] *Endoscope Reprocessing*, Queensland Government, <http://www.health.qld.gov.au/EndoscopeReprocessing/>, last viewed 11.01.2015.

[10] C. J. Alvarado, M. Reichelderfer, *APIC guideline for infection prevention and control in flexible endoscopy*, Association for Professioals in Infection Control and Epidemiology, 2000.

[11] *PDF ETD Double product broshure*, Available: <http://pdf.medicalexpo.de/pdf-en/olympus-medical-europa/etd-double/69587-87009.html>, viewed 11.01.2015.

Development of a level indicator for process chemicals of an automated endoscopy reprocessor

J. Markmann [1], B. Ottens [2] and S. Eschborn [2]
[1] Medizinische Ingenieurwissenschaft, Universität zu Lübeck, markmanj@miw.uni-luebeck.de
[2] Olympus Surgical Technologies Europe, Olympus Winter & Ibe GmbH, Benjamin.Ottens@olympus-oste.eu, Sascha.Eschborn@olympus-oste.eu

Abstract

The aim of the project is to develop a client software for the latest automated endoscopy reprocessor (AER) of Olympus which calculates the quantity of chemicals used and to create a graphical user interface (GUI). The new software should simplify the estimation of the remaining chemicals. Besides it should enable to obtain the current filling level of the chemical container of the AER from every computer using the same network. The requirements of the software are to include up to eight AERs and to have a GUI, which is compliant to the corporate product design (CPD) of Olympus. The software contains a server connection via hypertext transfer protocol secure (HTTPS) request, the processing of the generated data, the filtering of the chemical dosage information, the evaluation and a graphical representation. The software is going to be part of a customer survey, which examines, if the application would improve the reprocessing workflow.

1 Introduction

After treatment the endoscope has to be reprocessed, so it can be used again without risking the transfer of an infection to patients or operators. The Medizinprodukt Gesetz (MPG) § 26, Abs.1 and the Medizinprodukte-Betreiberverordnung (MPBetreibV) § 4, Abs.2 demand the reprocessing of medical products, which are used in intended almost sterile or sterile practices. There must be validated procedures, which can prove that the safety and the health of patients are not endangered [1]. The precise requirements can be read in the recommendation document by the Robert Koch-Institut in [2]. For the reprocessing of endoscopes Olympus developed a range of automated endoscopy reprocessor (AER), the Endo Thermo Disinfector (ETD) series. The work is accomplished using the example of the ETD Double, which is going to be launched in 2015. Based on the validated process, reprocessing operating parameters like the temperature profile, the dose, the pressure and the flow rate have to be within a specific range. According to the DIN EN ISO 15883, which contains the requirements for cleaning and disinfection devices all these critical process parameters have to be recorded [3]. For each reprocessing process a protocol is created, which contains the actual values. The last 150 reprocessing protocols are stored on a webserver as a part of the AER. The webserver is available via Transmission Control Protocol/ Internet Protocol (TCP/IP) connection, so a remote access via Extensible Markup Language (XML) protocol is possible. The ETD Double has a range of different reprocessing programs. At each reprocessing program the amount of used chemicals, the dosages and the kind of used chemicals vary. There are even programs, which do not use any process chemicals. Independent of the type of the reprocessing program in every process the water quality has to be constantly good. Therefore a small amount of peracetic acid (PAA) is used to inject the water to make sure the water is not contaminated. The injection is not mentioned in the protocol. The reprocessing chemicals are stored in containers inside of the AER, this can be seen in Fig. 1, so they have to have a specific size to fit in. The chemical containers have to be exchanged regularly.

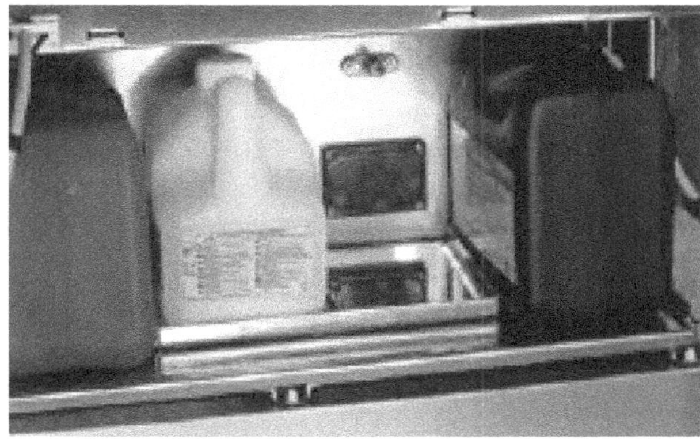

Figure 1: chemical containers inside the ETD Double

A client software, which shows the filling level of the containers and gives a warning when they have to be exchanged, could eventually help to optimize the workflow of reprocessing endoscopes in hospitals. For evaluation a first prototype of the client software has to be implemented.

2 Material and Methods

By now the filling levels of the chemical containers can only be seen at the graphical user interface (GUI) of the AERs, there is no option to see, if the containers should be exchanged, from another computer. The used chemicals are hazardous material, so the storage is subject of strict regulations. The depository is not necessarily next to the reprocessing room. Demand for a delocalized overview of the filling level of the chemical containers occurred, when hospital staff wanted to reprocess endoscopes, but had to go back to get new chemicals, because it was empty. This caused a delay in the workflow. An even worse scenario would be, if there are no more chemicals in stock, so no reprocessing is possible at all. To optimize the workflow with the ETD Double and so finally optimize the reprocessing process a client software should be implemented, which enables, the filling level values to be obtained from every computer and to implement a warning, when the chemical containers have to be exchanged. The main idea is to analyze the dosage information of the reprocessing protocols, which are stored on a webserver of the AERs.

The project can be split into several parts. The first step to do is to recall all of the data in report format from the ETD Double. To prepare the data for extracting the dosage information the multitude of protocols has to be processed. In the next step the desired dosage information have to be extracted. This information has to be transferred to the main function to be interpreted. To illustrate the data, a GUI has to be implemented. Finally there should be an additional function, which should calculate the chemicals in stock.

First of all the programming language has to be chosen. The client software is going to be a feature for the ETD Double; it is not implemented on the AER, but on the computer of the customers. Meaning a language, which is independent of the operating system, is needed. That is the main reason why Java is used.

2.1 Server connection and data requirement

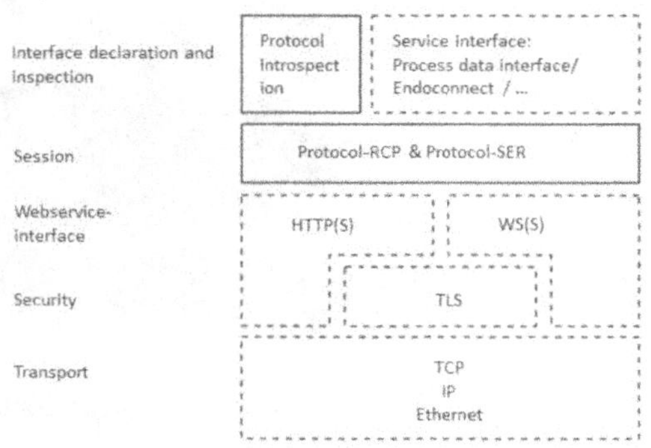

Figure 2: protocol stack

To get the data from the AER a connection to the webserver of the device is needed. It is implemented by using the IP on the network layer and the TCP on the transport layer of the Open Systems Interconnection Model (OSI)-model [4]. The ETD Double does not provide any other network or transport options. But you can choose between the hypertext transfer protocol secure (HTTPS) and a Secure WebSocket (WSS) connection [5]. The protocol stack can be seen in Fig. 2. In this project the HTTPS connection is used, because it is a singular method request, which means that there is one return value per request. It makes specific requests possible and does not slow the software, because of unnecessary constant data requirement, like the WSS connection would do. Every ETD Double has its own IP address. While using the IP address of the AER and the port where the data is saved a uniform resource locator (URL) address can be created. A "HttpsURLConnection" is generated [6]. Each HttpURLConnection instance is used to make a single request. The list of HTTPS header fields contains the parameters, which define the HTTPS transaction. The used request is HTTPS Post. The HTTPS message body contains an XML request. The specified request "GetAllProtocols" is sent to the webserver. It asks the AER to send all stored reprocessing protocols. There is no request option implemented, which offers the possibility to asks directly for specific information like the dosage information. An inputstream reads the data, including the HTTPS response message body, which needs to be analyzed, from the open HTTPS connection.

2.2 Protocol processing and filtering of the needed data

The inputstream has to be parsed to recover the XML format of the response message body. Therefore a Document Object Model (DOM)-oriented Java API application programming interface (API) is used. Although the whole data has to be fed to the memory, the advantage of getting specific information by searching for elements outweighs.

All of the reprocessing protocols are sent in one file, so they have to be separated before they can be used and individually be analyzed. The interface NodeList provides a function called getElementsByTagName, which returns a list of the elements with a given name, so you can search for a specific one. This can be used for splitting the protocols. The search for the protocol name returns a list of elements; these elements are the single protocols.

Because the XML response contains all protocols in one, the new single protocols do not have a XML header on their own, what means by splitting the protocols, the well-formed XML format gets lost. As the well-formed XML format is needed to get the actual wanted information it has to be recovered. This can easily be done by adding a XML header to every protocol. The split protocols have to be parsed to a XML file again, because the element search returns a string. There might be protocols, which are returned several times, because during the interval the AER might not produce as many protocols that all protocols are new. To make sure the dose of one process is not deducted more than once and sophisticates the results, the protocol number, which is part

of the protocol name and is onetime assigned, is saved on a stack. The protocol numbers of the single protocols are compared to the numbers on stack, if there is a match the protocol is already analyzed and is not used again. The data on the stack has to be serialized in a file otherwise they would get lost every time the software is closed. The number of new protocols is calculated.
When the new protocols are extracted, it has to be distinguished between two kind of protocols. On the one hand, there are the protocols of the thermal self-disinfection, which does not use chemicals besides the PAA injection, so no dosage information is obtained in the protocol. On the other hand there are the cleaning protocols, which describe the reprocessing of the endoscopes or minimal invasive surgical (MIS) instruments, so there is information about the dosage quantity.
Sometimes the reprocessing process terminates premature because of a device error. In this case there might be cleaning protocols, which have no dosage information. This could generate software problems and has to be treated differently. In the case of an abnormal termination a protocol including an error number is generated. If there is an error number including the protocol the following routine is started. It has to be checked, if the termination was before or after any kind of chemical was used, because the process did not necessary terminated before. To find the error protocol the same XML-searching method can be used by searching for the error number. The PAA injection is still considered. If these specific protocols are filtered, the dosage information of the standard protocols is extracted.

2.3 Interpretation of the dose

With the first start of the software the variables for the filling levels are initialized with the milliliter value of a full chemical container. That is why the software needs to be started, when all chemical containers are full. This situation can be forced artificially by replacing used chemical containers by new ones. At this point, all stored protocols are tagged as analyzed. The dosage of following reprocessing programs and the PAA injection according to the number of new protocols is subtracted from these values. This process occurs for every AER and chemical separately. The value is set to the initial value as well, if the user enters manually, that a container has been exchanged. At further software starts the calculation of the filling levels happens automatically, there is no user interaction needed.

2.4 Graphic user interface

To make sure all Olympus products have a similar design, there is a corporate product guideline (CPD), which describes the requirement of the products [7]. The GUI should show the costumer the current filling level of the chemical containers. The design should be CPD-compliant. As the software is for example written for the ETD Double the same colors should be used. The GUI of the ETD Double has a black background with white font as you can see in

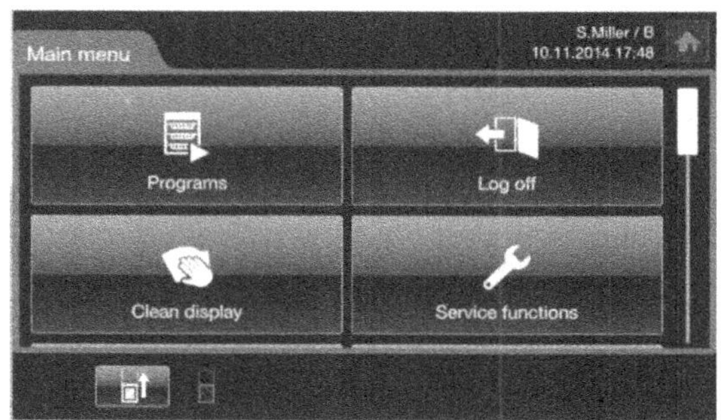

Figure 3: Customer Graphic User Interface

Fig. 3. The GUI should contain up to eight devices. The opportunity to delete and to add new devices should be given. To add devices there has to be an input field for the IP address, the port number has to be the same all the time. The filling level is presented in a bar chart. It shows the existing amount of milliliters as well as the percentage as related to the total content of the chemical containers.

2.5 Additional function

As an additional function it is required to show the current stock of chemicals. This also has to be visualized for the customers, so they can see if new chemicals have to be ordered. If new chemicals arrive in stock it has to be entered manually in a GUI text field as well as when chemicals are used from the stock.

3 Results and Discussion

The basic requirements are complied. The server connection via the HTTPS protocol works, so the reprocessing protocols can be retrieved from the AER, the processing of the protocols and extraction of the actual dosage information is implemented by using several XML-requests and the calculation of chemicals including the subtraction of the PAA dosage works. The visual realization is presented in a bar chart, which can be seen in Fig. 4. The calculation of chemicals in stock can be entered manually to the software and can also be seen in the GUI.

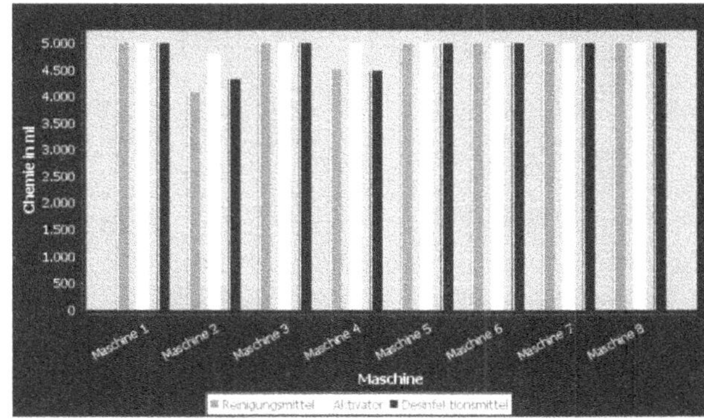

Figure 4: Barchart including 8 machines

But there are still some points, which might cause problems using the client software.
In the prototype version of the client software the exchange of chemical containers in the AER has to be entered manually to the software, because the software of the AER does not offer the possibility to see the change in the protocols. If the user forgets to do this, the dose is subtracted from the virtual empty chemical container, which means, that there is a negative amount of chemical in the container. To minimize the influence of the failure to the dosage calculation the value, which is bellow zero, is subtracted from the new container, after the container change was entered manually. This retains the data for getting lost.
The chemical containers have unique identifiers. By reading the identifier it can be recognized by the AER, if a used chemical container was exchanged. For the future a software update of the ETD Double would be useful, which offers this information on the webserver of the AER. This would help to reduce user failures.
A similar problem is the manual entering of new chemicals relating to the calculation of the chemicals in stock. Because of human failure it can be forgotten and the calculation of inventory would not work probably. If this error is to be avoided, a solution could be a scanning system. Olympus already uses scanning systems to read the preprocessed endoscopes, so there might be a possibility to extend these. It also could be possible to connect the software to an Enterprise-Resource-Planning (ERP) system, if one is used. The best way would be to send an indication automatically to the purchasing department, that new chemicals are needed.
Besides it is not possible to use containers which are half full at the beginning. If this situation would occur, the results would be wrong, because a full new chemical container is assumed. There should be a warning for the customers, that this causes errors. Even a hardware option like a measurement system, which weigh the chemical containers and calculates the volume, could be integrated.
Another problem is that there is no possibility to add new reprocessing programs, which uses other kinds of chemical, without changing the code. If there would be an update for the ETD Double which contains a new one, there would be a software failure. An improvement of the software would be to implement the search for chemicals in the reprocessing protocols in a dynamic way. The software could search for item numbers of the chemicals and evaluate and visualize the data depending on them.

4 Conclusion

The client software is not written with the aim to be sold to customers; it is implemented to show the possibilities of the administration and the handling of data. The primary function is to give the customer the possibility to try the software to find out, if features like this would improve the workflow. Based on the customer opinion a decision can be made, if a commercial use would make sense. Until now there has been no opportunity to do a customer survey, so there is no actual feedback. The main functions are implemented, so it could already be used for the customer survey. The client software shows that the analysis of the reprocessing data works. To get the software ready for the market the range of problems should be corrected, data integrity aspects should be verified and an appropriate method to deal with updates should be found.

Acknowledgement

The work has been carried out at Olympus Surgical Technologies Europe, Olympus Winter & Ibe GmbH; Kuehnstraße 61, 22045 Hamburg, Germany

5 References

[1] R-D. Böckmann, H. Frankenberg and H-G. Will, *Eine Vorschriftensammlung zum Medizinproduktrecht mit Fachwörterbuch.* TÜV Media GmbH TÜV Rheinland Group, Auflage: 4., Frankfurt, 2008.

[2] Bundesgesundheitsblatt, Gesundheitsforschung, Gesundheitsschutz *Hygieneanforderung bei Endoskopen.* Springer, 2002.

[3] DIN EN ISO 15883-04 1, *Reinigungs-Desinfektionsgeräte - Teil 4: Anforderungen und Prüfverfahren für Reinigungs-Desinfektionsgeräte mit chemischer Desinfektion für nicht invasive, nicht kritische thermolabile Medizinprodukte und Zubehör im Gesundheitswesen (ISO/DIS 15883-7:2014).* Deutsche Fassung pr EN ISO 15883-7, 2014.

[4] C. Facci, *Methodik zur formalen Spezifikation des ISO/OSI Schichtmodels.* Fakultät für Informatik der Technischen Universität München, 1995.

[5] S. Fuhrmann, *Funktions-Modul-Spezifikation für EndoThermal Disinfector Double Basisprotokoll.* intern document.

[6] C. Ullenboom, *Java ist auch eine Insel.* 7. Aktualisierte und erweiterte Auflage, Galileo Press, Bonn, 2008.

[7] Olympus, *Corporate product design guideline.* intern document.

Developing a Type Test for the Contamination-Monitor with Gamma Detectors with Focus on Detector Homogeneity - For Four Different Nuclides -

M. Zehlke[1], T. Bär [2], and H. Paulsen [3]
[1] Medizinische Ingenieurwissenschaft, Universität zu Lübeck, zehlke@miw.uni-luebeck.de
[2] Mirion Technologies (Rados) GmbH, Health Physics Division, tbaer@mirion.com
[3] Institute of Physics, Universität zu Lübeck, paulsen@physik.uni-luebeck.de

Abstract

The RTM750^{TM} monitor belongs to the CheckPoint: Laundry^{TM} family of Mirion Technologies (Rados) GmbH. It detects gamma radiation on clothing and gives an alarm in case of contamination. There are no existing DIN EN standard for this contamination-monitor. Due to this a new type test has to be formulated according to customer requirements. The focus of this paper is the detector homogeneity test, a part of the type test. Both gamma detectors of the monitor are tested for nuclides cobalt-60 (Co-60), barium-133 (Ba-133), cesium-137 (Cs-137) and americium (Am-241). The results of homogeneity are illustrated by a cartography for three planes. The results show compliance with the customer requirements. In any case the homogeneity is better than -50% and +50% of the detected gamma radiation.

1 Introduction

The RTM750^{TM} (figure 1) is designed to monitor suits, overalls, overshoes, towels and small items of clothing such as vests, socks etc. It is also well suitable to measure parts and gives an alarm in case a contamination above a pre-set threshold is detected. CheckPoint: Laundry^{TM} monitors are used in any place where gamma contamination has to be monitored for a certain limit value. This could happen at the exit of controlled areas, for example in nuclear facilities or laboratories. The monitor allows to measure objects with a maximum weight of 20 kg, a maximum width of 90 cm and a maximum height of 15 cm. The belt speed is calculated and set automatically. The measurement starts automatically after the monitor has been switched on and users can put some clothes on the conveyor belt for a contamination measurement.

There is no existing DIN EN standard for this kind of contamination-monitors like DIN EN 61098 2008-02 "Radiation protection instrumentation - Installed personnel surface contamination monitoring assemblies" for the HandFoot-Fibre^{TM}. This standard applies to contamination warning systems and monitoring devices, which are used for monitoring radioactive surface contamination of clothed or unclothed persons [3]. To allow RTM750^{TM} to execute standardized and reliable measurements a new type test has to be formulated according to customer requirements. These are based on the document "D455014018229, index 0" from 20.06.2014. This includes descriptions of modifications on the Automatic Conveyor-Monitor RTM750^{TM} and as well standards like DIN EN 60 068-2 "Measurement of sensitivity to shocks" with a pendulum steel ball [4].

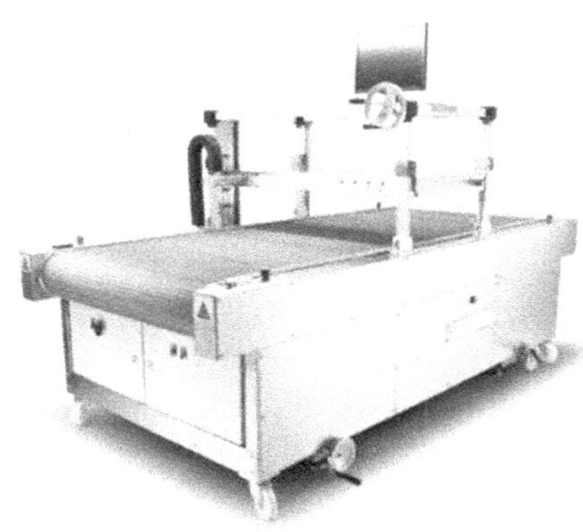

Figure 1: The CheckPoint: Laundry^{TM}Automatic Conveyor-Monitor RTM750^{TM}, Mirion Technologies(Rados) GmbH.

A type test is only valid for the special monitor version. In this case the tested CheckPoint: Laundry^{TM} monitor consists of Gamma Plastic Detectors which are protected against gamma background radiation by additional lead shielding. The conveyor changed in a plastic conveyor belt system and got software modifications. The goal of the type test is to present the procedure of the theoretical and practical tests, their results and evaluations. Because of the comprehensive type test and this limited number of pages of this paper will focus on the detector homogeneity test.

Both gamma detectors are tested for the nuclides cobalt (Co-60), barium (Ba-133), cesium (Cs-137) and americium (Am-241). The results of homogeneity are shown by a cartography for three planes. The theoretical and practical tests were carried out at Mirion Technologies (Rados) GmbH in 2014.

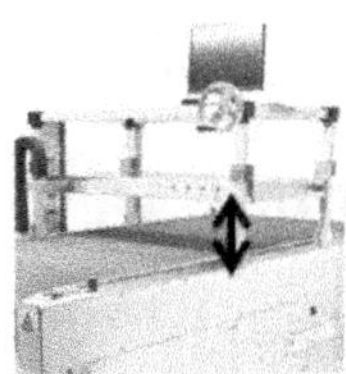

Figure 2: Height adjustment of the detector positions, detail of CheckPoint: Laundry^{TM}, Automatic Conveyor-Monitor RTM750^{TM}, Mirion Technologies (Rados) GmbH.

2 Material and Methods

Testing has been conducted in accordance to the document "D455014018229, index 0" from 20.06.2014 based on customer requirements. The Technical Handbook CheckPoint: Laundry^{TM}Automatic Conveyor-Monitor RTM750^{TM}, D310051, November 2014, has been used for the type test. The measurement mode is the standard state of the monitor. It starts automatically after the monitor has been switched on and a background measurement has been performed. In this mode the display shows "ready to measure" and users can put some clothes on the conveyor belt for a contamination measurement.

All tests in the type test, except of the environmental tests, were done at normal environmental conditions on a CheckPoint: Laundry^{TM}Automatic Conveyor-Monitor RTM750^{TM} with Gamma Plastic Detectors. Completeness of the specification and evaluation of the tests and their results are made by Mirion Technologies (Rados) GmbH. In this paper only the detector homogeneity tests are described. Equation (1) shows the activity (A) with the number of events (N) per unit of time (t). The unit of activity is Becquerel (1 Bq = 1 decay act / s) [5]. The measurements of the tests were done with different gamma emitters listed in table 1.

$$A = \frac{\Delta N}{\Delta t} \tag{1}$$

Table 1: Nuclides with Test Activity in Bq, used sources cobalt (Co-60), cesium (Cs-137), barium (Ba-133) and americium (Am-241) for practical performance tests, Mirion Technologies (Rados) GmbH.

Nuclides	Name	Test Activity (Bq)	Test Date
Co-60	OU381	15070 +/-1.5%	07.10.2014
Ba-133	OU380	24923 +/-1.5%	08.10.2014
Cs-137	OU382	30847 +/-1.5%	08.10.2014
Am-241	FS874	39123 +/-1.34%	08.10.2014

The RTM750^{TM} monitor consists of two identical gamma detector arrays. One is located on a fixed position under the plastic conveyor belt and the other parallel above the belt with manual height adjustment. The homogeneity of detection is measured in the volume between the detectors. The measurement is done in three positions (figure 2):
- lower: 30 mm distance (e.g. 'overshoes),
- middle: 75 mm distance and
- upper: 150 mm distance (maximum).

The spatial resolution of the measurement is in width 9.5 cm with a distance of 4 cm from the edges and in length 10 cm with a distance of 5 cm from the edges due to customer wishes (figure 3) .The Measurement is using a 24 points template. In this way all extreme cases were tested. The plastic conveyor belt is neglected in the measurements.

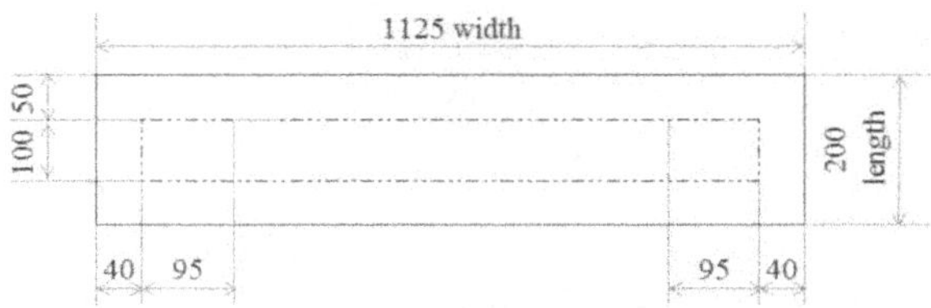

Figure 3: Spatial resolution of the measurement, Drawing in mm, Detector top view, Mirion Technologies (Rados) GmbH.

3 Results and Discussion

In the following the results of the practical tests are presented for the measurement of detector homogeneity for nuclides cobalt (Co-60), cesium (Cs-137), barium (Ba-133) and americium (Am-241). The homogeneity of detection is measured in the volume between the two detectors. The single measurement shall be considered using a 24 points template. The results are presented in cartography in the width beginning with 40 mm distance of the border to 1085 mm. The spatial resolution of the measurement in length is from 50 mm to 150 mm of the border (see figure 3). In this way all the extreme cases are obtained. The measured values are normalized over the two parallel detectors. The customer requirement was to detect better than -50% and +50% of the gamma radiation. Due to this, results are classified in three zones pictured in different gray shades. The values are normalized. The first zone is from 0 to 0.5 in dotted light gray. That area means no gamma radiation was detected up to one half of the gamma radiation. The second zone in plain light gray defines 0.5 to 1. This area includes 50% till all radiation from the gamma emitter. These zones are only found on the side due to the construction of the detectors. The last zone 1 to 1.5 in dark gray shows that 100% of the gamma radiation was detected and more up to 150%. This zone is in the middle area of the detector array. There the detectors are most sensitive and find gamma radiation definitely.

3.1 Measurement of detector homogeneity for the nuclide Co-60

In the following three measurements are shown for planes upper, middle and lower position for the nuclide Co-60. The first zone from 0 to 0.5 in dotted light gray does not exist. The light gray zone 0.5 to 1 is found on the side with a distance of 135 mm of the border left and right side in the upper and lower detector position (figure 4, figure 6). Only the middle plane has more of this zone in the width 230 mm and 895 mm. But this is approximately 100% (see figure 5). Because of the construction of the detectors they have a minimal deviation. These are within the valid range (-50%). The dark gray zone is detected in the middle area of the detector array in all three planes. The detector is more sensitive as mentioned before and finds the gamma radiation in any case.
The homogeneity of detection for Co-60 in the sensitive volume in all three planes is better than -50% and +50%. The tests performed upon variation of response with the source position of the CheckPoint: Laundry^{TM} automatic Conveyor-Monitor RTM750^{TM} show compliance with the requirements.

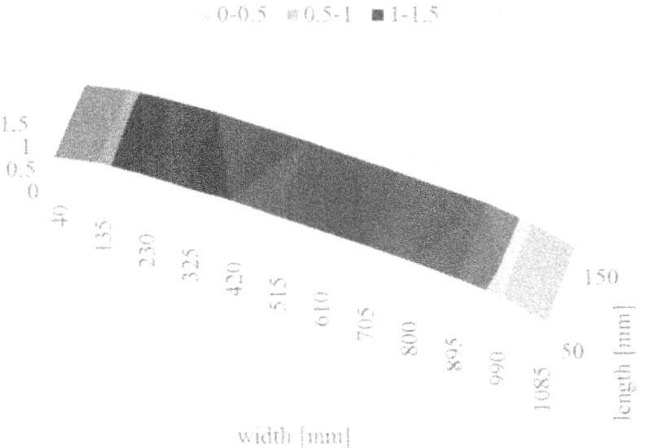

Figure 4: Measurement of detector homogeneity for Co-60, upper position (150 mm), normalized, Mirion Technologies (Rados) GmbH.

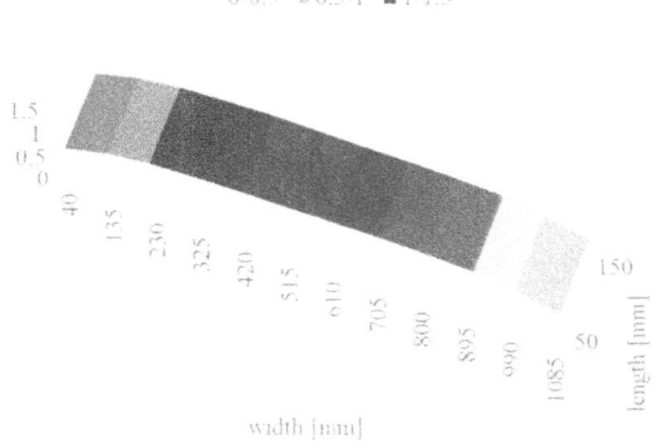

Figure 5: Measurement of detector homogeneity for Co-60, middle (75 mm), normalized, Mirion Technologies (Rados) GmbH.

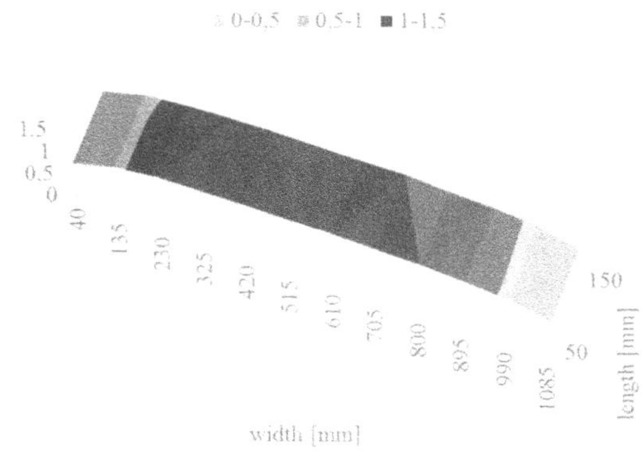

Figure 6: Measurement of detector homogeneity for Co-60, lower position (30mm), normalized, Mirion Technologies (Rados) GmbH.

3.2 Measurement of detector homogeneity for the nuclide Ba-133

The measurement of detector homogeneity for the nuclide Ba-133 were also performed for the three planes. Exemplary only the upper plane is illustrated. The results are similar to the tests with Co-60. In all planes there is no dotted light gray zone. The plain light gray zone 0.5 to 1 is obtained on the sides up to the measurement points (135,50) and (135,150) as well as (940,50) and (940,150). The dark gray zone is detected in the middle area of the detector array the same observation as for the nuclide Co-60. The three tests show compliance with the requirements. The homogeneity of gamma radiation detection in all three planes is better than -50% and +50% for Ba-133.

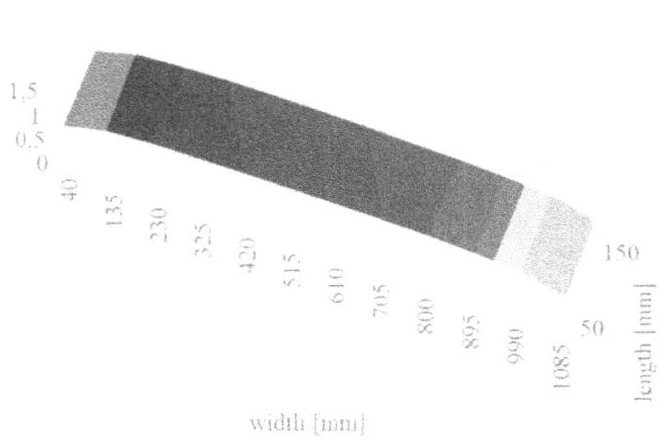

Figure 7: Measurement of detector homogeneity for Ba-133, upper position (150 mm), normalized, Mirion Technologies (Rados) GmbH.

3.3 Measurement of detector homogeneity for the nuclide Cs-137

Testing of detector homogeneity for the nuclide Cs-137 were executed as well. Only the middle plane is illustrated.

In all planes the dotted light gray zone does not occur. The light gray zone 0.5 to 1 which defines the lower tolerance limit -50% has been measured left and right border (figure 8). But these values are approaching 100%. The dark gray zone is detected in the middle area of the detector array. The homogeneity of detection for Cs-137 in all three planes is better than -50% and +50%.

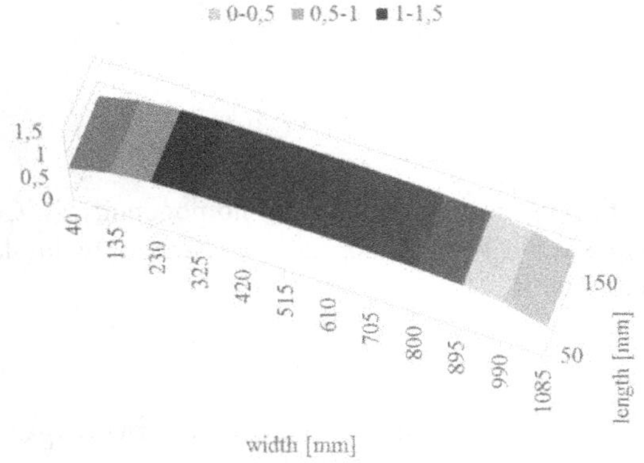

Figure 8: Measurement of detector homogeneity for Cs-137, middle position (75 mm), normalized, Mirion Technologies (Rados) GmbH.

3.4 Measurement of detector homogeneity for the nuclide Am-241

At last the test was performed with the nuclide Am-241 for the three planes. The lower plane illustrating the detector homogeneity is shown as an example. There is no dotted light gray zone in all planes. The light gray zone 0.5 to 1 is obtained, as the other nuclides Co-60, Cs-13, and Ba-133,left and right side in all three planes. The dark gray zone is detected in the middle area of the detector array. Due to this results of the homogeneity of detection for Am-241 in all three planes is better than -50% and +50%.

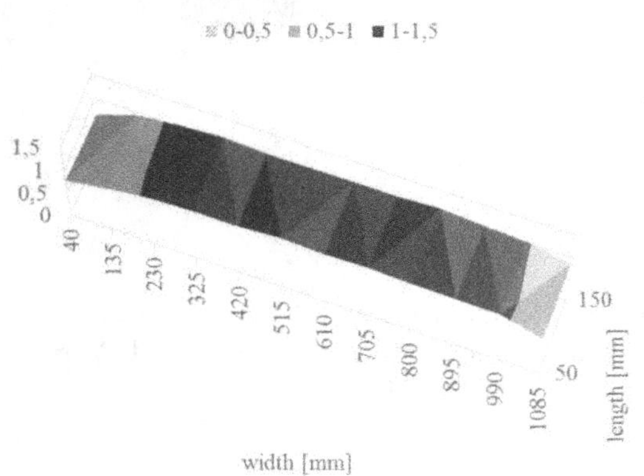

Figure 9: Measurement of detector homogeneity for Am-241, lower position (30mm), normalized, Mirion Technologies (Rados) GmbH.

4 Conclusion

The results for the measurement of detector homogeneity for the nuclides Co-60, Ba-133, Cs-137 and Am-241 measured in three planes show compliance with the customer requirements. In any case the gamma radiation detection was better than -50% and +50%. The zone 0.5 to 1 was only found on the side of the detector array. Because of the construction of the detectors they have a minimal deviation. These are within the valid range (-50%). It has been detected 100% and sometimes up to +50% of the gamma radiation. This zone is found in the middle area of the detector array. The detectors are more sensitive here and identify gamma radiation definitely. The results provide evidence that the "D455014018229, index 0" from 20.06.2014, is qualified for application and meets specification requirements.

Acknowledgement

I am using this opportunity to express my gratitude to everyone who supported me throughout the course of this project. The work has been carried out at Mirion Technologies (Rados) GmbH, Mirion Health Physics Division.

5 References

[1] Mirion Technologies (Rados) GmbH, *Customer requirements of Document D455014018229, index 0 from 20.06.2014*. Hamburg, Germany, 2014.

[2] The Technical Handbook, *CheckPoint: Laundry^{TM} Automatic Conveyor-Monitor RTM750^{TM}*. D310051, Hamburg, Germany, November 2014.

[3] DIN EN 61098:2008-02; VDE 0493-2-2:2008-02, *Radiation protection instrumentation - Installed personnel surface contamination monitoring assemblies.* (IEC 61098:2003, modified), German version EN 61098:2007, Beuth Verlag.

[4] DIN EN 60068-2-27:2010-02; VDE 0468-2-27:2010-02, *Environmental testing - Part 2-27: Tests - Test Ea and guidance: Shock (IEC 60068-2-27:2008) "Measurement of sensitivity to shocks"*. German version EN 60068-2-27:2009, Beuth Verlag.

[5] H. Bannwarth, B. P. Kremer and A. Schulz, *Physik, Chemie und Biochemie*. Springer, Berlin/Heidelberg, 2013.

6
Safety and Quality II

Development of a luminous field measurement station and comparison of a consumer LED headlight and a HEINE® LED LoupeLight

M. Fischer [1], B. Kabbeck [2], and O. Heine [2]
[1] Medizinische Ingenieurwissenschaft, Universität zu Lübeck, fischerm@miw.uni-luebeck.de
[2] HEINE Optotechnik GmbH & Co.KG, Herrsching a. Ammersee, {bkabbeck, oh}@heine.com

Abstract

Through automated measurements of luminous fields of optical medical diagnostic devices, it is possible to detect the inhomogeneity of different measurement values within luminous fields and to rate them quantitatively and reproducibly. A suitable positioning unit has been selected, on which the detector connected to a spectrometer, is fixed, which can be controlled by a programming software. Two LEDs were compared to one another for comparison purposes. Initially, the detector has to be calibrated and the constant accuracy of positioning unit determined. Results of the calibration are deviations of less than five percent and the accuracy of the positioning unit less than four microns. The comparison of the luminous field measurements shows a significant difference between the fields that cannot necessarily be detected by the human eye. This measurement station can measure luminous fields and evaluate quantitatively to improve products and to demonstrate the homogeneity over others.

1 Introduction

The idea of building a luminous field measurement station, is to create a test rig which can measure luminous fields photometrically and evaluate them. The luminous field of a diagnostic instrument is charaterized from the user-typical working distance. Thereby, homogeneity of colour and intensity should be rated and compared reproducibly and quantitatively with photometric quantities, such as the irradiance or illuminance and respective colour coordinates. A camera cannot be used for the project, as it cannot provide the required measurement values. It can only provide rough information about brightness and colour and not about photometric or radiometric values [1]. Instead, a spectroradiometer is used, whose sensitivity is high enough and which is able to measure all necessary and desired values in the required spectral range [2].
The challenge is to provide measurability for all HEINE instruments, for LEDs, as well as for xenon halogen (XHL) lamps in the spectral range. Instruments of HEINE mainly differ in dilatation and intensity of the luminous field. In addition, a detector has to be combined with a construction of apertures of different sizes and calibrations. Furthermore, the positioning of the detector, which is driven through the range of the luminous field, has to have a very good accuracy to make measurements reproducible. A suitable data structure to continue the handling of data is also of great importance. The graphical user interface of the software, programmed with LabVIEW should be easy to understand, so the handling is intuitive and even a layman could operate the test rig.

2 Material and Methods

The individual parts of the project and verification of the requirements of the measuring system will be described in the following section. For a better understanding of the whole project, figure 1 outlines the systematic structure of the luminous field measuring station to be constructed.

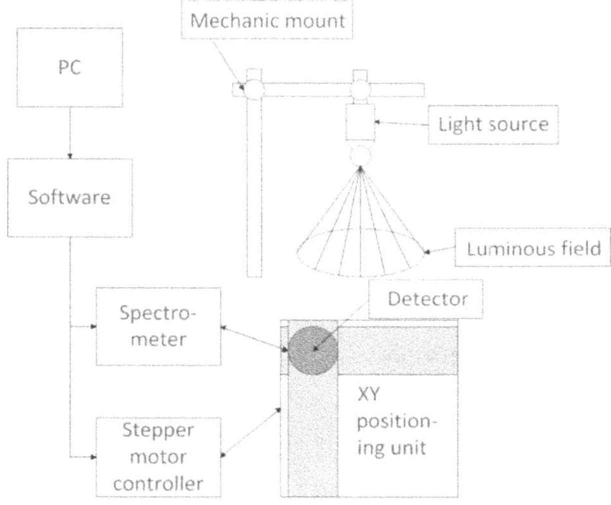

Figure 1: Schematic diagram of the luminous field measurement station.

2.1 Software and Automation

The software and automation part pertains to programming of the individual components.

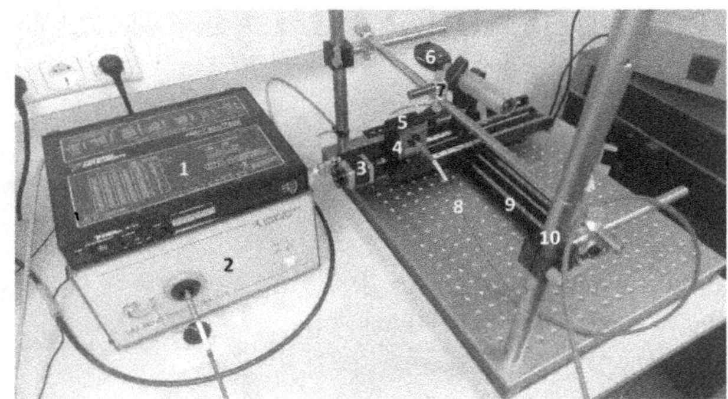

Figure 2: Part of the test rig with its components: (1) Stepper motor controler, (2) spectrometer, (3) stepper motor, (4) integrating sphere, (5) aperture construction, (6) device under test, (7) device mount, (8) optical fibre, (9) XY positioning unit, (10) bar system.

A LabVIEW Full Development System with device specific drivers for the spectrometer for a Windows PC was used. The XY positioning unit (Fig. 2 (9)), consisting of two connected linear stages (LTM80-300 from OWIS), and the measurement unit, consisting of the spectrometer (Fig. 2 (2)) (CAS 140CT from Instrument Systems), which is connected via an optical fibre (Fig. 2 (8)) to the integrating sphere (Fig. 2 (4)) (FOIS-1 from Ocean Optics), are controlled by the LabVIEW Software.
The positioning of the detector is moved gradually, so that finally, the entire luminous field is scanned. By controlling the already existing spectrometer and defining the measurement values, the single points of luminous field are measured and are gradually displayed in three dimensions which are stored for later rateability and comparability. The recorded measurement values are the illumination, respectively irradiance, spectra of each measuring point. Additionally the CIE chromaticity coordinates xy and u'v', the XYZ Tristimulus, colour rendering index R_a and R_1 to R_{16} - which all give information over the transmited colour - and the colour temperature in Kelvin [3].
Spectrometer and positioning unit have to be synchronized so that the measurement of a luminous field by the input of parameters such as dimension of the light field in the X and Y direction and scanning distance is automated. This means that a point is measured and the positioning unit is shifted after the subsequent measurement of each point by the desired sampling interval and the new point is measured until the entire luminous field is scanned and measured.

2.2 Positioning and Measurement

The measurement part of the test device contains the spectrometer, the stepper motor controller MID-7602 (Fig. 2 (1)) from National Instruments and the stepper motors (Fig. 2 (3)), which are controlled by the LabVIEW software. The two stepper motors in turn drive the XY positioning unit. The positioning unit has to be selected out of a variety of existing units. An important decision criterion is the price, although the following requirements for the positioning unit must not be neglected. The travel range of the two axis system should be about 300x300 mm, in order to examine the biggest luminous fields of HEINE diagnostic instruments. The minimal required incremental movement in an axis direction should be maximum 0.1 mm. The deviation of the position should not exceed 10 microns to avoid measurement errors caused by deviation in the position. The accuracy at various speeds and accelerations of the positioning unit, uniquely determined by its stepper motors through a laser distance measurement device (optoNCDT ILD2220-50 of Micro-Epsilon) determines the ideal acceleration and speed of the stepper motors.
The integrating sphere, connected to the spectrometer, is attached on the axis' system, which is moved by the XY positioning unit. Since the integrating sphere itself has just one aperture, i.e. the actual opening for measurements, an aperture was constructed, which is placed on the integrating sphere, and contains different sized apertures of 1 – 10 mm, which are placed in front of the opening (Fig. 2 (5)). For each aperture, a separate calibration must be created to ensure that the detector and the spectrometer measure correctly and not return falsified values. This calibration data was created with a calibrated lamp and an additional - also calibrated, but unsuitable for our purposes - illuminance measuring head. The illuminance measuring head could not be used, because it measures at the whole area of detection, which wouldn't be illuminated by most of the devices under test. An integrating sphere instead strays the light inside and focuses the light at one point, at which it is measured [4], [5]. For this purpose, the light source is measured with the calibrated sensor and then the same light with the integrated sphere to be calibrated first with a modified calibration file.
The correction factors depending on the wavelengths, respectively the values of sensitivity obtained with (2) must then be adjusted in the pre-modified calibration file. Any deviation of the measured values of the newly calibrated integrating sphere must not exceed five percent. The correction factors are calculated with

$$\frac{uncalibrated\ spectrum}{reference\ spectrum} = correction\ factors \quad (1)$$

or to show the dependance on the wavelength

$$\frac{E_{uncal}(\lambda)}{E_{ref}(\lambda)} = C(\lambda). \quad (2)$$

The verification of the calibration is checked with multiple HEINE instruments. All measurements are made at a distance of 250 mm. For one measurement, only one aperture size is used. For the aperture construction, it is important that no scattered light comes from the side of the sphere, only light entering through the aperture.

2.3 Distance control and device mount

The typical user working distances for HEINE diagnostic instruments can be different. The working distance of an otoscope lies in the millimetre range, while the working distance of an examination light is up to half a meter. The distance of the device, according to the light source of the measurement unit must therefore be adjustable. A bar system (Fig. 2 (10)) is used on which a mount (Fig. 2 (7)) is attached in which all HEINE instruments (Fig. 2 (6)) can be placed. A clamp for example fulfils that purpose. An examination lamp requires no additional mount, since it can be attached directly to the table.

3 Results and Discussion

Below are some results of the calibration from the measuring head, measuring the accuracy of the selected positioning unit. The comparisons are of the luminous field measurement between a consumer LED headlight and an HEINE® LED LoupeLight.

3.1 Calibration of the detector

The comparison of the measured values of a calibrated measuring head with the new calibrated integrating sphere (FOIS-1 from Ocean Optics), has shown that all measurement deviations of all apertures are within the tolerance of five percent. The Measurement has been done with six different devices, XHL devices as well as LEDs. The following table shows the average mean percentage deviation of the calibration for each aperture.

Table 1: Results of detector calibration

Aperture	Deviation [%]
10 mm	-0.42
9 mm	-0.14
8 mm	-1.14
7 mm	-1.18
6 mm	-1.07
5 mm	-0.92
4 mm	-1.17
3 mm	-1.30
2 mm	-1.81
1 mm	-1.21

It can be seen, that all deviations are negative, so the new calibrated detector measures always slightly less illuminance in comparison to the normal calibrated detector.
Inaccuarcies in this calibration measurement are caused by the lamps. Mostly they were not in a thermally stable condition, thereby causing fluctuations in the measurement. In addition, the indirect ophthalmoscope devices were not used with an external, constant power supply, but with a battery pack which has larger fluctuations due to the characteristic of the cell.

3.2 Accuracy of positioning

Using a decision matrix in which the specifications of the manufacturer and the price were weighted, it was decided that two linear tables LTM80-300 from the company OWIS would be used as the best option. The reproducible accuracy was tested again with different speeds and accelerations from the already connected stepper motors. The results showed that the stepper motors should not be accelerated faster than 20 rev/s^2 and that the speed should be between 200 and 1000 rev/min. Within these limits, all deviations are always less than or equal to four microns. The various accelerations and velocities were also tested with different micro-step operation modes. The operation mode of the stepper motor controller divides the full steps of a stepper motor further up to 51200 steps per revolution using the existing stepper motors. Corresponding to a spindle pitch of one millimetre the minimal incremental movement is about 20 nm. In micro-step operation mode 256, it is possible that the stepper motors "lose steps" due to the very small angular steps. Due to that, the stepper motors of the luminous field test site are controlled with a 64 micro-step operation mode. Thus 12800 steps per revolution are still possible, which corresponds to a minimum movability of about 80 nm.

3.3 Luminous field measurement

A measurement of a luminous field returns a large amount of data and at least five graphs. From the Excel output file, all measured values for every point can be displayed and for example, the spectrum of a given point can be shown.
Since not all data can be presented here, a comparison of a consumer LED headlight with a HEINE® LED LoupeLight, a loupe lamp for surgical and dental applications from HEINE is shown using the example of the photometric integral, the illuminance Lux.
The complete light field of the consumer LED headlight has a dilatation of 280 mm since a lot of stray light is deflected. The spot with the highest brightness has a diameter of about 60 mm from a distance of 150 mm. The luminous field of the LoupeLight, from the same distance, is clearly defined and has a diameter of about 50 mm.
The unit GU on the X and Y axis corresponds to grid units. The grid unit must be multiplied by the sampling interval to obtain the position in millimetre of the luminous field. Both light fields, the one of LoupeLight (Fig. 3) and the LED head light (Fig. 4) were sampled at five millimetre intervals in order to compare the dimension of the luminous fields with each other. The Z axis is represented logarithmically as the brightness of the eye sensation is also logarithmic. This gives a better impression of brightness. The well-defined, relatively homogeneous light field of LoupeLight has a maximum brightness of about 88.4 klx. The consumer LED headlight radiates the light, as mentioned above, very diffusely and reaches the maximum brightness at only one point. In the middle of the light field 187 klx is measured.
It can clearly be seen that on the edge of the light field of

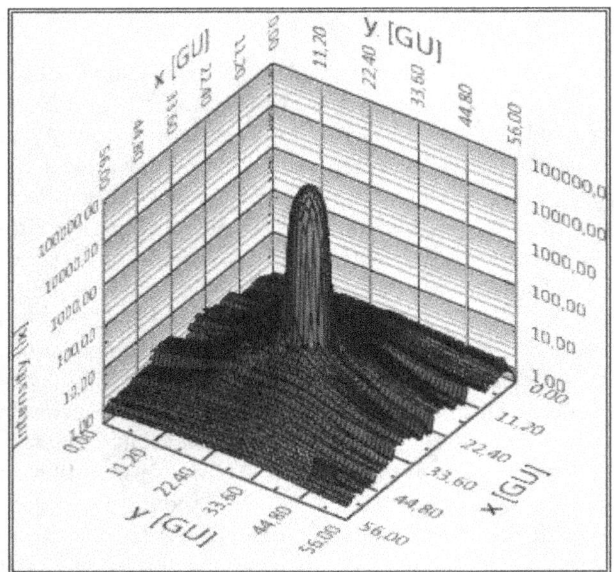

Figure 3: Luminous field of the HEINE® LED LoupeLight. X and Y axis show Grid Units [GU] and Z axis shows the illuminance in Lux.

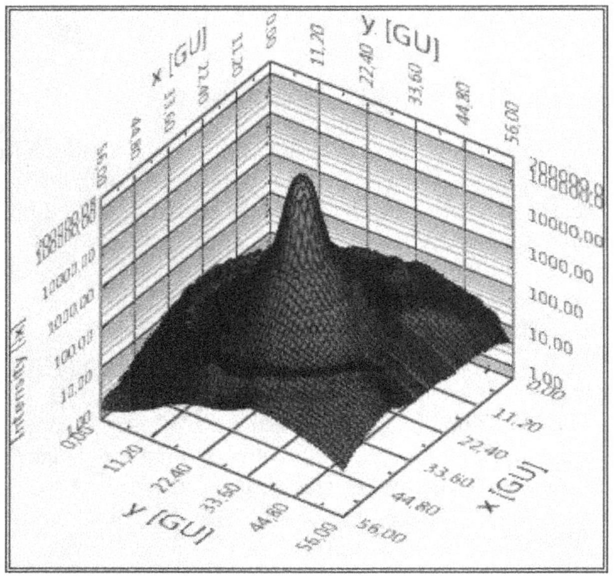

Figure 4: Luminous field of a consumer LED headlight. X and Y axis show Grid Units [GU] and Z axis shows the illuminance in Lux.

the LoupeLight, the graph quickly drops to about 25 – 50 lx. For the consumer headlight, the decrease is not as steep, the maximum brightness is only available at one point. From about 60 mm from the centre of the luminous field, illumination still amounts to 100 lx. Furthermore, it can be seen that in the LoupeLight, the brightness continues to flatten, but this is not noticeable to the eye. The consumer LED headlight increases the illuminance in rings several times around the centre. Through these large differences in illuminance in the luminous field of the headlight, other parameters vary widely, such as colour rendering indices or colour temperature, which in turn are very consistent with the HEINE® LED LoupeLight.

4 Conclusion

With the constructed luminous field measurement station, automated measurements of luminous fields are possible. It records a variety of data and smallest gradients of measured values can be seen to show inhomogeneities of luminous fields. This is shown in the example of the comparison of a consumer LED headlight and HEINE® LED LoupeLight (see 3.3).

A quantitative, reproducible evaluation of luminous fields is given through the data storage. In addition, data can be read again in LabVIEW and measurement points can be redefined.

The calibration of the apertures of the integrating sphere confirms that measurement errors of the self-calibrated measuring head are within the required tolerance of five percent. Likewise, the reproducible accuracy of positioning fulfils the requirements described by far.

For the future, the adjustment of the aperture-construction and the manual height adjustment of the measured light should be motorized to make the handling of the measuring station easier.

Furthermore, the test rig will be integrated into a darkened box to shield the measuring device from any stray ambient light, which can lead to large measurement errors.

Acknowledgement

The work has been carried out at HEINE Optotechnik GmbH & Co. KG, Herrsching am Ammersee.

5 References

[1] N. Bauer, *Handbuch zur industriellen Bildverarbeitung: Qualitätssicherung in der Praxis.* Fraunhofer IRB Verlag, Stuttgart, pp. 82–98, 2008.

[2] Instrument Systems GmbH, *Cas 140CT Array Spektrometer.* Available: http://www.instrumentsystems.com/fileadmin/editors/downloads/Products/CAS140CT_e.pdf [last accessed on 19.01.2015].

[3] M. Richter, *Einführung in die Farbmetrik.* de Gruyter, Berlin/New York, 1981.

[4] J. Nolting, *Grundprinzipien der Messung radiometrischer und photometrischer Größen,* Script of *Optische Messtechnik.* Technische Akademie Esslingen, Esslingen, 2006.

[5] T. Nägele, R. Distl, *Handbuch der LED-Messtechnik.* Company Magazine Instrument Systems, Münch, 1999.

Temperature dependencies in surgical lights – investigation and compensation concept–

F. Strahwald [1]
[1] Medizinische Ingenieurwissenschaft, Universität zu Lübeck, frederike.strahwald@miw.uni-luebeck.de

Abstract

Modern surgical light systems such as the Polaris 100/200 from Dräger are based on LED technology. Extended lifetime, low energy consumption as well as high luminance efficacy are only some of the benefits of LEDs. However LEDs also have a few drawbacks. A central issue in surgical lights is a stable illumination independent of ambient conditions. The intensity of LEDs is affected by temperature, in a way that an increase in temperature yields a reduction in intensity. In this publication we investigate the effect of temperature on a modern surgical light system and propose measures to compensate this undesirable effect.

1 Introduction

In the operation room surgical lights are necessary to illuminate the working area with a constant and homogeneous light field. According to technical norms, modern surgical light systems need to have an adjustable illuminance between 40 klx and 160 klx and a high colour rendering index to allow the surgeon to distinguish between different tissues [1] [2].

Light emitting diodes (LED) are solid-state semiconductor light sources [3] and are state of the art in surgical light systems. Their main advantages are the low energy consumption and an extremely long lifespan [4]. With 10-50 lm/W LEDs have a higher luminous efficacy than incandescent light bulbs (5-15 lm/W) or halogen lights (10-20 lm/W) [5], which makes them an ideal fit for surgical light systems.

The intensity of LEDs is modified by means of current control. Unfortunately LEDs react on temperature changes, i.e. increasing temperature leads to a decrease in the intensity of the LED and a widening of their spectral range [6]. In a surgical light there are many power electronic components, which will heat up during operation. Previous investigations state, that the relation between the temperature of the LED and the intensity is almost linear in the range between 20°C and 100°C [6]. The main goal of this work is to evaluate the influence of the ambient temperature on the intensity of a modern surgical light system on the working area and to conceptualise a temperature compensation to work against this effect.

The intensity is measured in illuminance, which describes the luminous flux on a predefined area. The corresponding unit lux (lx) is defined as lumen per square meter [7]:

$$[E] = 1\text{lx} = 1\text{lm/m}^2. \tag{1}$$

The luminous flux [Φ] in turn is the quantity of light emitted from the light source and is measured in lumen (lm).

2 Material and Methods

The surgical light system for which the temperature compensation is conceptualised is a modified Dräger Polaris 200. It is a surgical light that contains 66 LEDs arranged in 11 groups of 6 (compare Fig. 1). The specified life span of this light system is $> 30000h$, achievable due to the employed LED technology. Each LED is positioned behind specially designed lenses so that the overlap of all light beams results in a homogeneously illuminated working area. The light head is equipped with an handle in the centre to allow for positioning the light. A movable arm connects the light head with the ceiling. The surgical light provides a maximum output of 160 klx, which can be dimmed down to 40 klx. Thanks to the thermal management system the light head temperature will not exceed 35°C when operated at an ambient temperature of 20°C, which supports the compensation [8].

To investigate the effect of the temperature on the illumination, a TMP05 temperature sensor from Analog Devices Inc was used. This monolithic temperature sensor encodes the measured temperature in a modulated serial digital output (PWM). The low period (T_L) of the PWM is modified while the high period (T_H) remains static.

This sensor is connected to an Arduino Uno microcontroller board, based on an ATmega328 processor [10]. It is used to measure the length of the high and low period

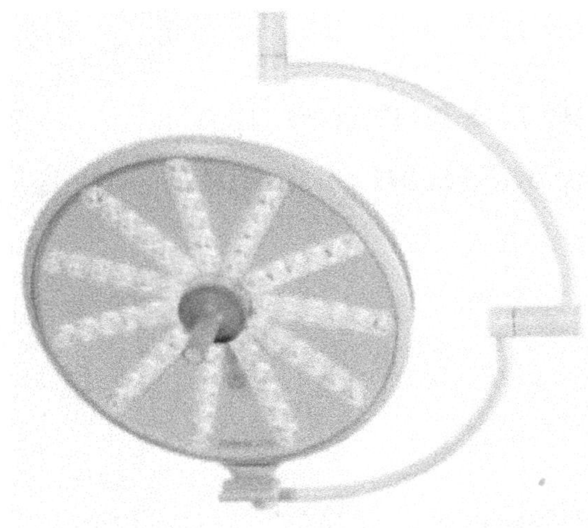

Figure 1: The Polaris 200 from below. It shows the 66 LEDs grouped in 11 stripes around the centre with the handle [9].

and to calculate the temperature in °C according to the following formula [11]:

$$\text{Temperature}(^\circ C) = 421 - (751 \cdot \frac{\mathrm{T_H}}{\mathrm{T_L}}). \quad (2)$$

The first step of this project is to measure the actual temperature of the surgical light in combination with the provided illuminance. To realise well specified ambient conditions an environmental chamber is used, allowing to control the temperature over a wide range. Therefore the surgical light, equipped with the installed temperature sensor, connected to the Arduino Uno, and the sensor to measure the illuminance, is placed in the temperature chamber. The data of both , the temperature and the illuminance sensor, are logged with timestamps to match the corresponding points afterwards. The temperature of the chamber is set to 5°C and increased by 5°C every two hours after it reached the target temperature. These 5°C steps every two hours are continued up to 45°C, which is far beyond the specified ambient temperature of the Polaris 200. Temperature and illuminance are logged during the entire procedure. During the measurement the surgical light is set to a high illumination level (155 klx) thus the increase of temperature of the light system is expected to be distinctly higher.

With these results the system response is analysed and a temperature compensation is derived. The mathematical analysis of the resulting data is done by correlation analysis and linear regression, for details see [12].

The resulting linear function allows to compute the expected illuminance of the surgical light for any temperature of the surgical light. This function can be used to calculate a compensation factors ($k_{\text{compensation}}$) by comparing the expected illuminance value (E_{intended}) with the realised ones (E_{realised}) for every temperature step:

$$k_{\text{compensation}} = \frac{E_{\text{intended}}}{E_{\text{realised}}}. \quad (3)$$

This compensation can be applied on the illumination control.

3 Results and Discussion

In Fig. 2 the complete logged data is shown. The chamber temperature is the dashed line, which shows that every step has at first a slight overshoot and then the temperature settles for the aimed value. After that the temperature of the chamber remains constant for two hours. The left y-axis shows the illuminance and the right one the temperature. The dotted line above the ambient temperature, shows that the temperature of the surgical light reacts smoother to the changes of the ambient temperature. It increases with a short delay after the chamber temperature, but converges against the next value. This step response behaves like a first-order lag element. The illumination is at its highest point at 5°C and decreases with increasing temperature. It declines at the beginning of every step but then also converges against the following value. To improve the analysis, nine points of interest were marked in Fig. 2. They mark the system at the settled state for each temperature step.

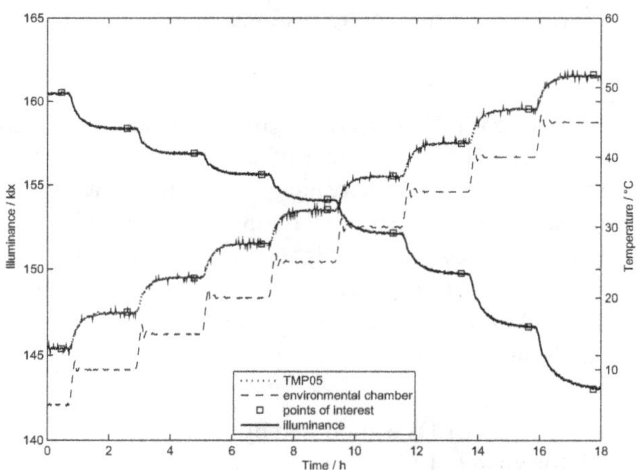

Figure 2: The complete measurement of the surgical light temperature, the temperature of the environmental chamber and the illuminance. The environmental chamber starts at 5°C and increases the temperature every two hours by 5°C. This goes up to 45°C. On the left y-axis the Illuminance in klx is shown and on the right one the temperature in °C. The points of interest mark the settled state of every step for the surgical light temperature and the illuminance.

To analyse this behaviour more closely the step between 5°C to 10°C is shown in Fig. 3. In this plot the overshoot and the settling of the chamber temperature is clearly recognisable. The drop of the illuminance seems to be logarithmic just like the increase of the temperature of the surgical light.

Therefore the linear connection between the two parameters is very probable. In Fig. 4 the corresponding illuminance and the temperature of the surgical light values are shown in a scatter plot. Additionally the correlation coefficient was calculated with $r = -0.9838$. Which is very near to the $r = -1$ of the perfect anti-correlation. So it is possible to find a linear function representing the connection between the two parameters by calculating the linear regression. The resulting function $y(x)$ is shown in the bottom left corner of the diagram and additionally plotted in the diagram. It allows to calculate a realistic illuminance for every surgical light temperature.

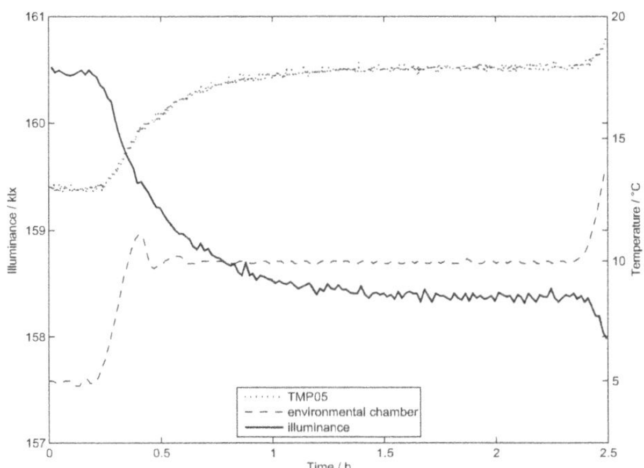

Figure 3: A detailed view on a single temperature step from the measurement of the surgical light temperature, the temperature of the environmental chamber and the illuminance to show the reaction on the step of the chamber temperature.

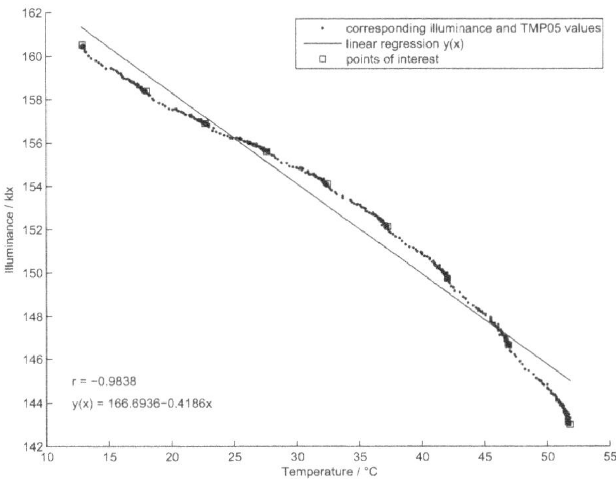

Figure 4: The corresponding illuminance and surgical light temperature values in a scatter diagram. Together with the correlation coefficient r and the result function $y(x)$ of the linear regression.

With these results it is now possible to calculate a linear compensation function by utilizing [(3)]. The intended illuminance is set to $E_{\text{intended}} = 155\text{klx}$ and for the realised one the formula for $y(x)$ is plugged in. Then it is possible to calculate for every surgical light temperature the compensation factor. The result is plotted in Fig. 5. The surgical light is calibrated at 20°C and so at the surgical light temperature of 27.6°C the compensation factor equals one.

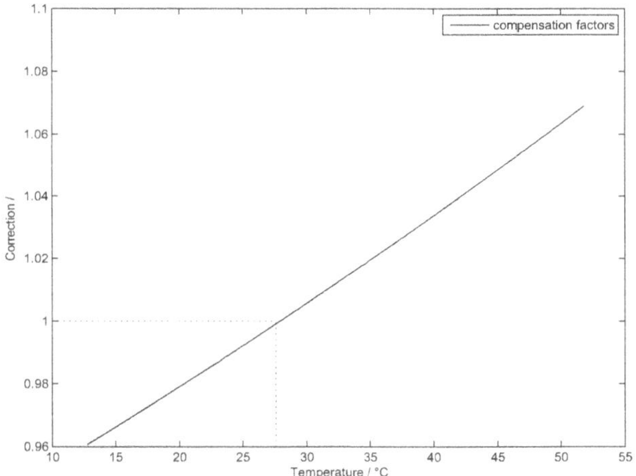

Figure 5: The calculated compensation factors. The point [27.6°C, 1] represents the aimed value of the compensation.

4 Conclusion

The goal of this project was to conceptualise a temperature compensation for the Polaris 200 surgical light system.

For that reason the illuminance and the temperature of the surgical light were analysed. They seem to have a similar reaction on stepping up the ambient temperature except that the illuminance decreases and the temperature increases. All eight steps of the temperature of the environmental chamber show logarithmic characteristics.

The relation between the measurements was analysed by calculating the correlation. The result shows, that there is a strong linear correlation. The linear regression was utilized to calculate a function that connects the illuminance and the surgical light temperature and its result was the base of the compensation.

The idea was to apply this compensation to all possible illuminance values but the compensation was measured only at one aimed illuminance. Further research is required to determine whether the compensation function is the same for all illuminance values or if it varies. For this the compensation for every possible illuminance value needs to be determined in the same way as shown above.

Acknowledgement

The work has been carried out at Dräger Medical GmbH, Lübeck.

5 References

[1] DIN Deutsches Institut für Normung e. V., *DIN 5035-3, Ausgabe: 2006-07, Beleuchtung mit künstlichem Licht - Teil 3: Beleuchtung im Gesundheitswesen.* http://www.fnl.din.de/cmd?artid=88503242&bcrumblevel=1&contextid=fnl&subcommitteeid=54746883&level=tpl-art-detailansicht&committeeid=54738975&languageid=de [07.01.2015].

[2] DIN Deutsches Institut für Normung e. V., *DIN EN 60601-2-41 and VDE 0750-2-41:2010-05, Ausgabe: 2010-05, Medizinische elektrische Geräte -. Teil 2-41: Besondere Festlegungen für die Sicherheit einschließlich der wesentlichen Leistungsmerkmale von Operationsleuchten und Untersuchungsleuchten (IEC 60601-2-41:2009) and Deutsche Fassung EN 60601-2-41:2009.* http://www.dke.din.de/cmd?level=tpl-art-detailansicht&committeeid=54738887&artid=126804475&languageid=de&bcrumblevel=3&subcommitteeid=54760626 [11.01.2015].

[3] A. Rockett, *The Materials Science of Semiconductors*, ch. 3.6.1, p. 120. Springer Science+Business Media, 2008.

[4] F. Wosnitza and H. Hilgers, *Energieeffizienz und Energiemanagement: Ein Überblick Heutiger Möglichkeiten und Notwendigkeiten*, ch. 7.10.13, p. 348. SpringerLink : Bücher, Vieweg+Teubner Verlag, 2012.

[5] F. Wosnitza and H. Hilgers, *Energieeffizienz und Energiemanagement: Ein Überblick Heutiger Möglichkeiten und Notwendigkeiten*, ch. 7.10.2, pp. 338 – 339. SpringerLink : Bücher, Vieweg+Teubner Verlag, 2012.

[6] E. Hering, H. Austmann, K. Bressler, J. Langner, W. Laveure, J. Gutekunst, R. Martin, J. Strauß, and W. Streib, *Elektronik für Ingenieure und Naturwissenschaftler*, ch. 6.3, pp. 247 – 248. Springer-Lehrbuch, Springer Berlin Heidelberg, 2005.

[7] E. Hering and R. Martin, *Photonik*, ch. 7.2, p. 318. Springer-Verlag Berlin Heidelberg, 2007.

[8] Drägerwerk AG & Co. KGaA, *Polaris 100/200.* http://www.draeger.com/sites/en_uk/Pages/Hospital/Polaris-100-200.aspx [11.09.2014].

[9] Drägerwerk AG & Co. KGaA, *Polaris 100/200 - Einfach gutes Licht.* http://www.draeger.com/sites/assets/PublishingImages/Products/inf_polaris_100_200/DE/9067047_PI_Polaris_100_200_6Seiter_DE_180214_fin.pdf [11.09.2014].

[10] Arduino, *Arduino - Arduino Board Uno.* http://arduino.cc/en/Main/ArduinoBoardUno [06.10.2014].

[11] Analog Devices, Inc., *TMP05/TMP06 $\pm 0.5°C$ Accurate PWM Temperature Sensor in 5-Lead SC-70 Data Sheet (Rev. C) - TMP05_06.pdf.* http://www.analog.com/static/imported-files/data_sheets/TMP05_06.pdf [08.01.2014].

[12] L. Fahrmeir, R. Künstler, I. Pigeot, and G. Tutz, *Statistik - Der Weg zur Datenanalyse*, ch. 3.4.1 – 3.6, pp. 134 – 158. Springer Berlin Heidelberg, 5. ed., 2004.

Implementation of Risk Management Report for Medical Ceiling Supply Units in IBM Rational DOORS®

G. Maltzen [1], A. Mess[2], and M. Leucker [3]
[1] Medizinische Ingenieurwissenschaft, Universität zu Lübeck, maltzen@miw.uni-luebeck.de
[2] Dräger Medical GmbH, R&D Line Organization Lübeck, Anke.Mess@draeger.com
[3] Institute for Software Engineering and Programming Languages , Universität zu Lübeck, leucker@isp.uni-luebeck.de

Abstract

This paper deals with the implementation of the risk management report for Dräger medical ceiling supply units in IBM Rational DOORS®. Supply units are medical devices with the purpose of supplying electric power, medical gases and load bearing. According to ISO 14971 medical devices are required to undergo a risk management process [5]. To improve usability, the risk management report has to be able to offer the possibility of integrating information from further documents. Consequentially, a transfer of the risk management report from Microsoft Excel to database IBM Rational DOORS® is desirable. IBM Rational DOORS® offers link modules which supports meeting the standard requirements of IEC 60601-1 Edition 3.1 [7] by referring standard requirements to risk management report. The result of risk management in IBM Rational DOORS® is the complete traceability, change tracking in all directions and ensuring the fulfilling of standard requirements in addition to an improved usability.

1 Introduction

This section introduces medical ceiling supply units, gives a short overview of the risk management process and presents the aim of performing the risk management report in IBM Rational Dynamic Object Oriented Requirements System®.

1.1 Medical Supply Units

Medical supply units are devices which consist of a ceiling fixation with movable arms and integrated modular components (Fig.1). Their purpose is the supply of medical gases such as oxygen or air, electric power or media data. Supply units have a wide range of load carrying capacity (Dräger devices from 25 kg to 270 kg). Therefore, they are able to carry anaesthesia devices (Fig.1, on the right side), multiple monitor holders, shelves and drawers and all kind of equipment holders in a customised design. In addition, there are integrated lights such as a reading light, an examination light or indirect light. The devices can be positioned exactly in accordance with where the clinical staff needs them. Hence, the supply units optimize the work space ergonomics and they are an important part of the workplace infrastructure. The integrated cable management and no contact to the ground improve the hygiene of the hospital by supporting easier clean up. The compatibility with modules makes the supply units individually applicable [1].
The described supply units are medical devices. As such, a complete risk management process is required and regulated in ISO 14971 [5].

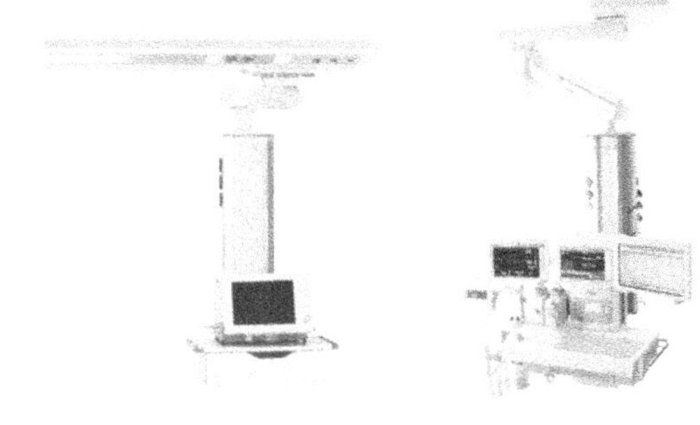

Figure 1: Dräger Ponta Ceiling Beam System and Dräger Movita with anaesthesia platform Perseus® A500 [2]-[3]

1.2 Risk Management

The risk management of medical devices such as supply units is specified in ISO 14971. Risk is defined as the possibility of damage or loss as a consequence of particular behaviour or event [4]. The aim of risk management is to systematically record and to evaluate risks and to build up an acceptable reaction to a possible risk [4]. The risk management involves different normative requirements depending on the type of the device. For medical ceiling supply units, the requirements ISO 14971 [5], ISO 11197 [6] and IEC 60601-1 3rd Edition [7] are of prime importance (Fig. 2).

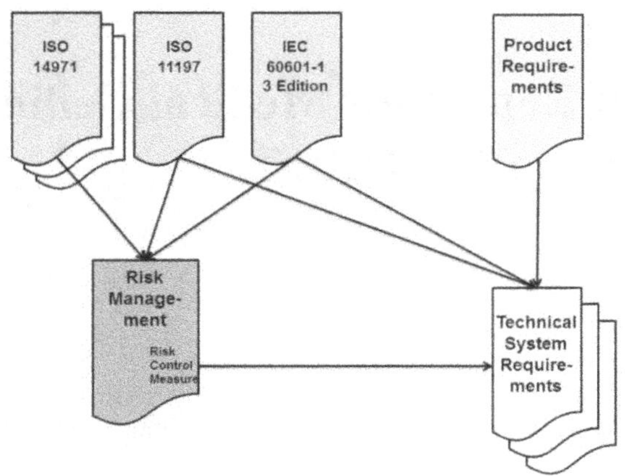

Figure 2: Connections between risk management of medical ceiling supply units and other standards/ requirements/ documents

The ISO 14971 specifies the process for the manufacturer in order to identify the hazards associated with medical devices for estimating and evaluating the associated risks, for controlling them and for observing the effectiveness of the risk control measures [5]. ISO 11197 specifies requirements and test methods for medical supply units intended for use in healthcare facilities which includes the supply of electric power, medical gases and/ or anaesthetic gas scavenging systems [6]. The IEC 60601-1 contains requirements concerning basic safety and essential performance that are generally applicable to medical electrical equipment [7].
The purpose of risk management is ensuring the compliance of all requirements. The result of risk management is an evaluation of possible risks associated with the medical device and especially risk control measures. The risk control measures are preventive measures to reduce the risk of damage for users and in particular for patients. Their aim is a reduction of the risk acceptance to an ALARP[1] or acceptable level. To implement the risk control measures, the technical system requirements (TSR), resulting from the general product requirements, are used (Fig. 2). The TSR are also have to meet certain standards and their requirements.

1.3 Requirements Management Tool IBM Rational DOORS®

IBM Rational DOORS® is a requirement management tool from manufacturer Telelogic. The tool was first published in 1991 [8]. The basic features are requirement management, traceability, scalability, a test tracking tool kit and integration [8]. For the risk management process, the IBM rational DOORS® tool offers the possibility of link modules. Requirements from separate documents can be linked showing one-to-one or one-to-many relationships. This is an important feature allowing traceability.
IBM Rational DOORS® also supports the import of Microsoft Excel files and Microsoft Word files. It has its own programming language called DOORS eXtension language "DXL". The property management can be done by allocating attributes and by using a unique identifier for each row in the file. The requirements are managed in a central repository for all users [8].

[1] As Low As Reasonable Practicable: Risk is acceptable as long as it cannot be further reduced by reasonable practicable measures [4]

2 Material and Methods

This section describes the available material, the used database and the procedure of transferring a part of the risk management report from Microsoft Excel to database IBM Rational DOORS®. Afterwards, the implementation of requirements from IEC 60601-1 Edition 3.1 [7] is demonstrated.

2.1 Set-up of a Risk Management Report

As already described, risk management is specified in ISO 14971 [7]. The requirements of this standard are implemented in an internal work instruction [4]. This secures that the risk management of each Dräger product is constructed in the same way. The work instruction manages the structure of risk management as well as how to start risk management, how to estimate risks, how to use risk chart, how to perform a risk/ benefit analysis, how to change risk management reports and more. If the instruction is strictly followed this equals meeting the requirements of ISO 14971.
The product risk management report includes all required informations. It is structured as follows:

1) Introduction and device information
2) Methods and criteria for risk assessment
3) Detailed result of the risk management
4) Overall residual risk
5) Risk/ Benefit analysis
6) Risk information for the customer/ user.

The content of this paper deals with the detailed results of risk management (section 3 of the internal work instruction) especially with the structuring of its subsection general hazardous situations. This subsection is shown as a table. Each row describes particular hazardous situation, names the evaluation of the risk and the risk control measures and finally evaluates the residual risk (Table 1). The evaluation of risk is performed by estimating severity and probability of a hazardous situation. Consequentially, the risk acceptance is calculated automatically with the help of the risk chart defined in the internal work instruction. If a hazardous situation results in a risk on an ALARP or not acceptable level, a risk control measure is required [4].
The table of general hazardous situations from Dräger

Table 1: Content of columns in general hazardous situations

Name of column	Description of content
ID	unique identifier of each row
Device	names the allocated device
Module	names the allocated module of the device
Functions	function or specification note of the device in combination with the module
Hazard	description of hazardous situation
Probable Cause(s)	possible cause(s) of hazard
Harm	description of harm for users or patients
Evaluation of Risk	severity, probability and automatic calculation of risk acceptance
Risk Control Measure	measures to reduce the risk
Residual Harm	description of residual harm for users and patients after implementation of risk control measure
Evaluation of Residual Risk	residual severity and residual probability and automatic calculation of residual risk acceptance

medical ceiling supply units is available in Microsoft Excel. The other documents (Fig. 2) are available in the database IBM Rational DOORS®. The tool IBM Rational DOORS® becomes important because its suitably for requirements management and its traceability through link modules. For optimisation of the risk management process, a transfer of the table of general hazardous situations from the risk management file to IBM Rational DOORS® is desirable.

2.2 Transfer from Microsoft Excel file to database IBM Rational DOORS®

First of all the Microsoft Excel file has to be prepared. The risk management reports from different types of supply units are merged because all types have nearly similar hazardous situations and should be treated in the same way. After some alignments, a template is formed containing all general hazards from Dräger medical ceiling supply units.
However, to separate one device from the others a device/ module based regulation is created. The separation is required in case of device or module changing. Consequentially, the associated risks have to be aligned. The device/ module based regulation is performed by adding three columns. The first column includes the allocation to the device (name of device), the second one supplements a module (e.g. light, lift and brake, electric/ gas fixtures) and the third column includes a specification note for particular devices with separate requirements or exceptions (for example Agila CC Indien, Agila lift).
Next, the Microsoft Excel template is transferred to a IBM Rational DOORS® template. Each row still describes a special hazardous situation and its risk evaluation. However, the risk control measures have their own subsection. The measures are sorted by different criteria such as hints in the instruction for use or installations instruction, electrical/ mechanical/ gas design and labelling. This is used to categorise and structure the section in a precise way. The direct reference to the row of hazardous situation is given by a link from risk control measures to each row they belong to. The positive aspect of this structure is shown in cases of an identical risk control measure which applies to several hazardous situations (e.g. four fold load test in accordance to IEC 60601-1 [7]). Hence, one risk control measure can be referred to different rows. In addition to implementing changes, there is only one alignment of the risk control measure necessary (e.g. change of a warning in the instruction for use). To improve usability, the risk control measures are automatically shown and updated in the rows of the general hazardous situation they belong to.

2.3 Requirements of IEC 60601-1 Edition 3.1 2012-08-20

The IEC is a worldwide organisation for standardization. The objective of IEC is to promote international cooperation on all questions concerning standardization in the electrical and electronic fields [7]. The IEC 60601-1 Edition 3.1 deals with general requirements for basic safety and essential performance of medical electrical equipment [7]. The standard is reviewed in regular intervals. In consequence, medical electrical devices have to conform to the modifications. The first step is preparing the standard in such a way that the already performed requirements are highlighted. Next, they are referred to the corresponding location in the risk management file by using IBM Rational DOORS® internal link module. The next step is to add data to the risk management file to meet the standard of the requirements from IEC 60601-1 [7]. The last step is linking the changed requirements to the adjusted location in the risk management file. This leads to a long-term management of the standard's compliance. In the end, two linked templates with the benefit of traceability and change tracking are created.

3 Results and Discussion

The results of the process of optimisation is demonstrated in Fig. 3. The risk management file is available in IBM Rational DOORS® and it is able to communicate with further documents through links.
The risk management file is prepared in Microsoft Excel in such a way that different device of Dräger medical ceiling supply units are modelled and integrated in one document. This unification ensures that similar aspects of different devices are regarded in context to each other. In consequence, the viewing of different devices is reduced to the relevant parts.
The implemented device based regulation enables with the help of modules to look at either one or more devices or

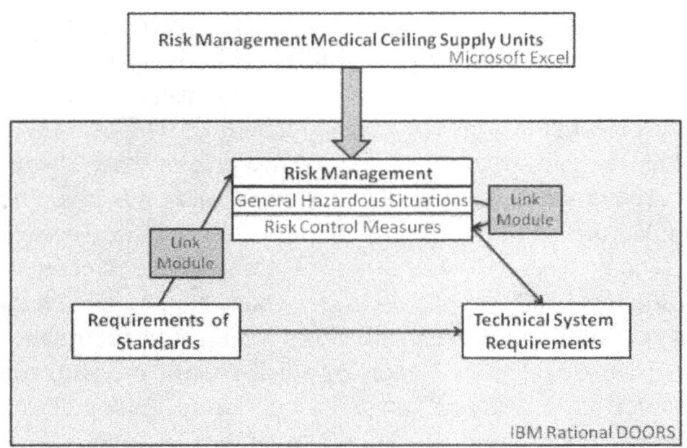

Figure 3: Benefit of process optimisation: improved handling with traceability and change tracking to other documents with the use of links

to look at modules such as light or electric fixtures which applies to all devices. This grants facilities to change one device or change modules (e.g. socket-outlet) relating to the corresponding adjustments of the hazardous situations. The tool IBM Rational DOORS® offers process optimisation by assisting with working on complex structures. In this case, the interaction of data, particularly the communication among the documents, is of prime importance.
The risk control measures have their own subsection and are referred to the rows with the general hazardous situations with the help of the IBM Rational DOORS® internal link module. The benefit of the link module is change tracking in both directions between risk control measure and hazardous situation. This leads to traceability. IBM Rational DOORS® enables a general improvement of handling the product risk management report. It produces a more custom-designed structure with traceability and change tracking in all directions inside the risk management report.
Additionally, the IEC 60601-1 3.1 is prepared in such a way, that changes between an old status and the updated status are visible. The changed requirements relating to risk management are added to the risk management report. In conclusion, all requirements of the standard IEC 60601-1 3.1 are referred to the suitable aspects of the risk management report by the IBM Rational DOORS® link module. The benefit of the link module is to track changes in both directions between the risk management report and the requirements of the standard. Finally, the link module secures the compliance of all requirements. In the end state 3.1 of the IEC 60601-1 is granted to the medical ceiling supply unit. In this content, the change tracking and traceability appear in another important role.
Fig. 3 demonstrates the benefit of the process optimisation of performing the risk management report in IBM Rational DOORS®.

4 Conclusion

All in all the transfer of the risk management report for Dräger medical ceiling supply units from Microsoft Excel to IBM Rational DOORS® has benefits in usability for the users of the documents and in consequence for the reliability of the medical device. Further steps would be the reference to the technical system requirements of Dräger medical ceiling supply units. At the moment, this document is designed in a module based structure.

Acknowledgement

The work has been carried out at Dräger Medical GmbH, R&D System Verification, Lübeck.

5 References

[1] Drägerwerk AG & Co. KGaA, *The Dräger Movita*, p.1, 2011, published in booklet, Available: http://www.draeger.com/sites/assets/PublishingImages/Products/inf_Movita/Attachments/movita_pi_9066662_en.pdf [last accessed on 10.02.2015]

[2] Drägerwerk AG & Co. KGaA, *Dräger Perseus ®A500 Ceiling-mounted version*, p.1, 2013, published in booklet, Available: http://www.draeger.com/sites/assets/PublishingImages/Products/ane_Perseus_A500/Modal/9068128_Perseus_A500_Ceiling_EN_fin.pdf [last accessed on 10.02.2015]

[3] Drägerwerk AG & Co. KGaA, *The Dräger Ponta*, p.1, 2012, published in booklet, Available: http://www.draeger.com/sites/assets/PublishingImages/Products/Architectural%20Products/Ponta-Beam-System-pi-9067217-us.pdf [last accessed on 10.02.2015]

[4] Norbert Pauli, Dräger Medical GmbH, *DMS IN4210 - Product Risk Management*, 2012-12-20, published as internal work instruction

[5] ISO 14971:2007, *Medical devices – Application of risk management to medical devices*, Edition 2, 2010-11-02

[6] ISO 11197:2004, *Medical supply units*, Edition 2, 2009-10-12

[7] IEC 60601-1, *Medical electrical equipment - Part 1: General requirements for basic safety and essential performance* , Edition 3.1 Amendment 1, 2012-08-20

[8] IBM, *Rational DOORS*, Available: http://www-03.ibm.com/software/products/en/ratidoor [last accessed on 13.01.2015]

Analysis of Coordinate Measuring Machines in Medicine especially in the Osteosurgery and Dentalsurgery

R. Saraei [1]
[1] Medizinische Ingenieurwissenschaft, Universität zu Lübeck, saraei@miw.uni-luebeck.de

Abstract

Rapid development in biomedical engineering generates the necessity of modern measuring devices with high accuracy. This work should give an overview about the most common used technology of CMM especially in medicine. Two main Applications in osteosurgery and dentalsurgery will be used for an review about CMM. In order to get information about these topic several papers which treats this have been analyzed and summarized. During the research it became clear that there a variety of different measuring techniques, but only a few of them could provide the needed accuracy. Therefore the main aspect in the medical metrology lies in optical measuring tools which are as accurate as the mechanical ones but does not need any contact to the samples which is important because of distorted measurement. It has been shown that there is enough to improve especially referring to the accuracy. The free-form shapes of the human anatomy makes it complicated to get results with high precision.

1 Introduction

The rapid development of modern metrology tools especially Coordinate Measuring Machines (CMM) and the demand of these in the biomedical engineering makes it an interesting aspect for the medicine to improve the quality assurance. Due to the fact of non-technical structures which are common in the medicine in consequence of the complex anatomy of human Body makes it necessary to measure the surface roughness for example artificial hips or joints with high accuracy. The process of creating artificial anatomic parts contains two stages namely Reverse Engineering (RE) and Rapid Prototyping (RP) which includes the use of Coordinate Measuring Machines and a Computer Aided Design Software for generating the Point Cloud Data from the physical Object [1].

Reverse Engineering contains three Steps: capturing significant Points of the Object, post-processing of these points and model manufacture. During the capturing process the surface of the physical object is scanned by a 3D-Scanner (for example CMM) in order to get a point cloud data which is used for generating a CAD Model. The Second Part incorporates the refinement with a Polygon-based technology such as sampling, filling, etc. The last process manufacturing serves the creation of CAD model or physical replicas from the refined data. In the following Figure three different modes of creating a physical model are presented [2].

In the first Path a 3D-Model is generated from the point cloud data and converted to a STL-File (Standard Tessellation Language). This file type only describes the surface geometry of a three-dimensional object without any representation of color, texture or other common CAD features. Afterwards it is sliced in order to generate a series of layers for Rapid Prototyping. On the second line the STL-File is directly generated from the Point Cloud data due to the fact of errors during the manual operation which is needed. The last strategy bypasses the creation of the CAD-Model and the STL-File generation. This step is possible because the initial scan data is reorganized and reduced to make the contour data. This can be used as a RP-Slice File due to the fact that contour data can be directly used for fabricating.

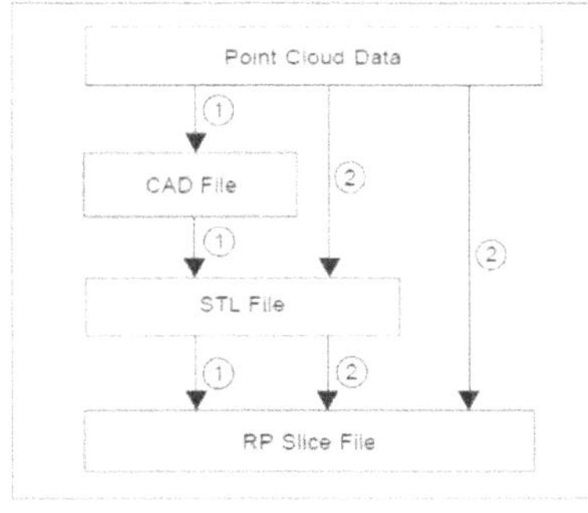

Figure 1: Linking process of Reverse Engineered data into a Rapid Prototype Model in three different strategies

In the following chapters two common applications will be described in order to illustrate the meaning of CMM's in medicine [3].

2 Application in Dentistry

A common application is the measurement of the tooth surface and creation of dental implants with CMM's. This belief lies in the fact of understanding how these devices per-

form in their functional environment. In order to develop for example implants it is necessary to adapt the measurement tools, data acquisition methods and the digital processing of the data which are associated with it [4].
In fact of surface roughness and precision not only the macroscopic but also the microscopic structure is necessary to guarantee a long-term bio-compatibility providing quality criteria. The implantation process is for every tooth individual and the manufacture is a hand made model. In the following Figure two work-flows describe once with the old method and the other with a new enhanced method [5].

As stated above the process is divided into two procedures

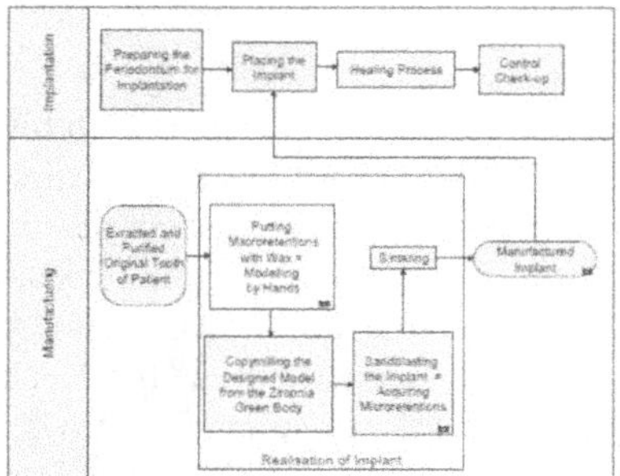

Figure 2: Process of the old Method of dental Implantation

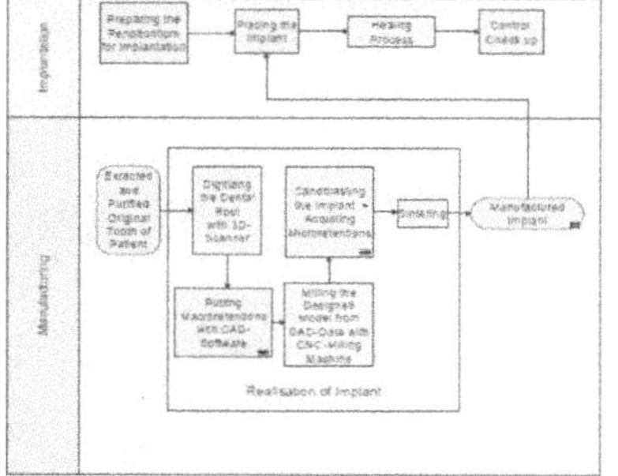

Figure 3: Work-Flow of the new way of dental Implantation

one for the implantation and one for the manufacturing of the tooth. In a first stage for the manufacturing the original tooth have to be extracted and cleaned up for modeling it with the hand. Afterwards the designed model is copy-milled from the Zirconia Green Body (an artificial diamond type with high tensile strength, high hardness and corrosion resistance) for the next stage the sandblasting for getting the microretention. In a last step it will be sintered and is ready for implantation [6].
The new method only differs in three steps. The hand modeling will be omitted and have been replaced by a CMM for digitizing the root of the tooth. Next macroretentions will be generated with a CAD Software. The milling will be done with a CNC-Milling Machine, the rest of the procedure is the same as before.
From the evaluated data through measuring there exists two forms of CMM, tactile and optical systems. In the following figures4 and 5 a CAD model and an active measurement with a CMM is shown [6].

The specifications of the measurement are rated with Geometrical Product Specifications (GPS) which includes not

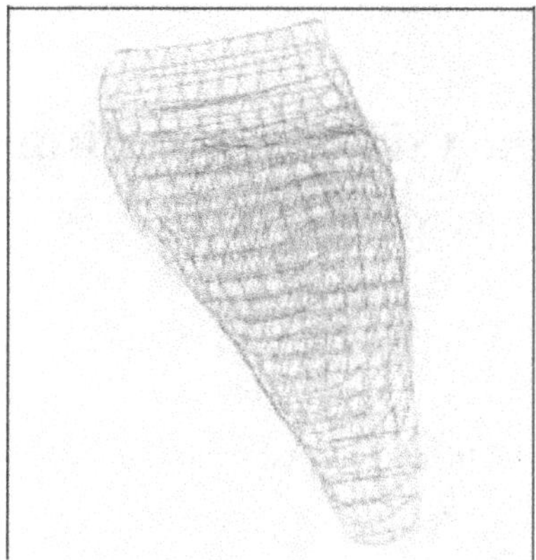

Figure 4: CAD Model of a tooth

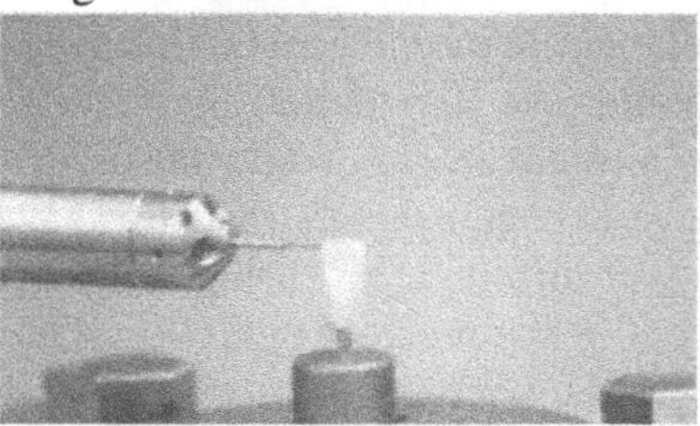

Figure 5: Process of measuring contours and surface of a tooth with a CMM

only size and dimension of the workpiece, but also geometrical tolerance and properties of the surface. The key parts of the GPS are shown in Figure 6.

One of the most important surface parameters is the sur-

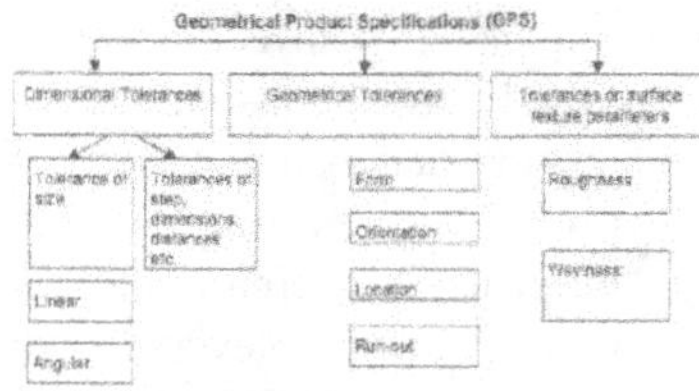

Figure 6: Overview of the General Product Specifications

face roughness which has two key parameters, arithmetical mean deviation of the assessed Profile R_a and the average maximum height R_z due to the fact that it is common by researchers and in the industry.
The use of a tooth serves the fact of differentiating between optical and tactile CMM because of its non-technical surface. The Stylus Profilometer which was used scans peaks and valleys of the tooth and the vertical motion is converted to an electrical signal [5] [7].

The optical part of the measurement is done with a medical CAD/CAM scanner in order to get the topographical features of the dental samples. It contains a scanning module and a computation module as shown in Figure 8.

Normally the surface roughness of a tooth lies in 4-9 μm. In the following section the use of CMM in the Osteosurgery especially in Reverse Engineering of the human femur is

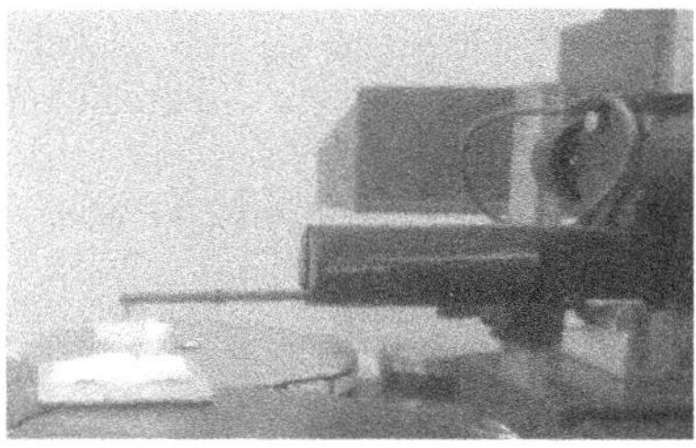

Figure 7: Contact-Stylus Profilometer during measurement of a dental sample

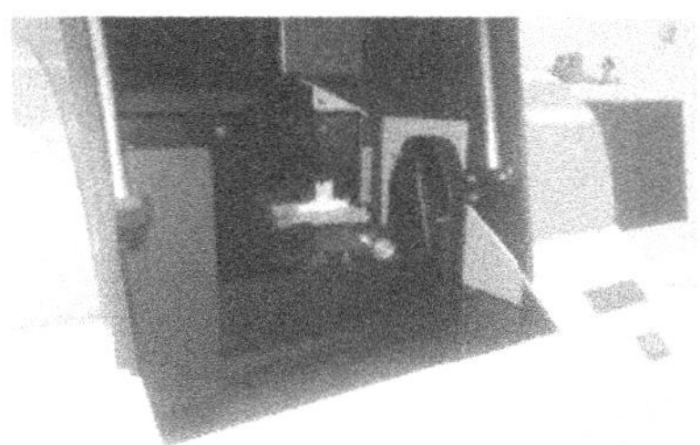

Figure 8: Medical CAD/CAM scanner with a dental sample

shown.

3 Application in Osteosurgery

Due to the fact that fractures of the femur is one of the most common injury it is necessary to analyse new methods not only of healing the damaged part, but to construct artificial femurs with nearly exact the same properties as an anatomically functional one. As stated before in the article the same procedure is used to generate a point cloud data with an 3D optical scanner (CMM) for generating a solid-state model. Afterwards this is used to produce a artificial femur. During this process the Finite Element Method (FEM) have been used to find stress distribution in different static loadings on half human femur model.

The Finite-Element-Method is a standard method for the computation of mechanical deformations and stresses. Mathematically it is a calculation method for solving partial differential equation. The main idea is to split up a complex problem into small pieces like the divide and conquer method in order to get the properties of the element and then describe this mathematically. The quality depends on the discretization level for the approximation later. Moreover the main problem which depends on the computation time is the discretization process. The degree of detail of the examined structure stands as a limitation factor. Therefore an interesting alternative is the Approximation method which replaces the surrounding area of the geometry through integral functions which will be then be evaluated to a stiffness matrix. This leads to smaller number of equations but more complex. The main advantage is that complex geometries could be calculated with standard hardware without any simplifications. The main procedure with detailed steps will be explained in the following part. In a first step the so called Preprocessing have to done in which a nearly exact mathematical model with finite elements have to be created. After approximation of the geometry through finite elements, the input of the geometrical constraints and the specific material properties loads with variety of direction vectors could be applied to the model. This results in a complex linear equation which allows the mathematical calculation of all deformations and allows conclusions referring to the strain and stress of the object. General types of Elements which are used in the FEM are triangles, rectangle and some other types.

A comparison of three different types of stress on the femur are shown in the next figures which shows that throughout this FEM a localization of displacements and strains can be detected [7] [8] [12]. As shown in Figure 9 and 10 three

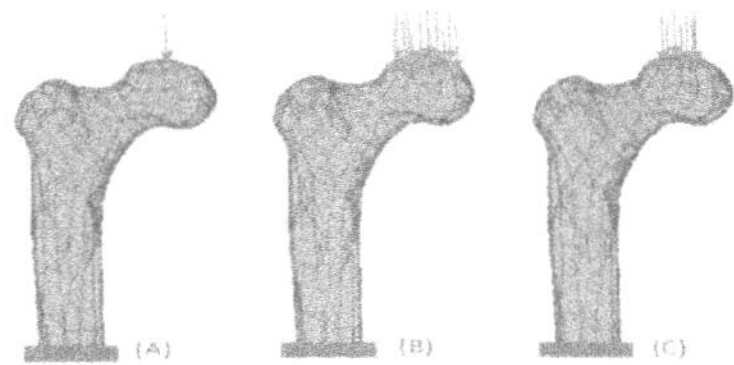

Figure 9: Different forces were applied on the surface of the femoral head while the middle part of the shaft has been fixed A: Single force, B: full distributed vertical force, C: partially distributed vertical force

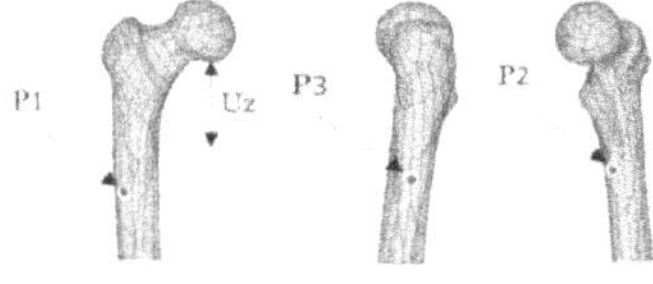

Figure 10: shows locations of displacement and strains because of the different forces

points have been selected at the surface of the femur for testing the stress and the resulting damage. In the following figures the stress distribution at 1500 N and strain distribution in Z-direction at 1500 N is shown [9] [10] [11].

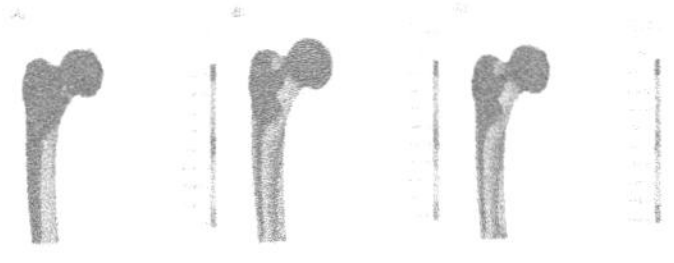

Figure 11: Stress Distribution at 1500 N A: Single loading, B: full loading, C: partially loading

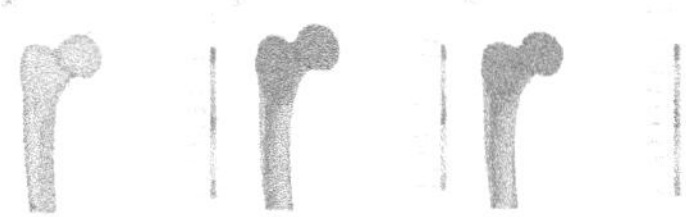

Figure 12: Strain Distribution in Z-direction with A: single loading, B: full loading and C: partial loading

4 Conclusion

All in all there exists a lot of variety in producing useful data for extracting features from anatomically parts of human body for manufacturing models, but also errors during this process can happen which leads to deviation in the precision of these parts like a tooth or a femur. The aim of this work was to show different methods in the metrology which are used in the medical technology for generating more precise models and implants. These examples only shows a little insight into this topic, but also make it clear that more work has to be done for better accuracy of the CMM. As shown above one common method the FEM is used very often in the medicine especially in the simulation of deformations for bones. The problem there is that the more constraints comes to the model the more complex it gets. Therefore one of the most important tasks is to improve the calculation of these equations in the FEM.

Acknowledgement

The work has been carried out at Carl Zeiss AG, Oberkochen in Germany.

5 References

[1] Gibson I, *Rapid Prototyping: From Product Development to Medicine and Beyond.* Virtual and Physical Prototyping, vol. 1, no. 1, 2006.

[2] T. Heimann and H-P. Meinzer, *Statistical Shape Models for 3D Medical Image Segmentation: A Review.* 2009.

[3] W. Sun, B. Starily, J. Nam and A. Darling, *Bio-CAD Modeling and its Applications in Computer-Aided Tissue Engineering*. Computer-Aided Design, Vol. 37, 2005.

[4] N. Vitkovic, M. Trajanovic, J. Milovanovic, N. Korunovic, S. Arsic and D. Ilic, *The Geometrical Models of the Human Femur and its Usage in Application for Pre-Operative Planning in Orthopedics – ICIST.* Kopaonik, Serbia, 2011.

[5] P.H. Osanna, K. Rezaie, N.M. Durakbasa and C.P. Heiss, *Form Measurements - A Bridge Between Production Metrology and Biomechanics*. Int. J. Mach. Tools Manufact. Vol. 35 (1995), No. 2, pp.165-168.

[6] P. Demircioglu and N.M. Durakbasa, *Investigations on machined metal surfaces through the stylus type and optical 3D instruments and their mathematical modeling with the help of statistical techniques*. Measurement 44 (2011), pp.611-619.

[7] P.H. Osanna and N.M. Durakbasa, *Concept for Computer Aided Non-contact Laser Roughness Evaluation of Engineering Surfaces.* in: Laser Metrology Applied to Science, Industry and Everyday Life - LM-2002, (2002), ISBN: 0-8194-4686-6; pp. 708 – 714.

[8] W.K. Gerhard Hugenholtz, R. Eibert Heerdink, P. Tjeerd van Staa, A. Willem Nolen and C.G. Antoine Egberts, *Risk of hip/femur fractures in patients using antipsychotics*. Bone (2005) Vol. pp. 864 - 870.

[9] L. Voo, M. Armand and M. Kleinberger, *Stress Fracture Risk Analysis of the Human Femur Based on Computational Biomechanics.* in: Johns Hopkins Apl Technical Digest (2004).

[10] S. Valliapan, N.L. Svensson and R.D. Wood, *Three dimensional stress analysis of the human femur.* Computers in Biology and Medicine, 7(4): pp. 253 - 264.

[11] V. Raja and K.J. Fernandes, *Reverse engineering : an industrial perspective.* Springer (2008).

[12] K. Doi, *Computer-aided diagnosis (CAD) and image-guided decision support.* Computerized Medical Imaging and Graphics, 31: pp. 195 - 197.

7
Medical Imaging

Novel Method to Measure Migration of Percutaneous Nerve Evaluation Leads

T. Tronnier [1], A. Rivard [2], and P. Falkner [2]

[1] Medizinische Ingenieurwissenschaft, Universität zu Lübeck, tronnier@informatik.uni-luebeck.de

[2] Medtronic Neuromodulation, Fridley, {adam.j.rivard, phillip.c.falkner}@medtronic.com

Abstract

Neuromodulation is deemed as one of the most important areas of the medical device industry. Sacral neuromodulation is approved to treat several chronic urological disorders including overactive bladder, non-obstructive urinary retention and fecal incontinence. For these therapies, well controlled stimulation current is delivered to the sacrum nerve area through implantable leads. To evaluate the therapeutic benefit, a temporary percutaneous nerve evaluation (PNE) lead is implanted for three to seven days. The current PNE lead does not have any fixation features, which may result to frequent lead migration. There is no exsiting method to measure in-vivo migration quantitatively. In this paper such a method was developed based on Mimics® software with computed tomography (CT) scans. The method was then used to assess 32 PNE lead in-vivo migration. The results show that this new developed lead migration method is successful in capturing and measuring the movement of the leads between day zero and day seven.

1 Introduction

For 20 years, sacral neuromodulation has been a successful therapy for several urological chronic diseases such as overactive bladder, urinary retention, non-obstructive urinary incontinence and fecal incontinence [1]-[3].

In 1997, the U.S. Food and Drug Administration (FDA) approved sacral neuromodulation for urgency incontinence, and in 1999 for refractory urgency-frequency syndrome and nonobstructive chronic urinary retention [4]. Additionally, Non-FDA approved uses are increasing. The sacral nerves control the bladder, bowel and pelvic floor [5]. In the late 1990s Medtronic developed the InterStim® system to treat the aforementioned diseases. Since then, more than 175,000 patients have been implanted worldwide [6]. The InterStim® system consists of a neurostimulator and a lead, technically comparable to a pacemaker [7]. The lead stimulates the sacral nerves, located near the sacrum, with mild electrical pulses (Fig.1).

While the exact mechanism of action is unknown, neuromodulation is thought to alter the pathological imbalance of sacral reflexes controlling bladder and bowel storage and emptying. Normally the S3 root is targeted through the foramen. Because it is difficult to predict the therapeutic response, a trial phase of sacral neuromodulation is performed before placement of a permanent InterStim® system. Two different testing methods are commonly used: the PNE method and staging implantation using permanent leads.

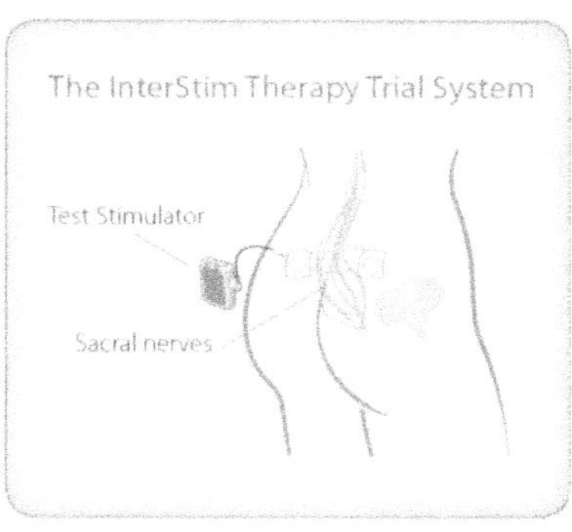

Figure 1: Location of the InterStim® system [8]

Before patients get a permanent InterStim® system, they have to go through a basic or advanced trial. The traditional PNE lead, or Basic trial (Fig.2), uses a temporary monopolar lead without a fixation feature placed through a 20 gauge needle, allowing for minimally traumatic deployment and retrieval. Most commonly, the lead is placed bilaterally via the S3 foramen under local anesthesia with or without the assistance of fluoroscopy. Correct lead placement is determined by a levator ani motor response, plantar flexion of the big toe, and sensory perineal stimulation. The temporary lead is retained for the duration of the trial phase by fixation to the skin surface with adhesive, and is connected to an external neurostimulator. The basic trial lasts from three to seven days and allows the patient and clinician to test the therapeutic effect.

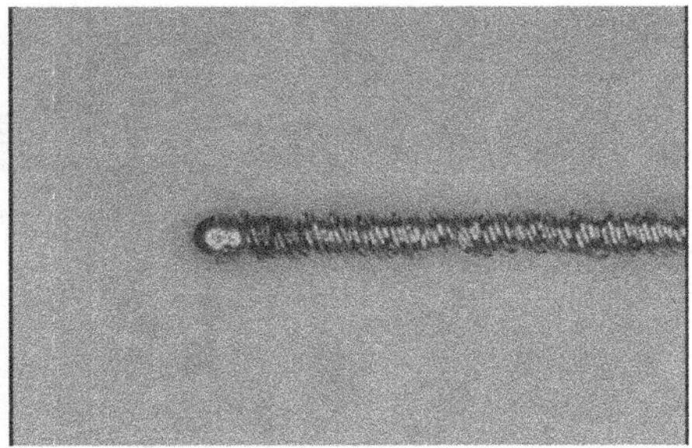

Figure 2: Current version of a temporary lead, which is used for the trial phase.

During the test period, the patient is supposed to perform all activities of daily living. If the patient shows a 50% or more reduction of the symptoms, they are considered a candidate for the permanent InterStim® system.

For a successful trial, the PNE lead has to stay parallel to the sacral nerve during the test period, but be easily removed at the end of the trial by the physician. The current PNE lead doesn't have any fixation features, which might lead to frequent lead migration. PNE lead migration is known to occur and result in a false negative test. There is no existing method to measure in-vivo migration quantitatively. It is desirable to develop a method to quantify in-vivo lead migration for future product development and optimization. In this paper such a method was developed based on Mimics® software with CT scans. The method was then used to assess in-vivo migration of 32 PNE leads. One sheep was used in the Institutional Animal Care and Use Committee (IACUC) approved study as required by the Animal Welfare Act. Three stainless steel screws and five stainless steel markers were implanted as reference points; 32 PNE leads were implanted in the lower back/ sacral area to assess in-vivo migration.

2 Material and Methods

2.1 Material

One sheep was used in this in-vivo study. A total of 32 PNE leads were implanted 6cm deep into the lower back/ sacral area of the sheep. The lead implant location is shown in Fig.3. Lead numbers 27-32 were implanted into the sacrum (S1-S3). Five stainless steel markers with a length of 2mm and three stainless steel screw (used as markers) with a length of 5mm (Fig.4) were implanted into the sacrum and gluteal muscles. To avoid migration of the markers in the muscle, small tines were used. The stainless steel screws were implanted into bones. Different lead configurations were developed. For intellectual property protection, design details will be hidden. Of the 32 leads used, two current PNE leads were used as controls.

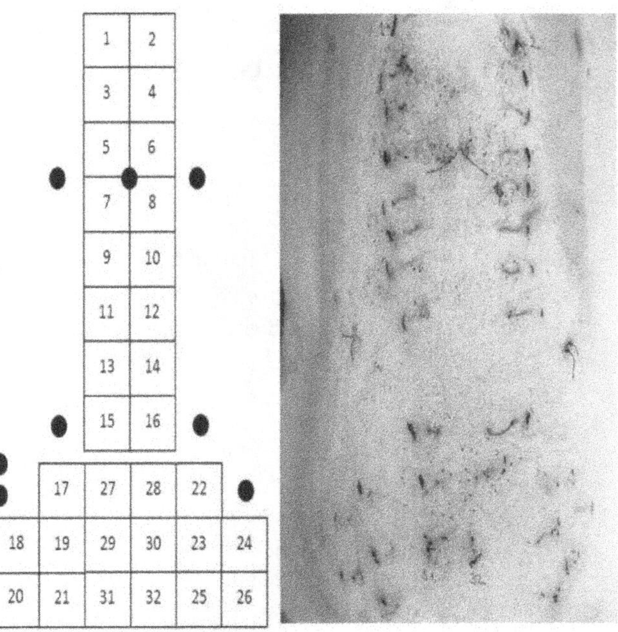

Figure 3: Placement of the leads (squares), markers and screws (black dots) in the lower back/sacral area(left). Back of the sheep with the 32 implanted leads (right).

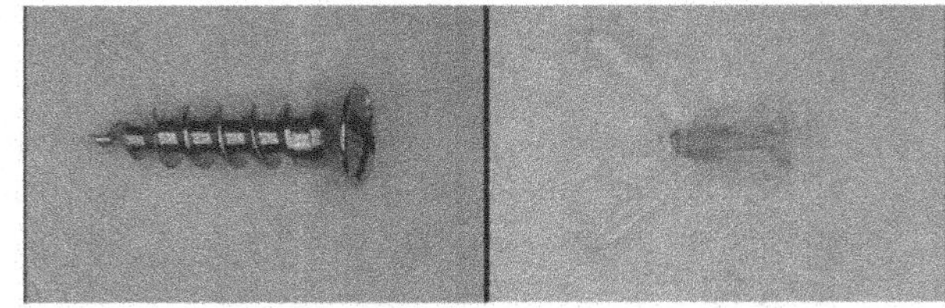

Figure 4: Stainless steel screw (left) and stainless steel marker (right).

2.2 Methods

A schematic description of the approach is shown in Fig.5. First, 32 leads were implanted into a sheep, using the typical needle entry/delivery method [9]. One CT scan was taken immediately after the leads were implanted (day 0) and another one after seven days (day 7). Both CT images were taken with a Siemens Definition CT scan. The resolution of the CT scans were 0.54mm. All scans were performed with the sheep resting on its belly, with legs pulled back and fixated. For the entire image processing and for measuring the migration of the leads, the software Mimics® Medical 17.0 (Medical Image Segmentation for Engineering on Anatomy™, Materialise HQ, Leuven, Belgium) was used. The Dicom files from both CT scans were imported into Mimics® for 3D reconstructions (Fig.6).The next step was to overlay the two 3D reconstructions (from day 0 and day 7) with a image registration method. The markers and screws were used to apply an image registration method called point-based registration. To do a point-base registration we used the function "N Points Registration" in Mimics®. Several points on the surface of the markers and screws of each CT scan were selected. Every point considers one registration point. The tip-to-tip distances of the leads were measured between day zero and day seven to calculate migration.

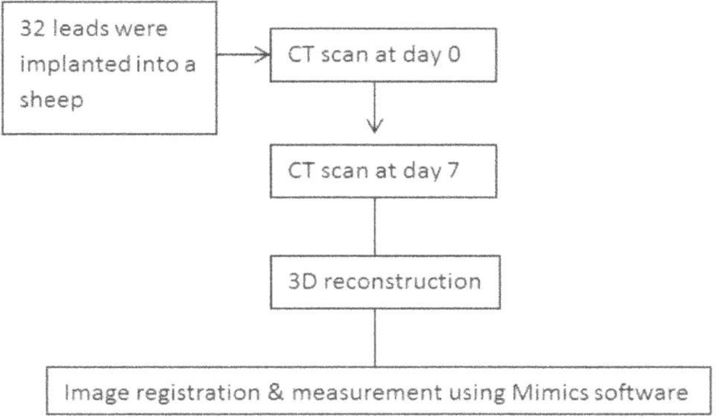

Figure 5: schematic description

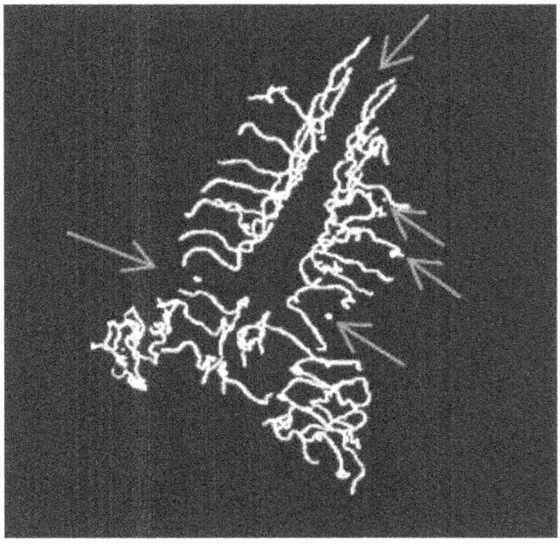

Figure 6: 3D reconstruction of the segmented leads; arrows show the reconstructed markers and screws.

3 Results and Discussion

Fig.7 shows the overlay of the two CT scans after registration. The migration of the 32 implanted leads were measured with Mimics and summarized in Table 1. Positive migration indicates the leads moved towards the skin surface. Negative migration means the leads moved deeper into the tissue away from skin surface. Leads with a fixation feature migrated a maximum of 6.5mm. Leads without a fixation feature migrated a maximum 32.0mm.
Two current PNE leads without fixation features were implanted. After seven days one PNE lead (lead number 16) migrated 6.1mm and the other PNE lead (lead number 25) migrated 32.0mm. This seems to indicate that the implant location might have significant impact on lead migration. Lead number 25 was implanted into the muscle of the leg, which represented the worst-case scenario, because of the significant sheep movement. Lead number 16, was implanted into the lumbar area, which is less affected by the sheep's movements. The absolute average migration of the 29 leads was 3.0mm. To get a good registration result, markers should only be implanted in the lumbar region.

Table 1: PNE leads Migration Measurement Summary

Lead number	Migration in mm at day 0	Migration in mm at day 7	Fixation (Yes/No)
1	0.0	-1.7	Yes
2	0.0	1.9	Yes
3	0.0	2.7	Yes
4	0.0	6.5	Yes
5	0.0	0.5	Yes
6	0.0	1.7	Yes
7	0.0	2.1	Yes
8	0.0	0.0	Yes
9	0.0	2.4	Yes
10	0.0	2.1	Yes
11	0.0	0.0	Yes
12	0.0	1.4	Yes
13	0.0	-3.9	Yes
14	0.0	1.7	Yes
15	0.0	0.0	Yes
16	0.0	6.1	No
17	0.0	-1.0	Yes
18	0.0	0.0	Yes
19	0.0	-1.9	Yes
20	0.0	*	Yes
21	0.0	-2.3	Yes
22	0.0	-1.3	Yes
23	0.0	3.7	Yes
24	0.0	*	Yes
25	0.0	32.0	No
26	0.0	4.4	Yes
27	0.0	1.1	Yes
28	0.0	0.0	Yes
29	0.0	0.0	Yes
30	0.0	0.1	Yes
31	0.0	2.8	Yes
32	0.0	*	Yes
Average in mm		3.0	

* were excluded from the measurement, because the migration was in lateral direction, which was not the focus of this study.

During the registration method the three makers in the sacral area migrated and weren't used for image registration. To improve the registration, markers should only be implanted in the lumbar region.

4 Conclusion

A method was developed based on Mimics®software with CT scans to measure lead migration. The method was used to evaluate in-vivo migration of 32 PNE leads. The results show that this new developed lead migration method is suc-

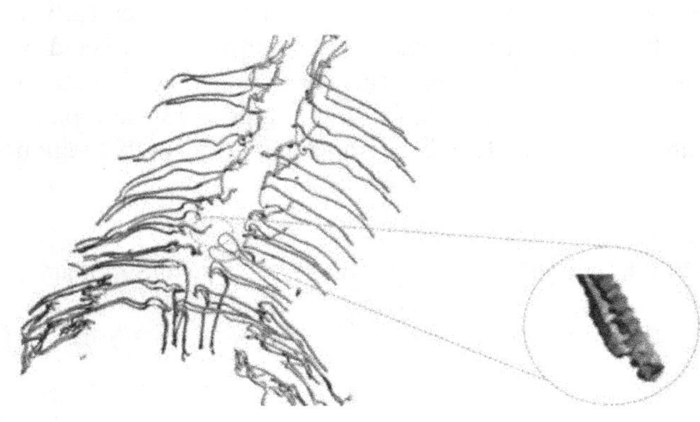

Figure 7: Alignment of the two CT scans on the left and zoomed in image on the right; tip of one lead at day zero (right) and the same lead tip at day seven (left).

cessful in capturing and measuring the movement of the leads between day zero and day seven.

Acknowledgement

The work has been carried out at Medtronic Neuromodultation, Fridley. I would like to express my gratitude to Medtronic for the support in carrying out this study, especially Haitao Zang and Jeevan Prasannakumar. I also want to thank the Institute of Medical Engineering, University of Lübeck for the opportunity to perform a study abroad and the German Academic Exchange Service for a travel grant.

5 References

[1] N. Kohli and D. Patterson, *InterStim Therapy: A Contemporary Approach to Overactive Bladder*, Reviews in Obstetrics and Gynecology, vol. 2, no. 1, pp. 18-27, 2009.

[2] M. Brazzelli, A. Murray and C. Fraser, *Efficacy and Safety of Sacral Nerve Stimulation for Urinary Urge Incontinence: A Systematic Review*, The Journal of Urology, vol. 175, no. 3, pp. 835-841, 2006.

[3] N. D. Sherman, M. G. Jamison, G. D. Webster and C. L. Amundsen, *Sacral Neuromodulation for the Treatment of Refractory Urinary Urge Incontinence after Stress Incontinence Surgery*, American Journal of Obstetrics & Gynecology, vol. 193, no. 6, pp. 2083-2087, 2005.

[4] Medtronic, *What Is Medtronic Bladder Control Therapy?*. Available: http://www.medtronic.com/patients/overactive-bladder/about-therapy/what-is-it/ [last accessed on 10.02.2015].

[5] National Hospital for Neurology and Neurosurgery, Queen Square London, *Sacral Neuromodulation in Pelvic FloorDisorders*. Available: http://www.neuromodulation.com/assets/documents/Fact_Sheets/fact_sheet_pelvic_floor_disorders.pdf [last accessed on 04.12.2014].

[6] Medtronic, *Questions and Answers: How long has Medtronic Bladder Control Therapy been around?*. Available: http://www.medtronic.com/patients/overactive-bladder/about-therapy/questions-answers/index.htm [last accessed on 10.02.2015].

[7] Medtronic, *What Is InterStim Therapy?*. Available: http://www.medtronic.eu/your-health/constipation/about-the-device/what-is-it/ [last accessed on 04.12.2014].

[8] Melbourne Bladder Clinic, *Sacral Neuromodulation- User Info*. Available: http://www.bladderclinic.com.au/printable-patient-literature/sacral-neuromodulation-user-info [last accessed on 04.12.2014].

[9] Medtronic, *INTERSTIM®THERAPY, Technical Manual*. Available: http://professional.medtronic.com/wcm/groups/mdtcom_sg/@mdt/@neuro/documents/documents/sns-testlead3065u-57man.pdf [last accessed on 12.02.2014].

The measurement of the peak kilovoltage across microfocus X-ray tubes by using K-shell radiation and K-shell absorption

A. Schu [1] and W. Niemann [2]
[1] Medizinische Ingenieurwissenschaft, Universität zu Lübeck, andre.schu@miw.uni-luebeck.de
[2] Yxlon International GmbH, wilhem.niemann@hbg.yxlon.com

Abstract

The difficulties of measuring the kilovoltages across a high voltage generator are that extra components for the system are needed and have to be integrated into the system or that you need a complex and expensive measurement setup. A simple measurement setup, which doesn't need expensive measurement equipment and reaches an acceptable accuracy would be desirable. One option to measure high voltages is to monitor the absorption effects of X-radiation in matter. There is the effect of additional emission of K-shell radiation and the effect of additional K-shell absorption. If you put these effects together the high voltage can be measured. Based on the method of J.R. Greening [1] measuring high voltage for standard X-ray tubes a method for micro-focus X-ray tubes in transmission geometry at low power is presented.

1 Introduction

The voltage affects the acceleration energy of the electrons and thereby the energy of the X-radiation. Therefore it is necessary to use a calibrated high voltage generator. The DIN EN 12544 standard to measure kilovoltages for X-ray systems currently involves three measuring methods. For a direct and absolute measuring of direct current kilovoltage values the voltage divider method [6] is used. This method requires that a voltage divider gets implemented between a X-ray tube and a generator and the partial voltage gets measured. Regular inspections of the kilovoltage stability of an X-ray system can be realised with the thick-filter method [7]. This method uses the dose behind a filter with defined thickness. In this way it is possible to measure voltage variations. One disadvantage of this method is that the output only verifies the stability of the kilovoltage. There are no information about the absolute values for the kilovoltage. The spectrometer method [8] measures the kilovoltage by using the energy spectrum of the X-radiation. This method has the best accuracy for measuring absolute kilovoltage values and there is no need to integrate measurement instruments into the system. A disadvantage is the complex measurement setup.

In 1954, Greening [1] described another method of measuring the kilovoltage of X-ray systems. At this the kilovoltage gets measured by using the ratio of additional emission of K-shell radiation and the additional K-shell absorption. The advantage of this method is that no measurement instruments have to be integrated at high voltage parts and that it is a simple measurement setup.

Because of the significant lower power of transmission X-ray tubes in comparison with standard X-ray tubes in this paper it is verified that the signal of the K-shell radiation at low power is high enough. Additionally it is shown that this measurement method is transferable to transmission X-ray tubes.

2 Material and Methods

At X-ray energies below 1MeV the photoelectric effect is the most significant interaction between X-radiation and matter. This effect is well known and described in the scientific literature. For this paper the references [2] and [3] were used. The incidental photon evolves its whole energy in form of kinetic energy to a shell electron. The photon itself gets absorbed at this interaction. This transfer of energy mainly happens in the inner shells (K- and L-shells). The released electron or photo-electron leaves an electron-hole. This electron-hole can be filled by an electron of a higher shell. At this process the electron releases the excess energy in form of a photon or it transfers its energy radiation-free to a third electron which gets emitted as Auger-electron or secondary electron. In the first case the emitted radiation is called X-ray fluorescence as shown in Fig. 1.

As described above the photoelectric effect is an effect which absorbs X-radiation. The probability of an interaction of this type can be described with the photo absorption coefficient. This coefficient is inversely proportional which means that the probability of an interaction between the X-radiation and matter drops with the increasing energy of the photons. At some areas this continuous decrease gets interrupted by the resonance effect. At this point the energy of the photon is equal to the electron shell binding energy. This state provides good conditions for an interaction be-

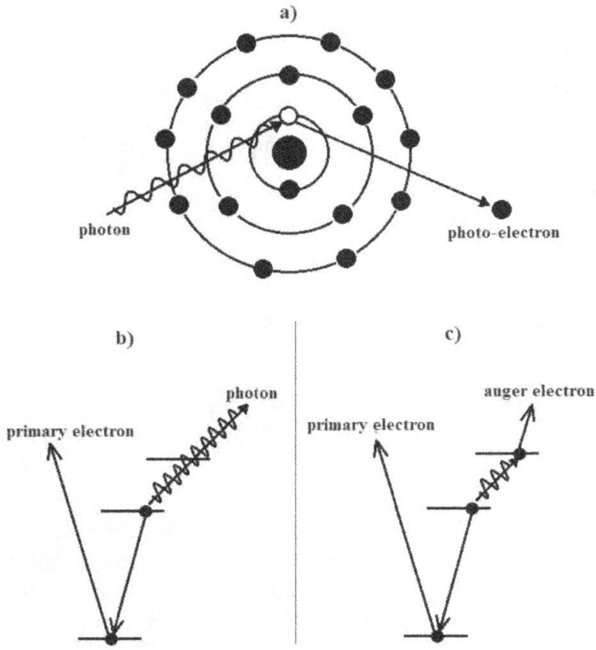

Figure 1: a) Principle of the photoelectric effect b) Emission of characteristic radiation c) Emission of secondary or Auger electrons

tween the X-radiation and the matter which leads to a sharp edge in the photo absorption coefficient which is called absorption edge. Based on the position of the edge the element can be identified because it is equal to the K-shell energy of the element. In Fig. 2 the absorption coefficient of lead is given as a function of the photon energy.

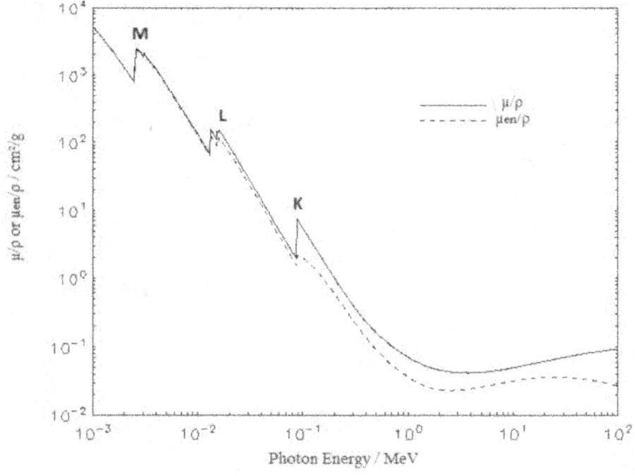

Figure 2: Absorption coefficient of lead as a function of the photon energy [5]

2.1 Detecting the threshold for K-shell radiation and K-shell absorption

The effect of the characteristic X-ray fluorescence radiation and the material specific absorption edge can be used to measure the high voltage. The measurement setup as shown in Fig. 3 was used to measure both signals. If you place the dosimeter in position A it is mostly shielded against the primary beam and the leakage radiation because it is positioned in a box B with about 2mm lead thickness. In this position the dosimeter can measure the specific fluorescence radiation of the test filter D and the scattered radiation which comes up in the test filter D itself. The scattered radiation overlaids the specific fluorescence radiation and has no useful contribution to the signal. Therefore a pre-filter with 0.5mm aluminium was implemented in position C to filter out the scattered radiation of low energy. As test filter a lead filter with a thickness of 0.1mm was used. The K-shell energy of lead is located at 88.005keV. For measuring the specific fluorescence radiation the voltage was increased in steps of 1kV from 70kV to 110kV. The dose in position A was integrated over 120s at each voltage-step. At voltages below 88.005kv the energy is too low to generate the specific fluorescence radiation. Because of this there is only a slight upward movement of the dose which is the result of the growing energy of the photons. At voltages above 88.005kV the signal of the specific fluorescence radiation is added to the scattered radiation. This leads to a knee in the dose graph at the K-shell energy of the test filter D.

To measure the additional K-shell absorption the dosimeter gets into position E. In this position the primary beam weakened by the test filter can be measured. Up to the energy of 88.005keV the absorption of the test filter drops with the increasing energy of the photons. By reaching the energy of 88.005keV the energy of the photons is equal to the K-shell energy of lead and this leads to an additional absorption in the K-shell. The result is a knee in the dose graph at 88.005kv. The intensity of this knee depends on the thickness and material of the test filter.

A typical energy spectrum of X-radiation from a tungsten anode has a high amount of radiation with low energy. If you set for example 88.005kV as voltage, only a few photons have the energy of 88.005keV. But this energy is needed to cause the effects of the fluorescence radiation and the additional absorption. The amount of the fluorescence radiation and the additional K-shell absorption in the transition area is very low. Therefore the knee in the graph is hard to localise. To intensify the knee in the transition area the signals can be put into ratio and plotted as function of the voltage. The graph is similar to two lines with an intersection at the K-shell energy of the test filter.

2.2 Calibration points available

In theory all elements can be used to calibrate the kilovoltage corresponding to the K-edge of each element. In practical use there are a lot of limitations. Most of the elements with a higher atomic number than uranium, the transuranic elements can not be used because of a too short half life. Others are rare and expensive. Because of this the highest verifiable kilovoltage is 115.602kV which corresponds with the K-edge of uranium. To calibrate the generator with a characteristic line with a step width of 10kV there are also

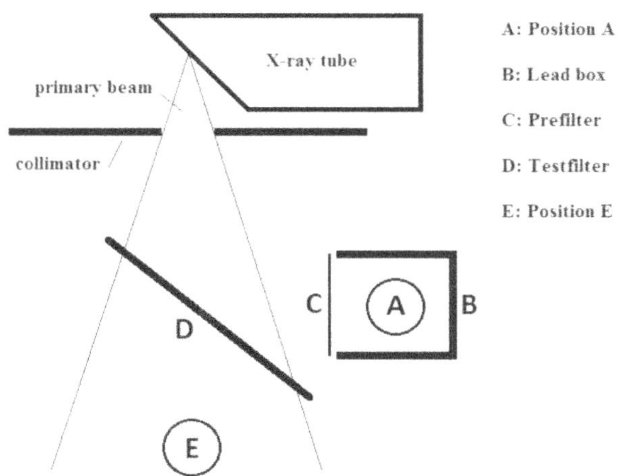

Figure 3: Measurement setup to measure the K-shell radiation and the additional K-shell absorption

limited elements for the lower kilovoltages. The elements with the atomic numbers between 58 and 73 (the K-edges of these elements correspond to the kilovoltages 35kV up to 67kV) belong to the rare earth elements which makes them rare and expensive. Some other elements are gaseous so they are difficult to use for this measurement. A list of elements which might be useful is given in the table 1. All these elements can be used as element, salt or oxide.

Table 1: List of elements of possible use for kilovoltage calibrations [4]

Atomic Number	Element	Kilovoltage of K-edge
92	Uranium	115.602
90	Thorium	109.650
83	Bismuth	90.526
82	Lead	88.005
81	Thallium	85.530
80	Mercury	83.102
79	Gold	80.725
78	Platinum	78.395
77	Iridium	76.111
74	Tungsten	69.525
73	Tantalum	67.416
58	Cerium	40.443
56	Barium	37.441
52	Tellurium	31.814
50	Tin	29.200
47	Silver	25.514
46	Palladium	24.350
42	Molybdenum	20.000

3 Results and Discussion

The generator was connected to a voltage divider of the company IMS. The voltage divider was calibrated before and had a precision of 0.5%. The result of the reference measurement was that the actual value was 2.45% higher than the set value. This difference was used as reference value for the actual kilovoltage.

3.1 Measurement of the K-shell absorption

In Fig. 4 the dose is shown as a function of the kilovoltage. The signal here shown is the primary beam which was weakened by 0.1mm lead. Both shown signals are the measurement results of the measurement at 100W with a standard X-ray tube and at 15W with a transmission X-ray tube. As expected the curves have a small knee downwards in area around 90kV. This is the effect of the additional absorption in the K-shell above the 88.005keV. At the beginning the curves are close which changes at 90kV. At this point the curves start to drift apart. In this case the effect of the additional absorption is even clearer in the 15W curve.

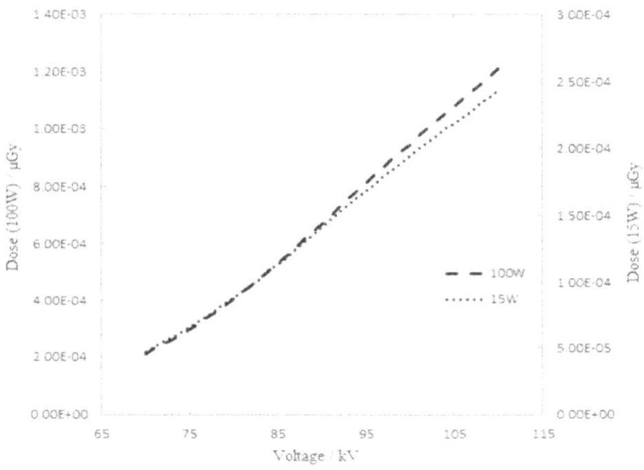

Figure 4: Measurement of the primary beam behind 0.1mm lead. Data at 100W recorded with standard X-ray tube. Data at 15W recorded with transmission X-ray tube.

3.2 Measurement of the K-shell radiation and scattered radiation

In Fig. 5 the dose is shown as a function of the kilovoltage. The signal which is shown in this figure is the characteristic X-ray fluorescence radiation which was measured in an angle of 45 degrees to the test filter behind a 0.5mm aluminium pre-filter. As before for the 100W signal the standard X-ray tube was used and for the 15W signal the transmission tube was used. Because of the additional fluorescence radiation we see a knee upwards in the area around 90kV. This was expected as well.

3.3 Method of detecting the K-shell threshold

The ratio of these two signals as function of the kilovoltage is shown in Fig. 6. At the beginning the ratios are close together. After the knee in the area of the K-shell energy of lead the ratios drift apart. If you put one line through the left and one line through the right part of the

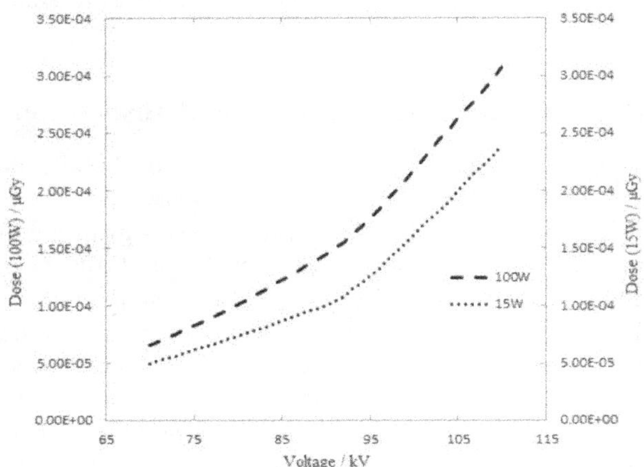

Figure 5: Measurement of the K-shell radiation. Data at 100W recorded with standard X-ray tube. Data at 15W recorded with transmission X-ray tube.

data these lines cross in both cases at 91kV. The material of the test filter was lead therefore we know that the knee should be at 88.005keV. This means that the actual value is 3.4% above the set value. In comparison with the reference value made with the voltage divider these values differ about 0.95%. The values of both tubes are equal which leads to the conclusion that this measurement method is transferable to transmission tubes.

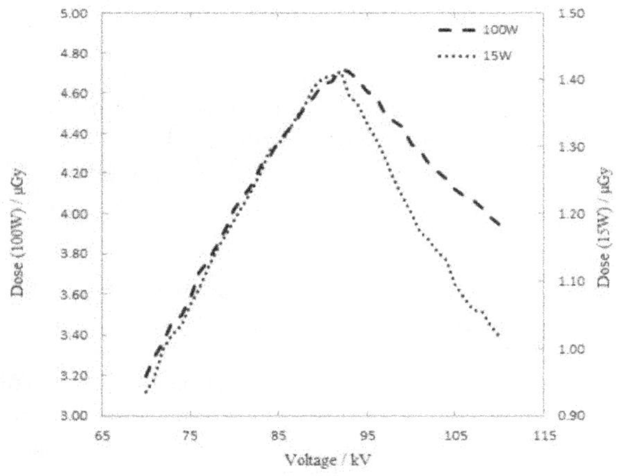

Figure 6: Ratio of the K-shell absorption to the K-shell fluorescence. Data at 100W recorded with standard X-ray tube. Data at 15W recorded with transmission X-ray tube.

4 Conclusion

The measurements have shown that it is possible to generate enough fluorescence radiation signal at a low tube power. In this case the effects of the K-shell radiation and K-shell absorption were even clearer at a low tube power. Additionally the location of the knee at 100W with the standard X-ray tube and the knee at 15W with the transmission X-ray tube where close together. This leads to the conclusion that this measurement method is transferable to transmission X-ray tubes.

So far the executed measurements are not sufficient to realize a complete calibration. To define a complete measurement setup to calibrate a generator several measurements have to follow. In this study the kilovoltage was calibrated at only one value. For a complete measurement setup a characteristic line has to be evaluated by using different elements (e.g. elements listed in table 1) as test-filter. This line could be used to calibrate a generator. The creation of such a test sequence with a characteristic line should be possible. Furthermore the measurement accuracy can be improved as well. So far the accuracy differs about 1% to the reference method with a voltage divider. An improvement of the accuracy should be possible by improving the signal output of the fluorescence radiation and the additional absorption. This might be achievable by using well-defined pre-filter and test filter.

Acknowledgement

The work has been carried out at Yxlon International GmbH in Hamburg. Special thanks to Prof. Dr. T. Gutsmann for being my supervisor.

5 References

[1] J. R. Greening, *The measurement by ionization methods of the peak kilovoltage across X-ray tubes*. London, British Journal of Applied Physics, 1954

[2] T. Laubenberger and L.Laubenberger, *Technik der medizinischen Radiologie*. 7. überarbeitete Auflage, Köln, Deutscher Ärzte-Verlag, S. 40-50, 1999

[3] H. G. Vogt and H. Schultz, *Grundzüge des praktischen Strahlenschutzes*. 4.aktualisierte Auflage, Kösel-Krugzell, Carl Hanser Verlag, 2007

[4] F. Kohlrausch, *Praktische Physik 2*. 24.Auflage, Stuttgart, B.G. Teubner, S. 467-468, 1996

[5] J. H. Hubbel and S. M. Seltzer, *Tables of X-Ray Mass Attenuation Coefficients and Mass Energy-Absorption Coefficients from 1 keV to 20 MeV for Elements Z = 1 to 92 and 48 Additional Substances of Dosimetric Interest*. URL(20.01.2015): http://physics.nist.gov/PhysRefData/XrayMassCoef /tab3.html

[6] DIN EN 12544-1 : 1999, *Spannungsteiler-Verfahren*.

[7] DIN EN 12544-2 : 2000, *Konstanzprüfung mit dem Dickfilter-Verfahren*.

[8] DIN EN 12544-3 : 1999, *Spektrometer-Verfahren*.

Analyzing the Impact of Different Path Termination Conditions in a Probabilistic Fiber Tracking Algorithm

S. Ariyamitr [1] and M. A. Koch [2]

[1] Medizinische Ingenieurwissenschaft, University of Lübeck, ariyamitr@miw.uni-luebeck.de

[2] Institute of Medical Engineering, University of Lübeck, koch@imt.uni-luebeck.de

Abstract

In diffusion tensor magnetic resonance imaging, fiber tracking algorithms that use Monte Carlo simulations still suffer from limitations. This work analyzes an algorithm and the impact of three parameters that cause it to terminate the pathway: the maximum number of jumps, the fractional anisotropy threshold and the angle of the forward cone restricting the jump direction. The criteria used to quantify the results are the length of the detected pathway, the width ratio and the number of branchings for one pathway along the corticospinal tract. The aim is to analyze the changes of these criteria depending on the chosen parameters. It is shown that the performance is massively influenced by how the parameters limit each other. As a consequence, modifying all three parameters slightly but simultaneously has the largest impact. It was found that the impact of the parameter modifications varies depending on the defined region of interest.

1 Introduction

Fiber tractography based on diffusion tensor imaging (DTI) data is a method used to analyze anatomical structures in human brains. It is capable of providing information about fiber bundle orientation in brain white matter which is not obtainable by using conventional magnetic resonance imaging (MRI) [1]. Similar to MRI, DTI is a non-invasive method to acquire in vivo data, i.e. to estimate the connectivity between different areas in the human brain. It was shown that a correlation exists between anatomical connectivity as estimated by fiber tractography and functional connectivity as assessed by MRI [2], [3]. Further fiber tractography provides us with apparent diffusion coefficients (ADC) [4] for each voxel. In fact what we get is an estimation of the fiber bundle pathways. One of our goals is to minimize the chances of indicating wrong connections. The other goal is to be able to track a fiber bundle in its entirety. In this paper we examine the impact of different parameters that cause the Monte Carlo simulation-based fiber tracking algorithm to terminate a pathway. The algorithm evaluates parameters such as fractional anisotropy (FA) [5], restricted propagation angle and maximum number of iterations to decide whether to continue a pathway or to terminate it (so called *jumps*). We analyze the influence on the results to verify the reliability of the implementation.

2 Material and Methods

Around the late 1990s several tractography methods had been proposed [6]. Here, one of the first probabilistic DTI fiber tracking algorithms [2] is used in a slightly modified version. The current study aims at evaluating the algorithm's limitations. The program called dconnect is written in C and called from a Matlab (The MathWorks Inc., Natick, MA, USA) routine providing a simple user interface. In order to use dconnect, the Matlab routine is supposed to be used in combination with statistical parametric mapping (SPM) [7] routines for data preprocessing and result display.

2.1 Data Used for Experiments

The DTI data for our experiments were acquired from a healthy volunteer using a whole-body MR system operating at 3 T (Achieva, Philips, Eindhoven). Diffusion-weighted echo planar imaging with a b-value of 800 s/mm^2 was performed. The b-value is a parameter that indicates the degree of diffusion weighting and reflects the strength and duration of the field gradients applied during data acquisition [9]. The voxel size is (1.75 mm $\times$ 1.75 mm $\times$ 2 mm).

2.2 Data Postprocessing

The data we used for the experiments are diffusion weighted image (DWI) data (see section 2.1). After applying a motion correction to the data the diffusion tensors are calculated. The diffusion tensor,

$$\mathsf{D} = \begin{pmatrix} D_{xx} & D_{xy} & D_{xz} \\ D_{yx} & D_{yy} & D_{yz} \\ D_{zx} & D_{zy} & D_{zz} \end{pmatrix}, \qquad (1)$$

is a symmetric 3x3 matrix, i.e. D_{yx}=D_{xy}, D_{yz}=D_{zy} and D_{xz}=D_{zx}. As a result, only six coefficients are needed to represent D. This matrix is used to describe the diffusivity in each direction [1]. Based on these values a FA map is calculated to describe the degree of diffusion. The FA is defined by

$$FA = \frac{\sqrt{(\lambda_1 - \lambda_2)^2 + (\lambda_2 - \lambda_3)^2 + (\lambda_3 - \lambda_1)^2}}{\sqrt{2}\sqrt{\lambda_1^2 + \lambda_2^2 + \lambda_3^2}} \quad (2)$$

where λ_i are the eigenvalues of the tensor. FA ranges from 0 to 1. A FA of 0 means the diffusion is isotropic, like in free water. So there is no restriction in mobility in any direction. A value of one means that diffusion is confined to one direction.

2.3 Monte Carlo Algorithm

The fiber tracking algorithm computes a map of values for the degree of connectivity between voxels by performing a Monte Carlo simulation. That means, by repeating a random experiment numerous times, we approximate fiber bundle orientations. Considering that, for each region of interest (ROI), a defined start voxel, a jump to an adjacent voxel is performed. From there on further jumps are performed until a termination condition is met. For the selection of the direction we calcute a probability distribution (see chapter 2.3.1). The number of visits for each voxel is an estimate for the strength of the anatomical connection between the voxel and the ROI. We will explain how the algorithm is implemented in dconnect and what the limitations are.

2.3.1 Workflow of the Analyzed Algorithm

The calculation of the connectivity map starts in a given ROI. Vertices of a tesselated sphere define 32 directions in which can possibly be jumped. The directions and the stepsize are used to define the adjacent neighbours which could be visited next. We assume that the probability of jumping in a certain direction is given by the ADC. That is a measure of interaction between a molecule and the surrounding tissue, i.e. the degree of mobility that is affected by the tissue. Probabilities for "forbidden" directions are set to 0. The conditions for a direction to be tagged as forbidden jump direction will be explained later in this chapter. Next up the probabilities are exponentiated with 7 to sharpen the distribution of probabilities. The jump direction is selected using a random number. The random numbers are generated with a distribution determined from the diffusion tensor: jumps along directions with high diffusivity are made more likely. The highest diffusivity direction mostly represents the main fiber direction. These jump calculations are repeated until the program meets a termination condition. The calculation for this ROI is finished when it was performed 4000 times (computed 4000 paths).
Every time a voxel is visited, it is checked whether the FA is below the threshold. In this case or if a tensor element is infinite the pathway is discontinued. A pathway is also discontinued if the fractional anisotropy is below the threshold. This condition prevents the algorithm from leaving the white matter. Depending on the last jump direction, all jump directions which are not in the forward cone angle are tagged as forbidden. Unless one of these conditions is met the algorithm stops the pathway when *n* jumps have been executed where *n* is the maximum number of jumps. The default conditions for terminating a pathway and the changes we applied are shown in Table 1. Parameters that were not changed during the experiments are not listed. For each voxel the maximum number of visits over the 4000 experiments is saved as result.

Table 1: Path Termination Conditions

parameter	default	1st attempt	2nd attempt
njumps	40	15	100
fa_thresh	0.2	0.1	0.4
halfcone	45°	30°	60°

njumps: maximum number of jumps per experiment, fa_thresh: fractional anisotropy threshold, halfcone: opening angle

2.3.2 Limitations

Terminating a pathway too early results in a wrong estimation as the fiber bundle is indicated to be shorter than it really is. We chose three crucial parameters in order to assess their impact on the outcome. The maximum number of jumps *njumps* per experiment is the first one. If this value is set too low the pathway will be terminated even if the end of the fiber bundle has not been reached. The parameter *fa_thresh* is the threshold which has to be exceeded not to terminate the pathway. Setting this value too low allows the algorithm to jump outside the white matter and reaching gray matter. This case have to be avoided since only in white matter diffusion tensors provide valid information about fiber bundle orientations. Choosing this parameter too high will allow only jumps to very coherent tissue. Crossing fibers that lower the FA in the current voxel would easily terminate the pathway. *Halfcone* restricts the jump direction to a certain forward cone. Depending on how this parameter is chosen the pathway avoids curves or could allow jumps perpendicular to the last jump direction. Our goal is not only to find parameters which grants better results but to figure out how reliable the algorithm is if these parameters change. Finding appropiate values is not the only challenge. Another problem comes with the resolution of DTI which is around 2 mm. Fibers in brain white matter have a thickness of only a few µm. The ADCs are calculated voxel-wise. Thus one tensor does not reflect the properties of a single fiber but of a collective of fibers. Particularly for voxels with crossing fibers it is hard to tell from the tensor how the fibers might be oriented [8].

2.4 Criteria to Quantify the Results

Two sets of experiments were executed. For the first set the ROIs were chosen near the motor cortex, for the second near the pons (Po). In both cases the aim was to follow the corticospinal tract (CST). After determining a reference output by using the default parameters, the termination conditions are modified as shown in Table 1. The two output images for the default parameters are shown in Figure 1. Three properties are examined in one specified coronal slice. The first property gives some indication of how far the algorithm was able to follow the pathway along the CST before and after the parameters were changed. The distance between the ROI area and the furthest end of the pathway was determined for the reference run and the experiment. The difference between these distances is δ. This value is measured in voxel size. It is 0 if modifying parameters has no impact on the result and the value is larger the more the pathways differ in length. The second property is the width ratio at the end of the estimated fiber bundle. Therefore we measure the width of the estimated fiber bundle's end for both the reference and the experiment. The ratio between these values is the width ratio ω. If the pathway of an experiment ends because the estimated bundle is thinning out the ratio decreases. That would suggest that it is not njumps that limits the tracking process. Otherwise a high width ratio indicates a larger spread at the end of the pathway which means focusing the jumps could help tracking a longer pathway in this direction. The last property is the spread and serves as an additional, more subjective criterion. That is the number of branchings outbounding from the main fiber bundle. If compared to the reference this number is decreased, we can assume that focusing parameters are massively influencing the outcome, e.g. if halfcone is too low.

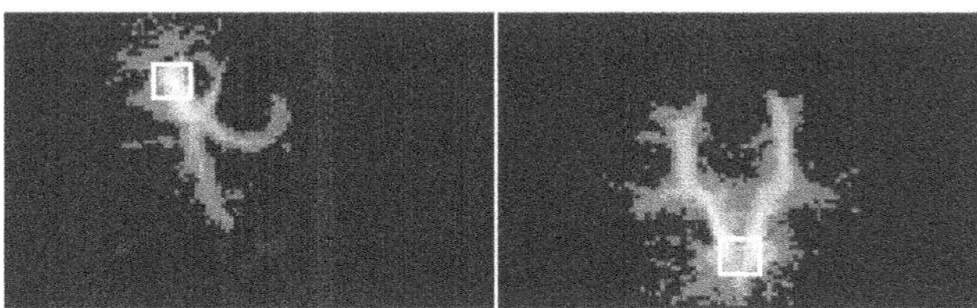

Figure 1: non diffusion-weighted image (background) for ROI (indicated by white boxes) at MC (left) and at Po (right) overlayed with the corresponding determined connectivity map for default parameters. The overlays depict the number of visits normalized to 32767 for better visualization.

3 Results and Discussion

The resulting properties for the two examined ROI areas are shown in Table 2 and Table 3.

3.1 Experiments

The results show that the impact of changing *njumps* greatly depends on the ROI. Varying *njumps* has a similar large effect on δ for both ROIs. In contrast to that, the influence on the count of branchings strongly depends on the ROI. Starting near the MC a change of njumps does not lead to more/less branchings. Whereas if we start fiber tracking near the Po modifying *njumps* leads to quite different results. The influence of the FA threshold seems to have the most significant impact on the results. When choosing a low value for *fa_thresh* the maximum tracking distance almost stays the same but the algorithm starts jumping out of the white matter. This is why there is a "X" in Table 3 in the last column. In this case the resulting pattern looks like there were no restriction to the jump directions so that it is not possible to properly identify branchings. For high *fa_thresh* the distance between the ROIs and the end of the indicated pathway increases a lot.

3.2 Discussion

The first thing we can infer is the most obvious fact that the FA threshold has the largest effect on the results. Independent from where you start tracking, the FA threshold has a large influence on how long the indicated fiber bundle can be, how precise (or focused) the proposed bundles are and how likely branchings are detected. Due to fact that lowering the FA threshold only slightly changes δ we can assume that another value is limitting efforts in tracking the CST. If raising njumps increases the maximum distance between the ROI and the end of the pathway (so that there is a new end of the fiber bundle) that indicates that the estimated fiber bundle does not end in this voxel because of reaching gray matter or the end of the pathway. Knowing that, one could attempt improving the algorithm by implementing njumps not as a fixed value but as a value derived from the FA in the current voxel or in the adjacent voxels. On the other hand decreasing halfcone considerably focuses the pathway preventing the thinning towards the end of a bundle. The results imply that the best way to improve the outcome when tracking the CST is to slightly decrease halfcone and increase *njumps* and *fa_thresh*. We started a new run with following parameters: *njumps=70, fa_thres=0.25 and halfcone=35°*. In Fig. 2 the result is shown right next to results of the reference outcome. We are able to gain more distance and a more focused bundle. The end of the determined fiber bundle is noticeably closer to the MC (Fig. 2, right) than in the reference image (Fig. 2, left). In addition, the indicated fiber bundle is more focused, meaning that the algorithm less likely jumps into gray matter. However, the results do not seem to offer an solution to the crossing fibers problem.

Table 2: Results of Trait Comparison for ROI at MC

parameter	value	δ	ω	branchings (current:default)
njumps	15	-19.93	1	3:3
njumps	100	19.93	0.51	4:3
fa_thresh	0.1	5.10	1.29	5:3
fa_thresh	0.4	-25.63	2.6	0:3
halfcone	30°	17.49	0.36	1:3
halfcone	60°	-3.1	0.80	4:3

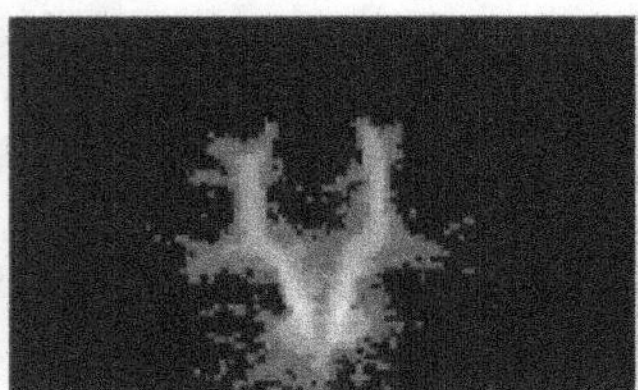
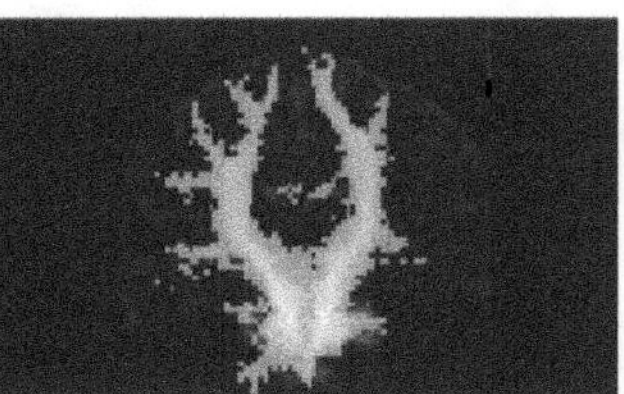

Figure 2: Results of performing dconnect for ROI at Po with default parameters (left) and slightly modified parameters as proposed in chapter 3 (right) overlayed on top of a non diffusion-weighted image(background). The overlays depict the number of visits normalized to 3276 for better visualization.

Table 3: Results of Trait Comparison for ROI at Po

parameter	value	δ	ω	branchings (current:default)
njumps	15	-11.00	2.78	3:7
njumps	100	13.75	0.54	10:7
fa_thresh	0.1	1	0.77	X:7
fa_thresh	0.4	-25.63	2.6	2:7
halfcone	30°	8.66	0.38	4:7
halfcone	60°	-3.1	0.80	7:7

4 Conclusion

The impact of the examined parameters on the result of a probabilistic tracking algorithm can hardly be evaluated one by one. It is necessary to know which parameter causes the pathway to be terminated. According to the anatomical structure it is important to adapt the parameters to the ROI and the pathway that is to be tracked. Hence, it is more promising to slightly modify not only one parameter. For tracking the CST starting in the pons it is advisable to constrict the angle of the forward cone slightly, increase the FA threshold and make sure the pathway is not terminated prematurely (e.g. in the internal capsule) due to reaching the maximum number of jumps. Additionally more insights could be provided if more systematic experiments were performed. For more insights a comparison to other algorithms could be considered.

Acknowledgement

The work has been carried out at the Institute of Medical Engineering, University of Lübeck.

5 References

[1] P. J. Basser, J. Mattiello, D. Le Bihan, *Estimation of the effective self-diffusion tensor from the NMR spin echo*. Journal of Magnetic Resonance, vol. 103, pp. 247–254, 1994

[2] M. A. Koch, D. G. Norris, M. Hund-Georgiadis, *An investigation of functional and anatomical connectivity using magnetic resonance imaging*. NeuroImage, vol. 16, pp. 241–250, 2002.

[3] C .J. Honey et al., *Predicting human resting-state functional connectivity from structural connectivity*. Proceedings of the National Academy of Sciences, vol. 106, pp. 2035–2040, 2009

[4] P. J. Basser, D. K. Jones, *Diffusion-tensor MRI: Theory, Experimental Design and Data Analysis - a technical review*. NMR in Biomedicine, vol. 15, pp. 456–467, 2002.

[5] P. J. Basser, C. Pierpaoli, *Microstructural and physiological features of tissues elucidated by quantitative-diffusion-tensor MRI*. Journal of Magnetic Resonance, vol. 111, pp. 209–219, 1994.

[6] P. J. Basser, S. Pajevic, C. Pierpaoli, J. Duda, A. Aldroubi, *In vivo fiber tractography using DT-MRI data*. Magnetic Resonance in Medicine, vol. 44 pp. 625–632, 2000.

[7] W. Penny, K. Friston, J. Ashburner, S. Kiebel, T. Nichols, *Statistical aarametric mapping: The analysis of functional brain images*. Academic Press, 2006.

[8] B. W. Kreher et al., *Connecting and merging fibres: Pathway extraction by combining probability maps*. NeuroImage, vol. 43, pp. 81–89, 2008.

[9] J. Graessner, *Frequently asked questions: diffusion-weighted imaging (DWI)*. Magnetom Flash, vol. 1/2011, pp. 84–87, 2011.

Measurement and Analysis of the respiration-driven Motion of the Pulmonary Artery

S. Malterer [1], J. Ehrhardt [2], A. Frydrychowicz [3], T. Oechtering [3] and H. Handels [2]
[1] Medizinische Ingenierwissenschaft , Universität zu Lübeck, stefan.malterer@miw.uni-luebeck.de
[2] Institut für Medizinische Informatik, Universität zu Lübeck, {ehrhardt, handels}@imi.uni-luebeck.de
[3] Klinik für Radiologie und Nuklearmed., UKSH Campus Lübeck, {Alex.Frydrychowicz, Thekla.Oechtering}@uksh.de

Abstract

4D-MRI allows for measuring involuntary motion of the human body while scanning. For example, using velocity-encoded phase contrast sequences, it is possible to measure blood flow inside of the respiratory system's blood vessels. Unfortunately, the measurement's quality itself is degraded by said motion. This project aims at the quantification of the respiratory-driven motion of the pulmonary vessels, especially the pulmonary artery. This is achieved by using displacement fields created by using non-linear image registration over multiple time-points. The motion of three points surrogating for the motion of the diaphragm, the heart and the pulmonary artery are extracted. Correlation analysis is conducted to link these motions to each other. Afterwards, regression analysis using a linear model is conducted. Two coronal 2D MRI datasets were used. They showed fairly reasonable correlation. Furthermore, the linear regression model held up better than expected despite of its heavily simplified character.

1 Introduction

When imaging patients or living subjects, whether employing MRI or any other given modality, involuntary motion is bound to cause complications. The problem especially persists in 4D image acquisition. Even though clinical applications of 4D imaging usually aim at measuring motion in a living system, the distortion caused by the patients' movements renders image-processing-based diagnosis more challenging than it would be in a motionless object. In the particular case presented, it is even more difficult.
The clinical motivation of this study is the analysis of the pulmonary vessel system's blood flow based on velocity-encoded phase contrast 4D MRI [1]. The problem at hand is, that while it is intended to measure the vascular blood flow, respiratory and heartbeat driven motion distort and move the pulmonary artery.
Up to date, the only way to reduce the influence of respiratory-driven motion or heartbeat is gated MRI acquisition which result in significantly longer acquisition times. A possible way to prevent long acquisition times would be, for example, to correct the motion of the pulmonary artery (PA) while imaging by using only a breath monitor to acquire the respiratory motion's influence without prolonging the image acquisition.
As a first step to reach this aim, one objective of this study is to measure the extent of motion of the pulmonary artery. Secondly, as the motion exerted by the pulmonary artery is influenced by both, heartbeat and respiratory motion, our work was an attempt to use statistical means to link these confounding factors.

2 Material and Methods

For the results presented in here, two datasets were acquired from volunteering subjects, by the Department of Radiology of the Universitätsklinikum Schleswig-Holstein in Lübeck. Both datasets consist of 2D coronal MRI slices through the thorax and show the internal organs in the mediastinum. They were part of an imageset containing various kinds of images. The images were acquired as a part of a study to analyze the intravascular bloodflow in 4D MRI. Regardless of the study's original purpose, these particular images were acquired to analyse respiration- and heartbeat-driven motion.
To be able to analyze the various motions in the mediastinum and their influence on bloodflow measurement, the images were acquired without any gating. Thus, the subjects were allowed to breathe freely and there was no ECG-triggering.
The first dataset consists of 45 images acquired with a temporal resolution of 1.6 seconds and a spatial resolution of 0.8 mm. The second dataset consists of 200 images with a temporal resolution of 0.2 seconds and a spatial resolution of 1.988 mm. Due to the need for high and diverse soft tissue contrast as well as speed during the acquisition of a single slice, two different balanced steady-state free precession (b-SSFP) [2] pulse sequences were used to acquire both datasets (first dataset: "WIP B-TFE_FB CLEAR", second dataset: "WIP sBFFE_RLT SENSE"). Both pulse sequences are implemented on a clinical 3T Philips Ingenia MRI scanner (Philips Healthcare, Hamburg, Germany).

2.1 Quantification of Motion and Image Registration

The acquired images $I_1, ..., I_n$ show movement over time due to being acquired at n different time-points. Thus, it is possible to track the motion of organic structures by measuring the structures' displacement from image to image. For this purpose, one image I_R is selected as a fixed image to be compared to all other images.
The quantification of internal motion was achieved using displacement fields created by a non-linear variational image registration algorithm [3]. This implementation uses a variational framework with interchangeable distance measures (D) and regularizers (S), solving for:

$$J[\phi_j] := D[I_R, I_j \circ \phi_j] + S[\phi_j] = min \qquad (1)$$

with $\phi_1, ..., \phi_n$ being the transformation of the image, at each of the n time-points, the moving image I_j at time-point $j (j = 1, ..., n)$ undergoes to match the reference image I_R. For I_R an image depicting a state of maximal expiration was selected. The optimization problem of the energy functional J is solved by analytically derivating (1) to formulate as an Euler-Lagrange-Equation. This way, a local minimum of J can be found by solving the partial differential equation (2) by using a gradient descent approach.

$$f(\boldsymbol{p}, \boldsymbol{u}(\boldsymbol{p})) - A[\boldsymbol{u}](\boldsymbol{p}) = 0, \boldsymbol{p} \in \Omega \qquad (2)$$

With $\boldsymbol{u} : \Omega \rightarrow \mathbb{R}^2$ being the actual displacement field to be calculated by the registration algorithm, A being a linear operator resulting from the regularization term and f denoting the force term derived from D. $\boldsymbol{p}$ denotes a single point of I_j, thus $\boldsymbol{\phi}_j(\boldsymbol{p}) = \boldsymbol{p} + \boldsymbol{u_j}$, with $\boldsymbol{u_j}(\boldsymbol{p}) = (x_j(\boldsymbol{p}), y_j(\boldsymbol{p}))^T$ where $(x_j(\boldsymbol{p})$ denotes the horizontal (right-left or x) and $y_j(\boldsymbol{p})$ the vertical (superior-inferior or y) component of $\boldsymbol{u_j}(\boldsymbol{p})$.
The different force terms include an SSD-based (Sum of Squared Differences) approach, the original Demon forces (3) and Normalized Cross Correlation (NCC). The regularizers available consist of diffusion based, gaussian and elastic approaches.

$$\boldsymbol{f}^{Demons}(\boldsymbol{\phi}) := \frac{(I_R - I_j \circ \boldsymbol{\phi}) \cdot (\bigtriangledown I_R)}{\parallel \bigtriangledown I_R) \parallel^2 + \alpha \cdot (I_R - I_j \circ \boldsymbol{\phi})^2} \qquad (3)$$

The Demon forces algorithm was introduced by Thirion and has been popular ever since. It is based on the SSD approach with alternate formulations in the force term. The parameter $\alpha \neq 0$ can be used to prevent errors in areas with low image contrast. This property is a huge advantage of the Demons algorithm in our application due to the numerous soft tissue types dealt with in cardiovascular imaging being confined in very limited space.
The evaluation of these methods has already been covered in length. Corresponding to the conclusions made in [4] we used the default parameters, Demons and diffusion based regularisation.

2.2 Correlation Analysis

To statistically connect the movements of two (or more) organic structures the linear dependency has to be quantified. This way, the relationships between those motions can be analyzed and estimated. As a means of quantification we used the Pearson correlation coefficient (4).

$$\varrho_e(r, s) := \frac{\frac{1}{n-1}\sum_{i=1}^{n}(r_i - \bar{r})(s_i - \bar{s})}{\sqrt{\frac{1}{n-1}\sum_{i=1}^{n}(r_i - \bar{r})^2} \cdot \sqrt{\frac{1}{n-1}\sum_{i=1}^{n}(s_i - \bar{s})^2}}. \qquad (4)$$

with r and s being the same component of two movements to be correlated.
By correlating those motions, the influences of respiratory-driven motion and heartbeat-driven motion concerning the pulmonary artery's motion can be estimated. This knowledge might give us the possibility to extract the influence of one of those motions mathematically to reach our aforementioned aim and correct the movement exerted by the pulmonary artery during image acquisition.

2.2.1 Image based Motion Tracking

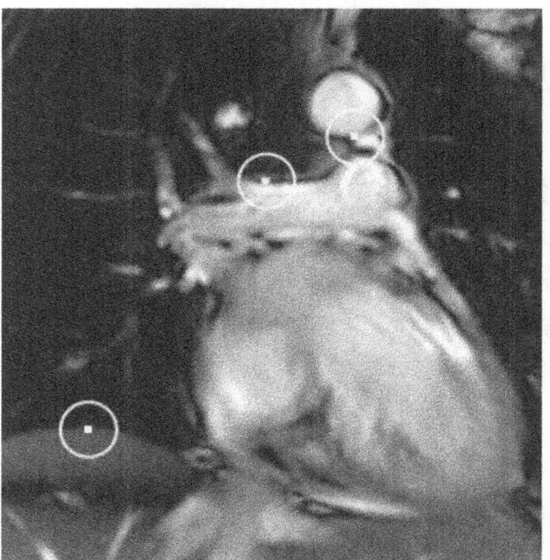

Figure 1: Pixels selected as surrogating points for organic motion

The three organic structures, the diaphragm as a surrogate for the respiration driven motion, the aorta, representing the heartbeat driven motion and the pulmonary artery are tracked. This is done by selecting single pixels surrogating each structure in the reference image I_R (Fig. 1). The pixels' motion can be extracted from the displacement field yielded by the image registration for each time point (see also Fig. 2).

2.3 Regression Analysis

After the motion of the aorta, the pulmonary artery and the diaphragm have been quantified using image registration and correlated using Pearson's correlation coefficient, the connection is further analyzed using regression analysis. We assumed a multivariant linear model to connect the motion of the aorta and the diaphragm to that of the pulmonary artery (5).

$$\boldsymbol{Y} = \boldsymbol{X}\boldsymbol{B} + \boldsymbol{E} \quad (5)$$

where $E(\mathbf{E}) = \mathbf{0}$ [5], assuming a normal distributed error, with $\boldsymbol{Y} = \begin{pmatrix} x_1(p_p) & y_1(p_p) \\ \vdots & \vdots \\ x_n(p_p) & y_n(p_p) \end{pmatrix}$, $\boldsymbol{B} = \begin{pmatrix} b_{0x} & b_{0y} \\ \vdots & \vdots \\ b_{4x} & b_{4y} \end{pmatrix}$

and $\boldsymbol{X} = \begin{pmatrix} 1 & x_1(p_d) & y_1(p_d) & x_1(p_a) & y_1(p_a) \\ \vdots & \vdots & \vdots & \vdots & \vdots \\ 1 & x_n(p_d) & y_n(p_d) & x_n(p_a) & y_n(p_a) \end{pmatrix}$.

The regression coefficients for x and y directions are denoted b_{jx} and b_{jy} respectively; $x/y_j(p_{a/d/p})$ denotes the x- or y-component of either the aorta's, the diaphragm's or the pulmonary artery's motion.

Thus, (5) is solved using a linear least-squares algorithm implemented in Matlab. Once the regression coefficients have been calculated, the model has been tested using the originally recorded movements $(x_j(p_d), y_j(p_d), x_j(p_a), y_j(p_a))$ to recreate ("predict") $y_j^*(p_p)$.

To assess the quality of the prediction of the pulmonary artery's motion, the rooted mean squared difference (RMS) between the actually measured motion and the estimated motion is calculated.

3 Results and Discussion

Since the image registration implementation used was not part of this research, the outcome of the image registration will neither be shown nor discussed here, though it has been visually inspected to ensure plausibility. The correlation analysis and all figures depicting movement in the following are only showing motion in the y/SI-direction (superior-inferior) as motion in the x-direction (lateral) was far smaller (± 2 mm).

3.1 Correlation Analysis

Table 1 shows the calculated Pearson's correlation coefficients for both datasets. All possible combinations of movement correlate highly, with the highest correlation between PA and diaphragm. Fig. 2 shows an exemplary plot of the movements exerted by diaphragm and pulmonary artery (extracted from dataset 2).

Table 1: Correlation coefficients

Correlated Structures (in SI-Direction)	C. Coefficients Dataset 1	C. Coefficients Dataset 2
aorta and PA	0.87	0.85
aorta and diaphragm	0.8	0.84
diaphragm and PA	0.92	0.94

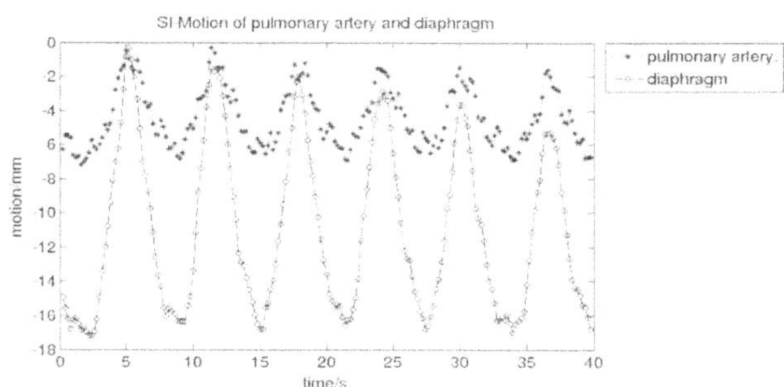

Figure 2: Motion of diaphragm and pulmonary artery in SI-Direction plotted over time

3.2 Regression Analysis and Prediction of Motion

Table 2 shows the estimated regression coefficients for both datasets in the Y-direction. Not only the coefficients' order (mostly) but also the coefficients' sign match their counterpart for the other dataset. The only noteworthy difference is the magnitude of both b_{4y} values.

Table 2: Regression coefficients

Regression Coefficients	R. Coefficients Dataset 1	R. Coefficients Dataset 2
b_{0y}	-0.206	-0.132
b_{1y}	-0.075	-0.107
b_{2y}	0.248	0.282
b_{3y}	-0.403	-0.229
b_{4y}	0.630	0.233

Fig. 3 a-b show the results of the prediction of the pulmonary artery's motion based on heartbeat and respiratory driven motion for both datasets. The RMS between the prediction of the first dataset ($y_j^*(p_p)$) and the actually recorded motion of the first dataset ($y_j(p_p)$) (Fig. 3 a) was 0.53 mm using 44 data points. The second dataset's prediction assessment (Fig. 3 b) yielded a RMS of 0.44 mm using 199 data points.

3.3 Discussion

The correlation analysis shows that all structures' movements are linked to each other and the acquired image sets seem eligible to depict motion in the mediastinum. This is supported by the temporal accordance both curves in Fig. 2 show. As Fig. 3 shows, the motion amplitude in SI direction of the PA is roughly 7 mm. This, with the PA having a diameter of roughly 18-28 mm, is too much to ignore and consequently needs to be compensated.

An omnipresent problem when attempting to compare multiple datasets acquired from multiple human sources are structural (pathological as well as physiological) differences.

To explain the differences in the regression coefficients, two aspects come to mind (beside structural differences). Firstly, the selection of the surrogating points is manual and

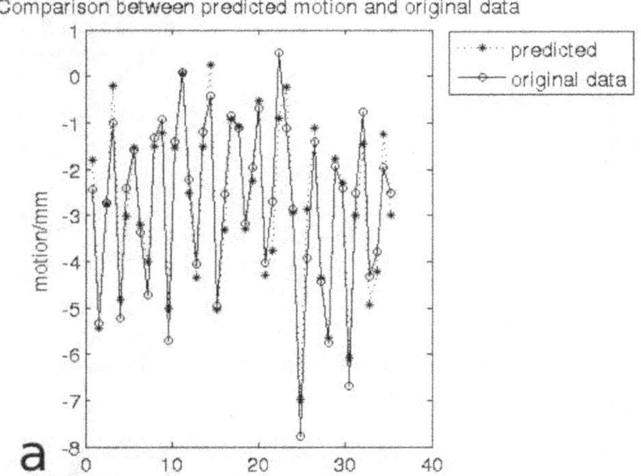

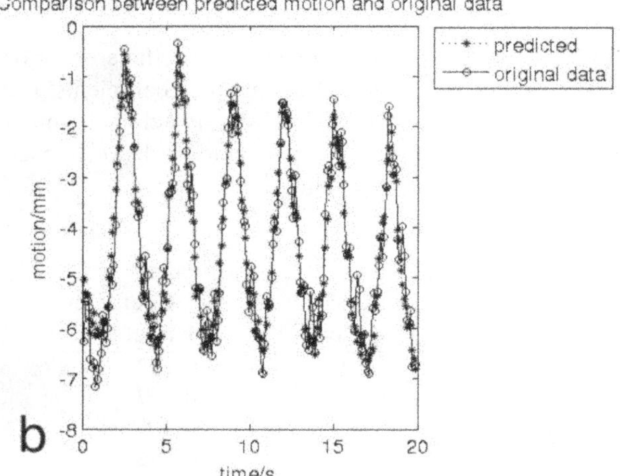

Figure 3: Comparison between the original movements extracted from the images and the predicted movements using regression analysis. Fig. 3a: Dataset 1, Fig. 3b: Dataset 2

thus prone to errors, especially when it is not necessarily given, that the slices of the datasets shows the exact same region (in the anterior-posterior (AP) direction). Secondly, the influence of the differences in the images in term of temporal and spatial resolution is at this state unclear.
Selecting the surrogate for respiratory driven motion was straightforward by placing the point on top of the liver while trying to keep as much distance as possible to other soft tissue structures. The point representing the pulmonary artery was placed on the cranial edge of the pulmonary artery due to the relatively desirable soft tissue contrast.
The surrogating point for the heartbeat, however, was far more challenging to select, as it is hard to tell from 2D images which structures move because of respiration or heartbeat. To keep the highest possible distance to the lung parenchyma, the aorta was selected to surrogate for the heartbeat driven motion, as there appears to be no physical tissue connection to the lungs and the aorta is known to exert strong motion during the heartbeat. However, the correlation analysis shows that the aorta's motion is influenced by respiration. Furthermore, the choice of single points for complex movements, such as the twist the heart undergoes while contracting, is one of the possible weak points of our model.

4 Conclusion

We have shown that there is a need for compensating the motion of the pulmonary artery in 4D MRI. However, to obtain more reliable results concerning correlation and regression analysis, acquiring more data is critical.
Even though the results of the regression analysis have been, so far, better than expected, the model we assumed is still heavily simplified and may be in need of further improvements once more data has been acquired. Other possible models may include polynomial models, sum-of-sine-based models and exponential models. Due to the asymmetrical character of both, respiratory and cardiac cycle, the need for combining multiple approaches might arise as well.

Acknowledgement

The work has been carried out at the Institute for Medical Informatics at the Universität zu Lübeck, in cooperation with the department for radiology and nuclear medicine of the UKSH Campus Lübeck.

5 References

[1] M. Markl, A. Frydrychowicz, S. Kozerke, M. Hope, and O. Wieben, "4D flow MRI," *Journal of Magnetic Resonance Imaging*, vol. 36, no. 5, pp. 1015–1036, 2012.

[2] O. Bieri and K. Scheffler, "Fundamentals of balanced steady state free precession MRI ," *Journal of Magnetic Resonance Imaging*, vol. 38, no. 1, pp. 2–11, 2013.

[3] A. Schmidt-Richberg, R. Werner, H. Handels, and J. Ehrhardt, "A flexible variational registration framework," *Available: http://www.insight-journal.org/browse/publication/917 [last accessed on 6.2.2015]*, 05 2014.

[4] R. Werner, A. Schmidt-Richberg, H. Handels, and J. Ehrhardt, "Estimation of lung motion fields in 4D CT data by variational non-linear intensity-based registration: A comparison and evaluation study.," *Physics in Medicine and Biology*, vol. 59, no. 15, p. 4247, 2014.

[5] L. Fahrmeir and A. Hamerle, *Multivariate statistische Verfahren*. de Gruyter, 1984.

Respiratory Surface Motion Measurement by Microsoft Kinect: Implementation and Evaluation of a clinical Setup

J. Ortmüller [1], R. Werner [2], M. Wilms [3], H. Handels [3] and T. Gauer [5]

[1] Medizinische Ingenieurwissenschaft, Universität zu Lübeck, ortmueller@miw.uni-luebeck.de

[2] Department of Computational Neuroscience, University Medical Center Hamburg-Eppendorf, r.werner@uke.de

[3] Institute of Medical Informatics, Universität zu Lübeck, {wilms, handels} @imi.uni-luebeck.de

[5] Department of Radiotherapy and Radio-Oncology, University Medical Center Hamburg-Eppendorf, t.gauer@uke.de

Abstract

In radiotherapy of abdominal or thoracic tumors, respiratory motion is a problem for an accurate treatment. Most motion compensation techniques require a breathing signal from the patient. The systems in clinical use usually work with 1D signals to describe the respiratory motion. Due to the fact that a 1D signal is not able to describe all breathing variations, in this work the Microsoft Kinect, which can record multidimensional breathing signals, is used. For the Kinect, a measurement setup is designed and measurements are compared to the Varian RPM system (clinical standard). The results show that both signals are temporally well aligned but with differences in the amplitude. A comparison of Kinect signals from different regions on the chest shows variations between these signals. This indicates that the use of a system, which provides multidimensional signals is worthwhile as related knowledge about breathing variations could be integrated into clinical tasks.

1 Introduction

Radiation therapy of tumors is – besides surgery and chemotherapy – one important component in tumor therapy. For tumors in abdominal or thoracic regions, respiratory motion is a major challenge during therapy. It leads to a movement of the tumor during the respiratory cycle up to two centimetres [1]. One way to compensate for tumor motion is to increase safety margins to cover the complete motion range. Technical solutions for motion compensation are tumor tracking [2] and gating [3]. Tumor tracking is an active process with the radiation beam following the tumor motion. Gating means that the radiation is only active when the tumor is located at a predefined position window. For the use of this technique, especially a breathing signal from the patient is required. Similarly, breathing signals are required for reconstruction of 4D-CT data, which often form the basis of treatment planning for abdominal and thoracic tumors. This can be an internal or external breathing signal. An example for an internal breathing signal is the movement of the diaphragm captured with fluoroscopy imaging. By fluoroscopy imaging, the patient is exposed to extra radiation, so mostly external breathing signals are used. External signals used in clinical practise are often one dimensional surrogat signals like spirometers, abdominal belts or the Varian RPM system. The RPM system captures the surface motion at one certain point of the chest and, a possible change from abdominal to thoracic breathing can not be captured. This kind of changes in respiratory motion is a problem during imaging and radiation. To describe these variations in respiratory motion, it is necessary to use multidimensional breathing signals [4]. Techniques to acquire multidimensional breathing signals are range image systems, which usually work with structured light [5] (e.g. the Microsoft Kinect) or with Time-of-Flight (ToF) [6]. Such systems do not need any additional marker on the surface and it is possible to extract signals from different surface regions simultaneously.

The equipment for recording respiratory surface motion in the University Medical Center Hamburg-Eppendorf is the RPM system. In this work a setup for recording multidimensional breathing signals with a low cost camera (Microsoft Kinect) is designed, evaluated and compared to the RPM system.

2 Material and Methods

2.1 Hard and Software Equipment

2.1.1 Microsoft Kinect

Camera System: The Microsoft Kinect is a low cost range sensor which is equipped with three different devices: a colour camera, an infrared camera and an infrared projector. The infrared sensor of the Kinect has a resolution of 1200x960 pixels but for further processing and bandwidth limitation of the USB port the resolution is reduced to 640x480 pixels. The opening angle of the camera is 43°

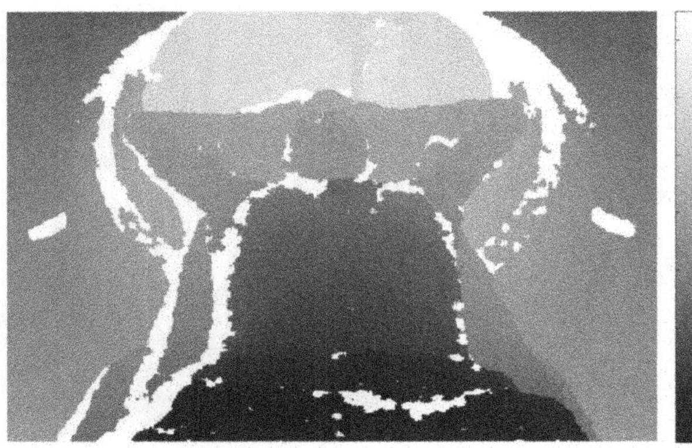

Figure 1: Depth map from a test person. In the back of the photo is the CT gantry. The test person is located in front of the CT on the CT couch. From areas that are coloured white, the Kinect does not receive any dot pattern, i.e. there is no depth information available from these areas.

vertical and 57° horizontal. The framerate of the Kinect is 30 frames/sec and the principle of the depth measurement of the sensor is structured light. The Kinect emits a dot pattern, that is reflected from an object in front of the camera and is captured by the infrared camera. By comparison of the received dot pattern to a reference pattern, the distance to the object can be calculated. For further information see [7].

To connect the Kinect with a computer, we used the libfreenect software from the *OpenKinect Project* [8]. Our in-house developed python program uses the libfreenect library to record the Kinect signals and the captured depth maps (see figure 1) are saved as Matlab matrixes. For the signal extraction, a Matlab program is used, which averages the distance values from a predefined region of interest in every recorded time step. It is possible to select several regions of interest of the entire Field of View for evaluation purposes.

Calibration of the depth measurement: For an accurate measurement it is important to calibrate the Kinect raw disparity value d_{raw} to the real distance D of an object to the camera. The mathematical model behind the conversion is described in [7]. There exists a linear relation between the inverse of the real distance D to the measured raw value of the Kinect:

$$D^{-1} = a \cdot d_{raw} + b \tag{1}$$

Thus, the real distance can be calculated by the inversion of equation 1. For determining the parameter a and b in equation 1, a linear regression is performed and therefore several known distances to the sensor must be measured. This is done for the Kinect and the results are presented in section 3.

2.1.2 Varian RPM System

The Varian RPM system is a clinical in used system to measure an external respiratory motion signal. For measurement, a marker block with six reflective markers is placed on the patient's surface and the movement of this block is captured in all spatial directions by an infrared camera. This infrared camera captures the reflected infrared light from the marker block. From the position of the markers over the time, a motion signal is calculated. For more details see [9].

2.1.3 4D Motion Platform

For an analysis of the potential of the Kinect as a respiratory motion sensor, a 4D motion platform is used [10]. This platform is computer–controlled and able to move in all three spatial directions whereby it is possible to simulate a reproducible motion trajectory. This motion trajectory can be a simple sinusoidal trajectory or a real patient trajectory, e.g. an extracted RPM signal.

2.2 Study Design

2.2.1 Measurement Setup

In the first part of our study, the measurement setup is installed in the CT room with relation to the potential application of the Kinect measurements in reconstruction of 4D-CT data or tumor gating (which also requires a 4D-CT dataset for planning). The goal was to find a camera position on condition that the setup does not interfere with the clinical work flow. One important clinical restriction to the setup is the RPM system, in so far as the RPM system should not get influenced by the Kinect camera. Furthermore, the Kinect itself has some restrictions which should be noted during the design of the setup. At first, the distance from the measured surface to the camera should be between 0.7 m and 1 m to get a signal with reasonable noise ratio. A second parameter is the angle between the optical axis of the Kinect to the measured surface because a large angle results in more reflected light from the surface to be captured by the camera. In literature, there are also some setups for recording respiratory motion with a Kinect or ToF camera [6, 11, 5], which had an influence on the design.

2.2.2 Experiments

At first, a calibration measurement series of the Kinect, as mentioned in section 2.1.1, is performed and the calibration parameters are computed. The second experiment is a comparison between the RPM signal and the Kinect signal for a sinusoidal movement of the 4D motion platform. In the third experiment, we compare Kinect signals, which are extracted from different regions on the upper body of a test person, e.g. one region at the thorax and one at the abdomen.

3 Results and Discussion

3.1 Measurement Setup

The first result in this paper is the developed measurement setup. The general conditions for the setup are described

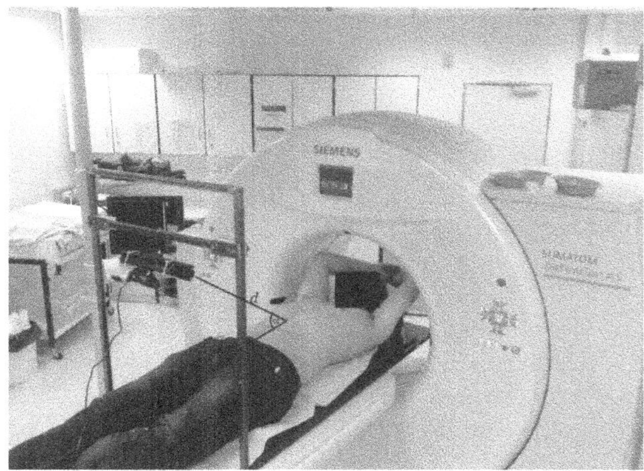

Figure 2: Photo of the experimental setup with a test person. The position of the camera and the test person is similar to the measurement setup. The CT gantry is located above the head of the test person. The angle α and the distance d to the chest are shown.

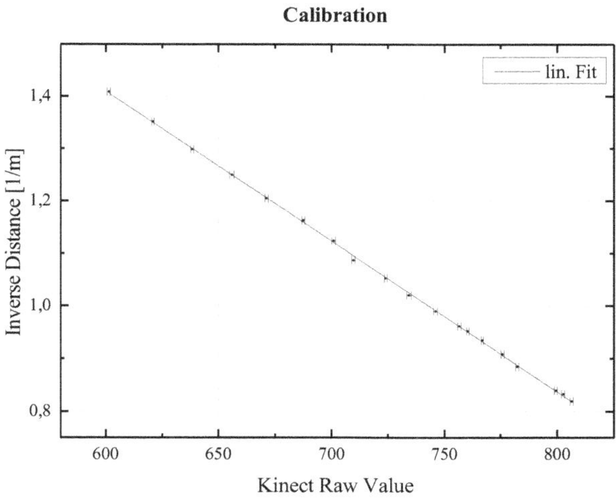

Figure 3: Plots of the linear fit through the calibration measurements and the corresponding standard deviation of the Kinect raw values in the selected ROI.

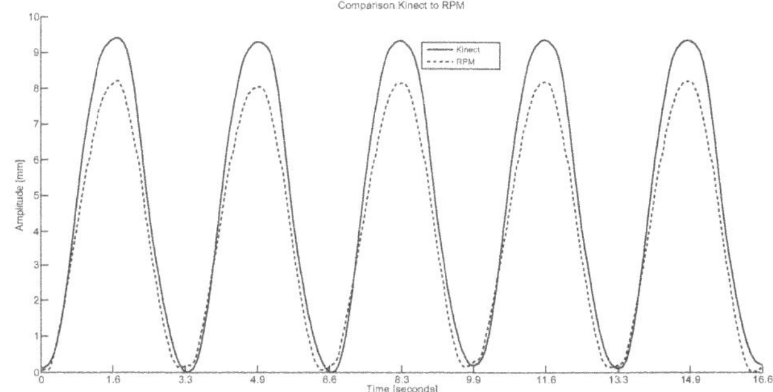

Figure 4: Comparison of the Kinect with RPM signal. The two signals are temporally very well aligned. The amplitude of the motion phantom was 8 millimeter.

in section 2.2.1. According to these, the Kinect is positioned centred over the CT table because in this way the field of view of the Kinect covers the whole chest of a person and the RPM system is not affected as apparent in figure 2. The field of view from the RPM system is always under the Kinect mounting. The construction is clamped to the table with the advantage that the table movement during a spiral CT must not be compensated. The height of the camera above the person is individually adjustable in that way that the gantry of the CT does not interfere with the field of view from the Kinect. The analysis of this chosen setup shows that the table movement has no influence on the image quality. Also the in room lasers that are used for positioning the person have no influence.

3.2 Calibration Results

The first experiment was the calibration of the Kinect. For the calibration, 19 well-known distances from 0.7 m to 1.22 m were measured. For the analysis of the calibration parameters the inverse of the real distance is plotted against the raw Kinect value (see figure 3). The Kinect raw value is the average of a selected ROI (regions of interest) in the Kinect depth map. The plots confirm the result of the literature that there exists a linear relation between the raw and the real distance. The analysis of the linear fitting delivers the two calibration parameters: $a = -2.86 \cdot 10^{-6}$ and $b = 0.0031$. These parameters are used in the subsequent experiments for conversion of the raw values to a distance in millimetres. Figure 3 also shows the standard deviation of the Kinect raw value in the selected ROI. The mean standard deviation over the whole measurement in the selected ROI amounts to 0.71 raw values.

3.3 Comparison Kinect to RPM System

The next experiment was the comparison between the Kinect and the RPM signal. For these measurements, the 4D motion platform is used. The platform trajectory was a sinusoidal curve in AP (anterior and posterior) direction with an amplitude of 8 mm. The comparison between the signal captured by the Kinect and the signal from the RPM system shows that both signals are temporally very well aligned in the turning points of the curve (see Figure 4). But there exists a difference in the amplitude at the turning points. The average difference from the RPM to the Kinect signal is 1.52 ± 0.11 mm. These values are on average over two measurements from the same sinusoidal curve. The results demonstrate that the movement, in this case in AP direction, can be captured temporally very similarly by the Kinect and the RPM system. Only the amplitudes of the two signals are different. A possible reason for the mismatch in the amplitude between the two signals could be the calibration curve. If there are inaccuracies in the calibration, they will have an influence on a correct measurement of the motion amplitude. Another possible error source could be

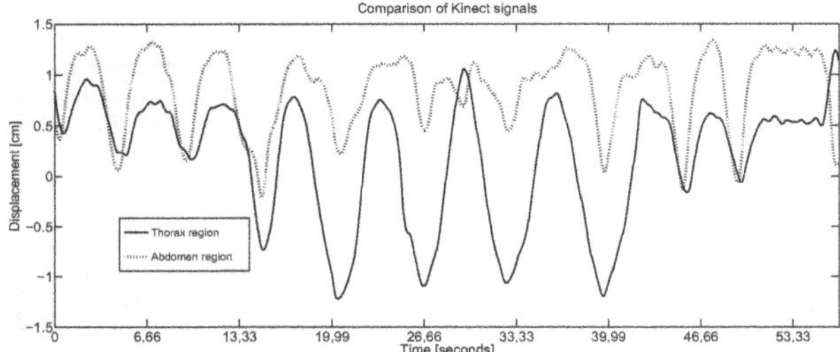

Figure 5: Comparison of two Kinect signals from thoracic and abdominal regions of the chest. The signal of the thorax has a lower amplitude than the signal from the abdomen with the exception of the time where the test person was asked to perform thoracic breathing.

the angle between the optical axis and the motion direction, which is important for the calculation of the AP movement.

3.4 Kinect Signals from a Test Person

One benefit of the Kinect is the possibility to extract breathing signals from different regions from a single measurement. For a setup like in figure 2, breathing signals from the thoracic and abdominal region of the upper part of the body are analysed. If the ROI are close together (e.g. side by side), the signals are nearly the same with a correlation coefficient of 0.99 to 0.97. But for regions with a larger distance like one ROI at the abdomen and one on the thorax, the correlation coefficient is only 0.55. Figure 5 shows the two different signals from the abdomen and the thorax. The most notable difference between the two signals is in the amplitude. In the first three breathing periods, the test person was asked to perform normal breathing. After that, the breathing pattern changes to thoracic breathing, which is observable in the strong increase of the amplitude of the signal from the thoracic region.

4 Conclusion

In this work, we analysed the implementation of a clinical setup for respiratory surface motion measurement with the Microsoft Kinect. The results of the second experiment the comparison Kinect to RPM system indicate that the Kinect has the potential to measure the respiratory motion on condition that the mismatch between the amplitude of the RPM system and the Kinect can be resolved in future work. The comparison of the signals in the third experiment show that breathing signals from different regions of the chest are not equal. This fact is important as the RPM system can only measure the motion at one single point of the chest and it is possible that the movement at this point changes during the measurement or treatment session. Future investigations will have the focus on a more detailed analysis of the variability and differences in breathing curves from different regions of the chest with the focus on the question if there is a phase shift between regions. Such a shift could have an influence on the 4D-CT reconstruction.

Acknowledgement

This work has been carried out at the University Medical Center Hamburg-Eppendorf, Hamburg, Germany. We would like to thank the test persons for their assistance.

5 References

[1] Y. Seppenwoolde, H. Shirato, K. Kitamura, S. Shimizu, M. van Herk, J. V. Lebesque, and K. Miyasaka, "Precise and real-time measurement of 3D tumor motion in lung due to breathing and heartbeat, measured during radiotherapy," *International Journal of Radiation Oncology*Biology*Physics*, vol. 53, pp. 822–834, 2002.

[2] A. Schweikard, G. Glosser, M. Bodduluri, M. J. Murphy, and J. R. Adler, "Robotic motion compensation for respiratory movement during radiosurgery," *Computer Aided Surgery*, vol. 5, pp. 263–277, 2000.

[3] H. D. Kubo and B. C. Hill, "Respiration gated radiotherapy treatment: a technical study," *Physics in Medicine and Biology*, vol. 41, no. 1, p. 83, 1996.

[4] J. R. McClelland, D. J. Hawkes, T. Schaeffter, and A. P. King, "Respiratory motion models: A review," *Medical Image Analysis*, vol. 17, pp. 19–42, 2013.

[5] F. Tahavori, M. Alnowami, and K. Wells, "Markerless respiratory motion modeling using the Microsoft Kinect for Windows," *Proc. SPIE*, vol. 9036, pp. 90360K–90360K–10, 2014.

[6] T. Wentz, H. Fayad, J. Bert, O. Pradier, J. F. Clement, S. Vourch, N. Boussion, and D. Visvikis, "Accuracy of dynamic patient surface monitoring using a time-of-flight camera and B-spline modeling for respiratory motion characterization," *Physics in Medicine and Biology*, vol. 57, pp. 4175–4193, 2012.

[7] K. Khoshelham and S. O. Elberrink, "Accuracy and resolution of kinect depth data for indoor mapping applications," *Sensors*, vol. 12, pp. 1437–1454, 2012.

[8] "Openkinect." `http://openkinect.org/wiki/Main_Page`. Accessed 2015-01-12.

[9] *Varian Medical Systems: RPM Respiratory Gating System Reference Guide, Version 1.7, 2012.*

[10] C. Grohmann, T. Frenzel, R. Werner, and F. Cremers, "Design, performance characteristics and application examples ofa new 4D motion platform," *Zeitschrift für Medizinische Physik*, vol. Available online, 2014.

[11] P. J. Noonan, J. Howard, D. Tout, I. Armstrong, H. A. Williams, T. F. Cootes, W. A. Hallett, and R. Hinz, "Accurate Markerless Respiratory Tracking For Gated Whole Body PET Using the Microsoft Kinect," in *Nuclear Science Symposium and Medical Imaging Conference (NSS/MIC), 2012 IEEE*, pp. 3973–3974, 2012.

8
Signal Processing I

Single-trial variability of non-invasively recorded high-frequency somatosensory evoked potentials

M. Scheuermann [1], G. Waterstraat [2], and G. Curio [2,3]

[1] Medizinische Ingenieurwissenschaft, Universität zu Lübeck, scheuerm@miw.uni-luebeck.de
[2] Klinik und Hochschulambulanz für Neurologie Charité-Universitätsmedizin Berlin, {gunnar.waterstraat, gabriel.curio}@charite.de
[3] Bernstein Center for Computational Neuroscience Berlin, gabriel.curio@charite.de

Abstract

Peripheral nerve stimulation leads to somatosensory evoked potentials (SEPs) in the brain. Whenever recorded non-invasively, trials including SEPs needed to be averaged to gain a satisfying Signal-to-Noise Ratio (SNR). SEPs include high-frequency (hf) oscillations (>400 Hz). Here, we established a method to preserve hf-SEPs in its single-trial form to analyse the variability of the so called σ-burst, an hf-SEP component ranging from 400 – 800 Hz. Therefore, we used optimized neurotechnology combined with offline spectral analysis and spatial filtering to increase SNR. The change of amplitude, absolute deviation from the median amplitude (absolute variability) as well as the variability divided by the median (relative variability) was taken into account to analyse characteristics of the σ-bursts. All observations were checked for significance. In 9 of 10 subjects an increased amplitude and absolute variability were observed in the time-frequency window of the bursts, whereas the relative variability showed to decrease in 6 of 10 subjects significantly.

1 Introduction

Non-invasive electroencephalography during peripheral nerve stimulation contains functional information about the processing of the stimulus. It has been shown that the clinically established low-frequency EEG (< 100 Hz) is mainly sensitive to synchronised cortical postsynaptic potentials, i.e. to the input of neuronal computation.

In contrast, somatosensory evoked potentials (SEP) contain an additionally oscillatory high-frequency EEG burst ($\approx$ 600 Hz), here denoted as 'σ-bursts', which is concomitant with the first cortical low-frequency component (the "N20" for median nerve stimulation) and can be isolated by high-pass filtering above 400 Hz. Simultaneous macroscopic subdural EEG and microscopic cortical single-cell recordings in behaving non-human primates revealed that the σ-bursts is synchronous [1] and co-variable [2] with cortical single-cell spike bursts. Hence, σ-bursts can be regarded as a non-invasive correlate of cortical population spikes, hereby complementing the information content of the established low-frequency EEG and providing access to the very output of neuronal computation, i.e. spikes.

To increase the SNR, the average EEG response to multiple repetitions of peripheral nerve stimulation (labelled as 'trials') is commonly calculated, hereby presuming an invariable 'static' sequence of SEP-waves. Using this technique allowed to localize the generator of the σ-bursts to the primary somatosensory cortex (S1) and to thalamocortical radiation fibres [3] and revealed valuable physiologic information about the correspondence of burst-amplitude to sleep, sedation and certain diseases [4]. However, averaging across trials precludes studying the single-trial variability of SEP, which is a key feature of a functional description of mechanisms underlying the temporal variability in somatosensory processing.

Here, we combine custom-built low-noise amplifier technology and spatial filtering of multichannel EEG to increase the SNR of high-frequency SEP recordings evoked by median nerve stimulation. This enables us to characterize the extent of trial-to-trial variability attributable to σ-bursts (population spikes).

2 Material and Methods

2.1 EEG recordings

EEG was recorded from 3 female and 7 male subjects, with a mean age of 35 and a range from 22 to 56 years. Measurements were performed using a custom-built low-noise EEG amplifier with a set of 8 Ag/AgCl-plated ring electrodes on the scalp. Their placement was chosen to preferentially cover areas above the left pre- and post-central cortex. The EEG reference electrode was placed at Nasion. Careful preparation of the EEG electrodes ensured impedances at or below 2 kΩ, which was checked repeatedly between the recording sessions and corrected if necessary. The EEG was digitized at a sampling frequency of 10 kHz and an acquisition bandpass of 0.016 to 5000 Hz. SEPs were evoked by electric median nerve stimulation at the right wrist of each subject with no consideration about handedness. The intensity of the boxcar-shaped stimulus, with duration of 0.2 ms and a stimulus frequency of 4 Hz, was set to 1.5 x motor-threshold so that a twitch of the thumb was visible for every stimulus. Subjects were placed on a comfortable chair in upright position. They were instructed to keep their eyes open, blink rarely, and to avoid any movements. The recordings consisted of three 10 min blocks during median nerve stimulation. Consequently, approximately 7200 trials were recorded in each subject. The time interval corresponding to the stimulus artifacts (-8 to 5 ms) was interpolated using monotone cubic Hermite spline interpolation to prevent ringing of the applied digital filters and to prevent the prominent stimulus artefact from dominating the results of the subsequent analysis steps.

2.2 Outlier Rejection

Outlier segments of the recordings were identified by the departure of their power spectral density (PSD) in channel Fz from baseline. The similarity to other channels was assumed. The baseline-PSD was defined by a logarithmic fit to the median block-wise PSD (non-overlapping blocks of 1 sec duration) in channel Fz, estimated using Welch's average periodogram method. Subsequently, the Euclidian distance between each block-wise PSD and the baseline-PSD was determined and all segments with a distance above the 75th percentile + 1.5 $\times$ interquartile range were rejected from further analysis.

2.3 Spatial filtering

Each channel of the recorded multi-channel EEG contains the activity of a multitude of neurons. However, only a minority of these neurons contributes to the activity of interest; hence, it is desirable to 'focus' the EEG recording by using a spatial filter maximizing the contribution of cortical regions involved in the generation of σ-bursts. Here, we employed a variant of Canonical Correlation Analysis (CCA) denoted as "Canonical Correlation Average regression" (CCAr). CCA finds filters w_x and w_y maximizing the correlation between two multivariate datasets X and Y. CCAr directs this filter optimization towards stimulus-evoked activity by using the average SEP as dataset Y. Hence, spatial filters are optimized by maximizing the correlation between single trials and their respective average, as shown in 1, where ρ is the correlation coefficient:

$$\arg\max_{w_x w_y} \rho = \frac{w_x^T X Y^T w_y}{\sqrt{(w_x^T X X^T w_x)(w_y^T Y Y^T w_y)}} \quad (1)$$

To optimize spatial filters with respect to σ-bursts, the dataset was band-pass filtered utilizing Butterworth with cut-off frequencies at 450 and 1200 Hz. The filter order was chosen as the lowest order guaranteeing a maximal loss of 3 dB in the pass-band and a minimal attenuation of 8 dB in the stop-band, with a transition width between these bands of 15 % of the respective cut-off frequency. CCAr was subsequently applied to the segment ranging from 10 ms to 30 ms post-stimulus. The two spatial filters with the highest canonical correlations were applied to the unfiltered broad-band EEG recordings for subsequent analysis.

2.4 Time-frequency transform

σ-bursts are confined in their spectral band ($\approx$ 600 Hz) and temporal range (around 20 ms). While the time domain cannot represent the spectral characteristics of the signal the Fourier domain does not resolve its temporal signature. Hence, a combined time-frequency representation (TFR) was sought to optimally represent the recorded single-trial SEPs.

The Short-Time Fourier Transform (STFT), an approach to extend Fourier analysis to the analysis of non-stationary signals, does not offer a satisfying compromise to deal with the uncertainty principle: uniform temporal and spectral resolution is assumed in all frequency bands. Advancing upon that, the Wavelet transform (WT) adds the concept of progressive resolution. However, the WT is non-linear and reference to absolute phases is lost.

Here, we adopt a version of the S transform which combines globally referenced phases and progressive spectral and temporal resolution in one TFR [5]. The formulation of the ST

$$S(\nu,\tau) = \int_{-\infty}^{+\infty} g(t)\, \frac{|\nu|}{2\pi} e^{-\frac{(\tau-t)^2\nu^2}{2}} e^{-i2\pi\nu t} dt \quad (2)$$

illustrates that it is a Fourier transform extended by a Gaussian window function to obtain time resolution, where ν and τ are the transform time and frequency. Progressive resolution is achieved by a frequency-dependent window-width. The discrete ST algorithm developed by [5] permits to sample from the time-frequency plane of the ST in a freely chosen manner. If the sampling scheme in the time-frequency plane is chosen appropriately, the computational complexity and memory requirements traditionally associated with the ST are therefore significantly lowered. Here, we sample from the time-frequency plane of the ST in a regular grid in steps of 2 ms and 30 Hz in a temporal range from -10 ms to 100 ms post-stimulus and a frequency range from DC to 1500 Hz.

2.5 Analysis of single-trial amplitude and variability

Three distinct time-frequency resolved single-trial measures were calculated for each subject: (i) amplitude, (ii) absolute variability, and (iii) relative variability. Amplitudes were determined as the absolute values of the single-trial ST coefficients and absolute variability as the absolute deviations from the median amplitudes across trials. The absolute deviations were divided by the median amplitude across trials to yield a the measure of relative variability. Significance testing against the null hypothesis (i.e. ,the measures of single-trial amplitude und variability are equally distributed in the evoked and in the background EEG) was performed using the non-parametric Mann-Whitney U test. Specifically, N (N equaling the number of trials) 110 ms long segments were randomly drawn from the spatially filtered broad-band EEG (omitting the -8 ms to 5 ms post-stimulus intervals containing the interpolated stimulus artifacts). For fair comparison, the stimulus interpolation algorithm was also applied to the same time window as in the true evoked EEG trials, and subsequently the time-frequency resolved measures of amplitude and variability were calculated for these randomized 'background trials'. The Mann-Whitney U statistic for the comparison between true evoked trials and background trials was standardized to z scores using a normal approximation. To ensure proper generalization of the results, this procedure was repeated 10 times with randomly re-drawn background trials and the z score with the smallest absolute value was retained. If the sign of the 10 z scores was equivocal, the respective z score was set to 0. The p values were calculated using the standard normal cumulative distribution function and the family-wise error rate was kept below 0.05 using Bonferroni correction (in total 5500 time-frequency resolved z scores were present for each measure). For visualization, the z scores were interpolated onto a finer time-frequency grid using nearest neighbor interpolation and illustrated as grayscale images.

3 Results and Discussion

Figure 1 exemplarily illustrates the determination of outlier seconds in subject S02, hereby effectively guarding the analysis from being influenced by large artifacts stemming, for example, from movements, blinking and swallowing.

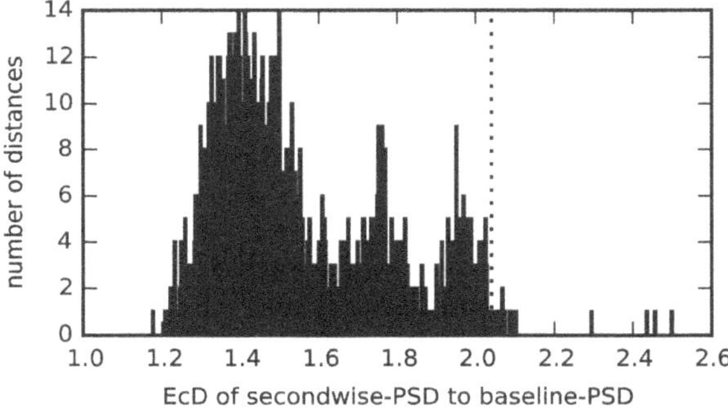

Figure 1: Determination of outlier seconds by calculating Euclidean distances of their PSDs to an optimal logarythmic fit. The outlier threshold (dotted vertical line) was set to the 75th percentile plus 1.5 × interquartile range.

CCAr was used to obtain an optimal projection of all EEG channels. The two spatial patterns corresponding to the highest canonical correlations are shown in Figure 2. For all subjects, a monopolar and a bipolar pattern were obtained, most likely representing the different generators of the SEP, as there are radially oriented dipoles from thalamic and thalamocortical sources and a tangentially oriented dipoles from generators in area 3b of the somatosensory cortex [3] [6].

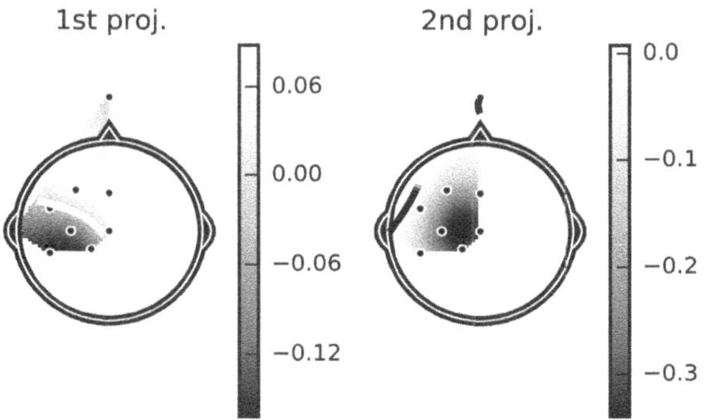

Figure 2: Patterns corresponding of the CCAr analysis. For all subjects, a monopolar and a bipolar pattern were derived. Due to the low number of electrodes, the patterns cannot be resolved over the complete head surface. The white (black) line left (right) panel indicates the change of polarity. The scale of values is arbitrary.

Subsequently, for each subject and both spatial projections the single-trial amplitude, absolute variability, and relative variability were determined. Significance testing was done against EEG segments of equal length which were randomly drawn from the dataset without fixed relation to the median nerve stimulation. The non-parametric Mann-Whitney U statistic was standardized to z-scores and illustrated as grayscale images. Exemplary results for subject S02 are shown in Figure 3.

At around 20 ms, when SEP activity is expected, highly significant increase (amplitude and absolute variability) or decrease (relative variability) is present in the low frequency band (0-400 Hz) and in the high frequency band (500-1200 Hz)

4 Conclusion

As a main result, we were able to show that by using custom-build low-noise EEG amplifier technology it is possible to characterize the single-trial amplitude and variability of evoked high-frequency oscillations (σ-bursts) by using non-invasive surface EEG. In contrast to former studies, we were not forced to calculate the average across measured trials to obtain a satisfactory SNR. Here, optimized neurotechnology and offline analysis were combined to increase the SNR of the high-frequency SEP recordings to permit single-trial analysis, even outside a specialized electromagnetically shielded recording chamber [7]. Hence, we can provide direct evidence that the SEP is not a sequence of static EEG components, rather it shows significant tem-

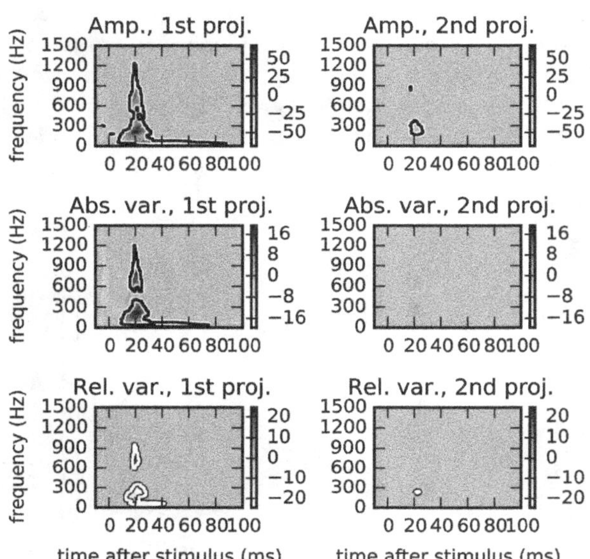

Figure 3: Comparison of amplitude (top), absolute variability (middle row) and relative variability (bottom) against background EEG in Subject S02 for the projection with the highest (left) and 2nd highest (right) canonical correlations. The grayscale corresponds to z-scores obtained by normal approximation of the Mann-Whitney U statistic. Enframed segments of the time-frequency maps indicate significance with a family-wise error rate below 0.05 (using Bonferroni correction).

poral, i.e., trial-to-trial, variability.

Confirming previous results [8], it was shown that σ-bursts are accompanied by an increase of the single-trial amplitude in the respective time-frequency segment. Secondly, the present study provides non-invasive evidence for a single-trial amplitude variability that can directly be attributed to σ-bursts. Reference [4] investigated the amplitude variability of σ-bursts in sub-averages of 3 minutes in comparison to the amplitude variability of the N20. The present study differs in examining single trials and guarding the analysis against the influence of frequency dependent changes in SNR by comparison to background EEG in equivalent time-frequency segments. As third finding, it could be shown that the relative variability of σ-bursts is smaller than the relative variability of background EEG, which confirms the expectations when an evoked EEG component is added onto a comparatively variable background process.

With this approach it was possible to detect the variability of σ-bursts using non-invasive EEG. This variability can be presumed to reflect the non-stationary process of somatosensory stimulus processing in the human brain. Questions for future studies using this methodology could address the source of this variability, whether it depends on the pre-stimulus brain state and the consequence of variable σ-bursts responses for the subsequent processing of the stimulus.

Acknowledgement

The work has been carried out at Klinik und Hochschulambulanz für Neurologie Charité-Universitätsmedizin Berlin. M.S. acknowledges mentoring supprt from Prof. Alfred Mertins, Institute for Signal Processing Universität zu Lübeck. The authors acknowledge support from BMBF Bernstein Center for Computional Neuroscience Berlin, project B1.

5 References

[1] S. N. Baker, G. Curio and R. N. Lemon, *EEG oscillations at 600 Hz are macroscopic markers for cortical spike bursts*. in: J Physiol, 550.2, pp. 529-534, 2003.

[2] B. Telenczuk, S. Baker, A. Herz and G. Curio, *High-frequency EEG covaries with spike burst patterns detected in cortical neurons*. in: J Neurophysiol., Jun 2011.

[3] P. Ritter, F. Freyer, G. Curio and A. V. M. Villringer, *High-frequency (600 Hz) population spikes in human EEG delineate thalamic and cortical fMRI activation sites*. in: Neuroimage, vol: 42, pp. 483–490, 2008.

[4] F. Klostermann, G. Nolte and G. Curio, *Independent short-term variability of spikelike (600 Hz) and post-synaptic (N20) cerebral SEP components*. in: Neuroreport, vol. 12, no. 2, pp. 349-352, 2001.

[5] R. A. Brown, M. L. Lauzon and R. Frayne, *A General Description of Linear Time-Frequency Transforms and Formulation of a Fast, Invertible Transform That Samples the Continuous S-Transform Spectrum Nonredundantly*. in: IEEE Transactions on Signal Processing, vol. 58, no. 1, 2010.

[6] G. Curio, B. Mackert, M. Burghoff, R. Koetitz, K. Abraham-Fuchs and W. Haerer, *Localization of evoked neuromagnetic 600 Hz activity in the cerebral somatosensory system*. in: Electroencephalogr Clin Neurophysiol, vol.91, no.6, pp. 483–487, 1994.

[7] G. Waterstraat, T. Fedele, M. Burghoff, H.-J. Scheer and G. Curio, *Recording human cortical population spikes non-invasively – An EEG tutorial*. in: J Neurosci Methods, pii: S0165-0270(14)00297-0, 2014.

[8] G. Waterstraat, B. Telenczuk, M. Brughoff, T. Fedele, H.-J. Scheer and G. Curio, *Are high-frequency (600 Hz) oscillations in human somatosensory evoked potentials due to phase-resetting phenomena?*. in: Clin Neurophysiol, vol. 123, no. 10, pp. 2064-73, 2012.

Evaluation of a Skin-to-Electrode Impedance Measuring System

J. P. Diesing [1], T. Moszkowski [2], R. Ruff [2] and A. Mertins [3]

[1] Medizinische Ingenieurwissenschaft, Universität zu Lübeck, diesing@miw.uni-luebeck.de
[2] Fraunhofer Institut for Biomedical Engineering, St. Ingbert, {tomasz.moszkowski, roman.ruff}@ibmt.fraunhofer.de
[3] Institute of Signal Processing, Universität zu Lübeck, mertins@isip.uni-luebeck.de

Abstract

Neuromonitoring by stimulating with invasive electrodes can damage the nerve tissue. Surface electrodes on the skin do not have this disadvantage, but have to be placed properly, need good electrical connection and the spatial resolution is inferior. To determine the quality of the placement, the skin-to-electrode impedance can be measured – a low impedance means a good connection and therefore safe stimulation. This paper evaluates an impedance measurement system of an intraoperative neuromonitoring setup, developed at Fraunhofer Institute for Biomedical Engineering (IBMT), using three experiments. The setup was tested on its dependency on different frequency and voltage configurations of the input signal; a comparison with two existing impedance measuring systems was done to determine the accuracy and reproducibility of results. The results suggest that an accurate measurement is possible in the frequency range between 100 Hz and 10 kHz. However, mathematical errors in the software should be identified and corrected.

1 Introduction

63000 patients with rectal carcinoma were under medical treatment in German hospitals in 2012 [1]. The main therapy is to excise the diseased tissue through surgery, which often leads to damaging the nerves in the surrounding tissue and thereby postoperative complications for the patient, such as anorectal or sexual dysfunction [2]. By stimulating the nerves in question and observing the responses of innervated muscles, the damage to the nerve may be identified or prevented during the surgery. This technique is called intraoperative neuromonitoring [5]. In the case of cancer treatment in the lower pelvic area the relevant nerves are the inferior hypogastric plexus and the pelvic splanchnic nerves [3], [4].

The stimulation in this application, can be done through penetrating, and thereby harming the nerve with a needle electrode and applying the current directly. Alternatively, surface electrodes can be placed on the skin surface. This technique, however, requires good positioning of the electrodes and a good connection to the skin, since the electric field has to reach the nerve through several tissues. Measuring the impedance, which is the complex ratio of voltage to current at a particular frequency in an alternating current circuit, can serve to evaluate the quality of skin-to-electrode connection. The impedance can be described by an absolute value and a phase angle, which is the phase difference between the voltage and the current [6]. A low impedance can be a sign of a good electrical connection. A neuromonitoring system based on transcutaneous stimulation can evaluate the placement of the electrodes, by measuring the impedance between them and the skin. This is done by measuring the amplitude of the voltage drop between the anode and cathode placed on the patient's body while applying a fixed AC current with a specific frequency. The current can have a sinusoidal, a rectangular or a triangular waveform. The devices in this experiment are using the sinusoidal waveform.

The aim of this paper is to evaluate an impedance measuring system for intraoperative neuromonitoring developed at Fraunhofer IBMT. Therefore, we determine the behavior of the evaluated setup in a controlled setting and we compare the setup to two other available systems by analyzing the results of two experiments with regard to their accuracy and reproducibility.

2 Material and Methods

2.1 Measuring setups

To evaluate our system we compared it to two other impedance measurement devices. An overview of the three systems follows. All three devices use a sinusoidal waveform for their measurement signal.

Evaluated setup The setup we wanted to evaluate consists of a personal computer where the user can define stimulation parameters in an interface built using LabView by National Instruments. This software communicates via USB with an external multifunctional data acquisition module – NI USB-6225 (DAQ card).

The DAQ card is attached to a demultiplexer and a neurostimulator, provided by inomed Medizintechnik GmbH, both connected to the experimental setup. The demultiplexer switches between 64 available channels, with each one representing one electrode used for stimulation using the neurostimulator. The voltages needed to compute the impedance signal are recorded by the DAQ card and passed to the software on the computer. Here the raw signal is processed and presented in NI LabView.

Solartron Frequency Analyzer The Solartron Frequency Analyzer consists of a computer for control and user interaction, a function generator (1255 by Solartron Instruments) and an electrochemical interface (1287 by Solartron Analytical) used as a potentiostat connected to the experimental setup. The results of the measurements are presented in a graphical user interface as real and imaginary parts of the complex impedance. The complex results can be saved into a file. The user enters the parameters of measurement into the software.

EIMS Multichannel Box This electrical impedance measuring system (EIMS), which originates from another project, consists of a multichannel box, where the experimental system can be attached to, and software, where the user can choose the sampling frequencies and the amplitude of current. A NI USB-6225 DAQ card controls the box via a computer.
The results are presented as a plot of absolute impedance and phase, where the values of the impedance are given in kΩ and the raw data are not accessible. This leads to difficulties in the interpretation of the data, as described in section 3.

2.2 Experiments

We designed three experiments to cover a range of possible use cases for the impedance measurement using two-terminal setting. The first was only done with the evaluated setup, with the next two we compared the three devices.

Dependence of the system accuracy based on the input voltage and input frequency To get an overview of the measurement characteristics of the evaluated setup, such as the changing in results using different frequencies and voltages and to detect possible systematic errors, we designed an experiment using multiple resistors, measurement frequencies and voltages. A decade resistor was tested using a 10 Hz- and 30 Hz-sinewave signal and a voltage of 20 mV and 50 mV for resistor values between 1 Ω and 5 kΩ, and 100 mV to 200 mV for the range between 30 Ω and 7 MΩ. Each measurement was done 20 times and a median value was calculated. This median was then compared to the true value of the resistor.
Additionally, a 1 kΩ resistor was tested with sine wave signals in the range between 40 Hz and 10 kHz to clarify the frequency dependence of the evaluated setup.

Comparison of the three devices One experiment to compare the three devices consisted of measurements of five resistors, with values of 500 Ω, 1 kΩ, 5 kΩ, 10 kΩ and 50 kΩ, of a decade resistor, using a constant frequency of 20 Hz and a constant current of 0.5 mA. The limiting 500 Ω resistor was imposed by the EIMS system, which could not measure values below this. Each resistor was measured ten times to gain statistically significant results.

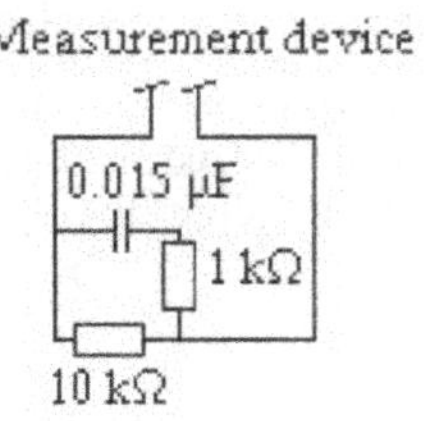

Figure 1: Electrical scheme of the setup used in the measurement of the skin impedance model. It consists of a 0.015 μF capacitor and two resistors with 1 kΩ, respectively 10 kΩ.

Additionally, we tested a basic skin-electrode impedance model, described in [7], in respect to the accuracy of the measurement (see Fig. 1). The model consisted of a 0.015 μF capacitor, connected in parallel to a 1 kΩ resistor, and a 10 kΩ resistor serially connected to both. The model has a specific frequency-dependent impedance curved, which we tested over the frequency range between 10 Hz and 10 kHz using an ammeter and Solartron frequency analyzer. A median of 10 measurements was calculated and the systems were compared against each other. Due to system specifications, a current of 5 mA was used for the evaluated setup, 50 mA for the Solartron frequency analyzer, and 5 μA for the EIMS system. While the Solartron frequency analyzer is not suitable for in vivo measurements, the other two settings would be not noticeable by the patient.

3 Results and Discussion

Dependence of the system accuracy based on the input voltage and input frequency The results in this experiment can be evaluated by comparing the measured resistance to the reference value provided by the decade resistor and determining the relative error (Fig. 2 and 3). For the measurements with 20 mV and 50 mV, this error is high for a resistance between 1 Ω and 10 Ω. The rest of the range up to 3 kΩ can be measured correctly. Here, the higher voltages show lower error. The relative error of the measurement with 100 mV (Fig. 3) is under 10% for both used frequencies of 10 Hz and 30 Hz. The latter can provide results for resistors up to 70 kΩ with an accuracy of 95%. The error in the range above 10 kΩ could be due to the maximal impedance the stimulator can handle.
Another problem can be observed in Fig. 3, which shows the relative error of the measurement with a potential of 200 mV and frequencies of 10 Hz and 30 Hz, respectively. The relative error rises from 10% for the 10 kΩ resistor to nearly 100% for the 30 kΩ one. Here the measured resis-

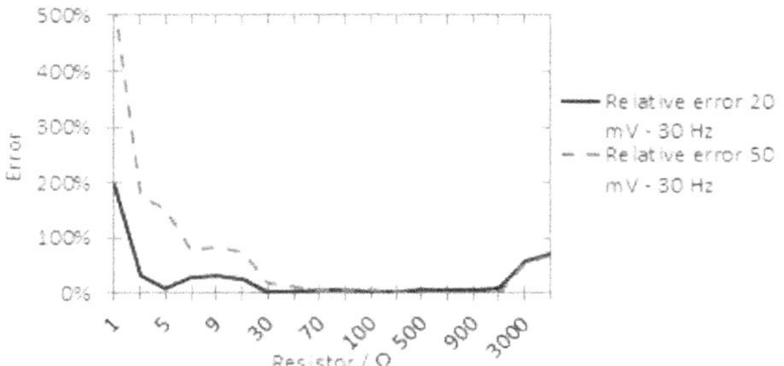

Figure 2: Comparison of the relative error of the measurement with the evaluated system, using voltages of 20 mV and 50 mV and a frequency of 30 Hz. Very low resistor values cannot be measured correctly. The lower voltage shows lower error. (n=20)

tance for the 30 kΩ resistor was 900 Ω, which is far too low. The same applies to all the following resistors. This error can be due to an internal safety circuit of the neurostimulator in the setup, which limits the applied voltage by changing the measurement current.

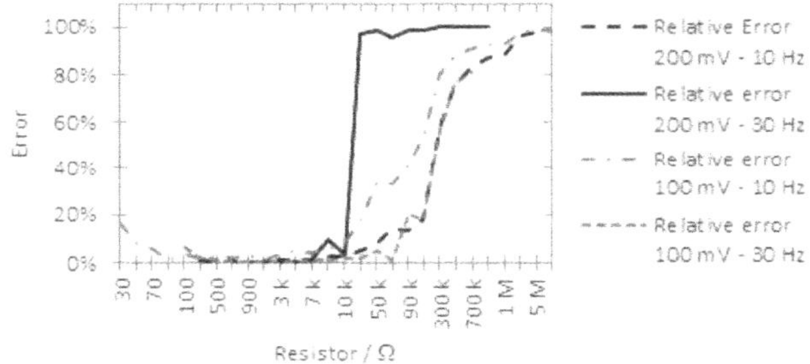

Figure 3: Comparison of the relative error of the measurement with the evaluated system, using voltages of 100 mV and 200 mV and frequencies of 10 Hz and 30 Hz (n=20). The 200 mV / 30 Hz measurement shows a systematic error, due to the safety circuit in the neurostimulator.

The measurement of the 1 kΩ resistor shows that the evaluated setup can give the true value of the resistor with a frequency between 40 Hz and 10 kHz. We observe an error for frequencies lower than 20 Hz (Fig. 4).

Comparison of the three devices The software of the EIMS Multichannel Box provides the results in kΩ, while rounding to one decimal place. This leads to unknown accuracy, especially concerning small resistors. The comparison of the results of the three setups are given in tables 1 and 2, and Fig. 5.

The tables tables 1 and 2 show a low variance in the results of the measurements with the Solartron Frequency Analyzer and the EIMS system. The evaluated setup can measure resistors up to 10 kΩ reliably with 20 Hz and 50 mA, but fails at the 50 kΩ resistor. This error may be equalized with an adjustment of the used frequency, as the first experiment showed, but also a modification of a multiplication factor in the software may be helpful, as seen in the next paragraph. The design of this experiment demanded a constant frequency over all three devices, so we expected an error at this high-value resistor.

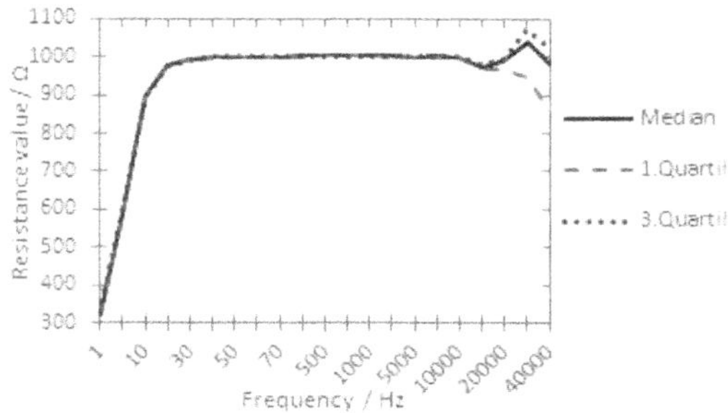

Figure 4: The measurement of a 1 kΩ resistor with the evaluated system, using frequencies between 1 Hz and 40 kHz (n=10). Low (< 40 Hz) and high (> 10 kHz) frequencies cannot give the correct value.

Table 1: Median of the measurement of five resistors (n=10). While the Solartron Frequency Analyzer and the EIMS setup can measure all resistor values correctly, our setup fails at the 50 kΩ resistor. The EIMS setup only gives the kΩ values and rounds to one decimal place.

Resistor value: in kΩ	IBMT setup in Ω	Solartron in Ω	EIMS in kΩ
0.5	495	500	0.5
1.0	979	1004	1.0
5.0	4740	5013	5.0
10.0	9116	9974	10.0
50.0	32336	49912	49.9

Table 2: Standard deviation of the measurement of five resistors with the three setups (n=10). The results of our system are good for all resistors but the 50 kΩ one. The EIMS setup seems to have no variance, due to the rounding procedure.

Resistor value: in kΩ	IBMT setup in Ω	Solartron in Ω	EIMS in kΩ
0.5	51.33	0.007	0
1.0	12.77	0.064	0
5.0	72.23	0.075	0
10.0	148.31	0.302	0
50.0	2078.72	3.59	0

The difference between the measured values of all resistors and the desired ones are lower than the given error of the components of the decade resistor, which is ±1%.

The results of the experiment with the skin impedance model are shown in Fig 5. The course of the plot is as expected equal to the value of the 10 kΩ resistor at first and drops for higher frequencies towards the value of the 1 kΩ resistor. This is due to the capacitor, which behaves like an infinite resistor for small frequencies and has no impact on higher ones. All three devices are capable to make these properties recognizable. The problems of the evalu-

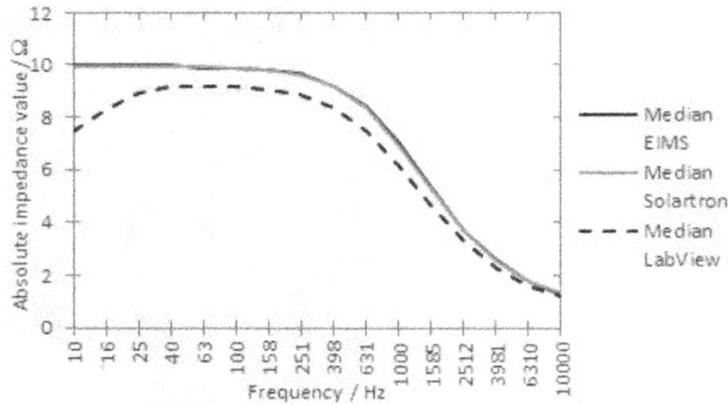

Figure 5: Measurement of the skin model (n=10). The evaluated system has a systematic error and is incorrect at low frequencies.

ated setup with low frequencies are already discussed in the first paragraph of this section. The high value resistor cannot be measured correctly at low frequencies of the input signal.
Additionally, there seems to be a systematic error since the results of the evaluated setup are constantly 10% lower than the ones of the reference setup and the EIMS. This can be patched by adjusting a factor in the code of our setup.

4 Conclusion

The intention of these experiments was to evaluate the usability of an impedance measurement system developed at Fraunhofer IBMT and get reliable results. The outcome of the comparison between the evaluated setup, the reference system and the EIMS multichannel box looks promising. The evaluated setup could produce reliable results and is nearly on the same level of accuracy, if some adjustments are made. In particular, the safety circuit of the neurostimulator prevents the correct measurement of impedance values above 10 kΩ. The differences between our system and the two others can be attributed to systematic errors, like inaccurate coefficients in mathematical calculation of the impedance, or system components, which impact the recorded data.
Additionally, the frequency dependence of the accuracy of the evaluated setup can be balanced by choosing recording frequencies in a spectrum between 100 Hz and 10 kHz. The results gained in this span have the lowest error with respect to unknown impedance in the region between 1 kΩ and 30 kΩ. These frequencies also offer the ability to reproduce results consistently. Generally, at low resistance values a lower voltage leads to lower error compared to a measurement with a higher voltage and the same frequency. At high resistor values, a higher frequency can give lower error. However, linked to a higher voltage, this can lead to triggering the safety circuit of the neurostimulator. The settings would allow for safe usage of the system on a human patient due to internal safety circuitry.
The next step is to eliminate the mathematical errors in the algorithm, and identify the problems with the setup components, such as shielding of the cables and lowering internal resistances. A more powerful replacement for the used neurostimulator should be taken into consideration.

Acknowledgement

The work has been carried out at Fraunhofer Institute for Biomedical Engineering, St. Ingbert.

5 References

[1] Federal Statistical Office, *Diagnostic data of the hospitals starting from 2000.* in: www.gbe-bund.de (Search by topics: C20 hospital data, Diseases/Health Problems → Diseases in General → document type: tables). [Date of retrieval: 22.01.2015].

[2] C. P. Maas et al., *Radical and nerve-preserving surgery for rectal cancer in The Netherlands: a prospective study on morbidity and functional outcome.* in: Br J Surg, vol. 85, no. 1, pp. 92–97, 1998.

[3] W. Kneist et al., *Selective Pelvic Autonomic Nerve Stimulation with Simultaneous Intraoperative Monitoring of Internal Anal Sphincter and Bladder Innervation.* in: European Surgical Research, vol. 46, no. 3, pp. 133–138, 2011.

[4] W. Kneist et al., *Total Mesorectal Excision with Intraoperative Assessment of Internal Anal Sphincter Innervation Provides New Insights into Neurogenic Incontinence.* in: Journal of the American College of Surgeons, vol. 214, no. 3, pp. 306–312, 2012.

[5] R. Kramme, K. P. Hoffmann and R. Pozos, *Springer Handbook of Medical Technology.* Springer, Berlin/Heidelberg, 2011.

[6] C. Alexander and M. Sadiku, *Fundamentals of Electric Circuits.* McGraw-Hill, New York, 2006.

[7] U. G. Kyle et al., *Bioelectrical impedance analysis – part I: review of principles and methods.* in: Clinical Nutrition, vol. 23, pp. 1226–1243, 2004.

Quantitative evaluation of online signal processing for fMRI-based neurofeedback

A. Lanfermann[1], M. Zvyagintsev [2], K. Mathiak [3] and A. Mertins [4]
[1] Medizinische Ingenieurwissenschaft, Universität zu Lübeck, Andrea.Lanfermann@miw.uni-luebeck.de
[2] University Hospital Aachen, {mzvyagintsev, kmathiak}@ukaachen.de
[4] Institute for Signal Processing, Universität zu Lübeck, mertins@isip.uni-luebeck.de

Abstract

Neurofeedback is a learning process which allows subjects to self-regulate their brain activity. It bases on operant conditioning. This means a special behavior is requested and the subject is rewarded with a positive feedback. This feedback is the main challenge of neurofeedback. To give a feedback in real time the data given by the MRI scanner have to be prepared in a few seconds and the standard analysis is not suited to do this. This paper validates the recently developed approach for feedback. On the one hand we make a standard offline analysis, which has no special time conditions, and on the other hand we make online analysis which is used for feedback and have to be performed within a few seconds. The aim of this paper is to compare the analysis quantitatively – whether they come to similar results which will further suggest that the online analysis can be used for neurofeedback.

1 Introduction

Neurofeedback is often used in psychological cases. Usually the patient lays in a magnetic resonance tomography and the brain is scanned. Over a screen the patient sees diverse stimuli and has to react to these and according to his reaction a feedback is calculated. The feedback is often given in form of percentage, as a bar or similar illustrations. A desired reaction will be rewarded with a positive feedback, otherwise a negative feedback will be provided.
In this paper the data from one of the actual feedback studies are analyzed. Eleven humans, with the average age of 28.7 and all right-handed, participated in this study. All participants had normal or corrected-to-normal vision, normal hearing, no contra-indications against MR investigations, no history of neurological or psychiatric illness and no history of psychopharmalogical therapy. The study was realized under the instructions of the declaration of Helsinki and the participants were informed about the whole study and all experimental procedures. In addition they had to read the informed consent.
For the experiment a 3-Tesla Siemens Trio Scanner (Siemens, Erlangen, Germany) with a standard 12-Channel head coil was used. The anatomical data were T1-weighted. A MPRAGE sequence with following properties was used: TE = 2.98 ms; TR = 2300 ms; TI = 900 ms; flip angle = 9°; FOV = 256 x 256 mm^2; voxel size = 1 x 1 x 1 mm^3; 176 sagittal slices. For the functional data an EPI sequence was used. (TE = 28 ms; TR = 2000 ms; flip angle = 77°; voxel size = 3 x 3 x 3 mm^3 ; gap = 0.75 mm; FOV = 192 x 192 mm^2; matrix size = 64 x 64; 34 transverse slices)
The experiment starts by finding a suitable region of interest (ROI) in the left ventrolateral prefrontal cortex. Therefore a functional localizer session with up to 29 blocks is used, consisting of 15 baseline blocks, 7 auditory and 7 visual imagery blocks. Every block takes 20 seconds. During the baseline blocks the participants shall count backwards from 100. While the auditory and visual blocks they have to imagine either auditory or visual stimuli. With the scanner information of these localizer data a suitable region of interest can be selected. Then the real time fMRI-based neurofeedback started. The experiment itself consists of four sessions with the previously defined ROI. Each session consists of 17 blocks, whereby 9 blocks are baseline blocks and 8 blocks belong to the neurofeedback. Every block takes 30 seconds. During neurofeedback the participants have to upregulate their brain activity using mental imagery.
During the neurofeedback the data is processed with an online technique, which is explained later. Afterwards the data are analyzed using an offline technique. For the present study the results of online and offline analysis will be compared.

2 Material and Methods

All image data on which operations are performed come from the real-time functional magnetic resonance imaging. This technique is able to show blood flow changes in brain areas. This works by the help of the so called "blood-oxygen-level dependent" (BOLD) signal. The magnetic properties of the oxygenated and the deoxygenated blood are used to detect brain activity. When a brain area is active the metabolism and the blood flow increase. Thereby the concentration of oxygenated hemoglobin increases, too, relatively to the deoxygenated hemoglobin. Since this change of concentration the transversal relaxation time of the nuclear spins changes and the signal of the fMRI changes too. This way a signal is created, which can describe the activity in the brain [2]. In the following two processing methods for fMRI data are explained. In addition several ways to compare online and offline signals are shown.

2.1 Online feedback

The temporal conditions on online feedback are very strict since the participant needs to obtain the feedback information as quickly as possible to be able to learn how to regulate his brain activity. The signal processing consists of three subsequent stages: Exponential moving average filter, Kalman filter, normalization. Every stage ensures that the data from the fMRI scanner approaches to the values of the offline feedback and by that an optimal feedback for the participant is created.

Exponential moving average filter (EMA)
There are two different kinds of moving average filter. The exponential moving average is a special kind of the simple moving average, which only calculates the average of the data points whereby all data points are weighted equal. The EMA filter calculates also the average of all data points but it weights the latest points less than the newer ones and so changes in the data row can be recognized easier.
In this online feedback the EMA filter is used as a high-pass filter with a cut-off frequency of 0.003 Hz. The smoothing factor α can be chosen between the values zero and one, in this case it is chosen as $\alpha = 0.98$. With this factor the time-constant amounts $\tau = 49$ s with a sampling interval TR = 1 s [1].

Kalman filter
The Kalman filter is applied to remove artifacts from the fMRI signal and filters out the high frequency noise. By means of estimations the filter can prognosticate how a system with measurement errors would behave without these errors. Due to this property the Kalman filter is a recursive filter, whereby the mathematic structures of the dynamic system and the measurement errors have to be known to get a good result [3]. In this process a linear Kalman filter has been used to detect spikes and remove high-frequency noise. The filter is also used to remove outliers from the BOLD signal of the fMRI. To control the spike detection in real-time a threshold (Ths) has to be chosen, in this case Ths = 0.9*std(y_0,y_1,...), whereby std is the standard deviation of the measurement data y. The cut-off frequency for the Kalman filter as low-pass filter rests with 0.01 – 0.12 Hz [1].

Normalization
The normalization stage is designed to normalize the filtered signal to another interval. This step does not change the measurement data, it only scales it to the interval [0,1] in this case, to adapt the signal to the display [1].

2.2 Offline feedback

The offline signal processing is considered here as a gold standard for the analysis. This should provide the optimal signal, but it cannot be used in real time neurofeedback, because the processing time is too long. The processing consists of four stages: Slice time correction, motion correction, smoothing and filtering. The offline feedback is done by the program "Brainvoyager" [4].

Slice time correction
The problem of different slice scanning times can lead to a suboptimal statistical analysis. For example if a functional volume of 30 slices and a volume TR of 3 seconds are measured, the last slice is measured almost 3 seconds later than the data of the first slice. This is caused by the hemodynamic response function, which is very indolent. One possibility to cope with slice scanning time differences is to measure a reference slice and shift the data of a slice to the same time point the reference was scanned. So it seems that the whole volume has been measured at the same time [4].

Motion correction
Head motion is the biggest error source in fMRI studies, so that the motion correction is the most important step in the process. In general the motion correction uses one reference volume to compare the incoming data. Does the position of the data deviate extremely from the reference position the motion correction filters this and tries to estimate the true position of the data [4].

Smoothing
For smoothing a spatial smoothing is used. This means that the data points are averaged with their neighbors so that the high frequencies are removed from the data while the low frequencies are enhanced [4].

Filtering
The filtering was performed by using a MATLAB-based routine after the processing in Brainvoyager was done. The filter was a bandpass filter with the same cut-off frequencies like in the online feedback. The lower cut-off is 0.003 Hz and the upper one 0.1 Hz.

2.3 Comparison methods

There are diverse ways to compare online and offline analysis. In the following the used comparison methods are explained.
The easiest way to compare both methods is to compare directly the different signals in a plot. This method is used mainly, because it is the easiest way to see the direct differences between both signals. Additional, the general linear model (GLM), a statistical linear model, is used. It is written as a usual linear equation

$$Y = XB + U \quad (1)$$

whereby Y is the measurement data, X is a design matrix, B a matrix with parameter, which have to be estimated, and U a matrix with error or noise. The estimated matrix B gives information about how similar the matrices Y and X are [5]. The measurement data is compared with a so called predictor, which is an example how the data has to look in an optimal case. By using the GLM the offline and online analysis can be compared since both beta values can be compared. The similar they are, the better the online signal processing approach.

3 Results and Discussion

The aim of this project was to show that the online signal processing used for the feedback is good enough and can further be widely recommended for future real-time fMRI neurofeedback studies. First the result of the experiment is shown to see how the neurofeedback worked generally and the online signal is comparable with the optimal result. Second, the single steps of the online method are analyzed. Finally we show how the signal changes with each step of online processing and how the signal looks like when each single step is left out.

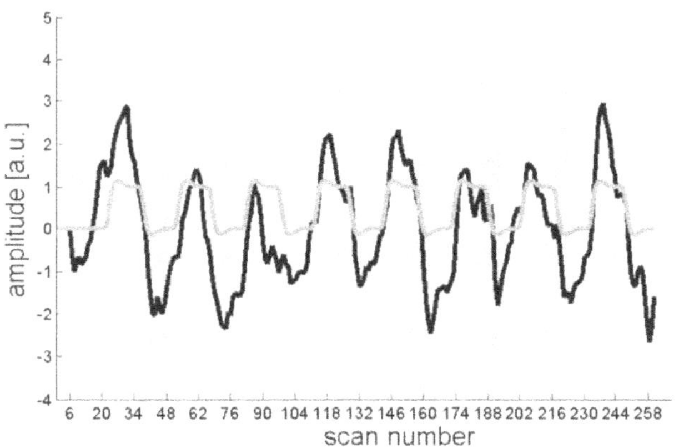

Figure 1: Results of the experiment of the study in 2009. In black the true data, averaged about all subjects and all four sessions, are shown. In gray the hemodynamic response function as optimal result is demonstrated. The background is divided into up regulation and down regulation parts. [a.u. = arbitrary units]

Fig. 1 shows the general result of the experiment. In the background the up- and down regulation parts are highlighted in different colors. During every up regulation the signal increases clearly and so the characteristic peaks are recognizable. Fundamentally, the true results correspond to the optimal results, represented by the hemodynamic response function. Fig. 1 only shows the averaged data, so that it must be taken that there are some subjects who handle the task very well and some who not.

In the following the online signal processing method is compared with the offline signal processing method. As an example one single data set of one subject at the first session is used for the tests. The GLM demonstrates that both techniques provide very similar results, since the GLM parameter for offline feedback is 2.0890 and for online feedback 2.057. Fig. 2 shows the processing of online feedback after each step and demonstrates what each filter is doing. At the same time the data is compared with the offline data to show how the results approach more and more after each step.

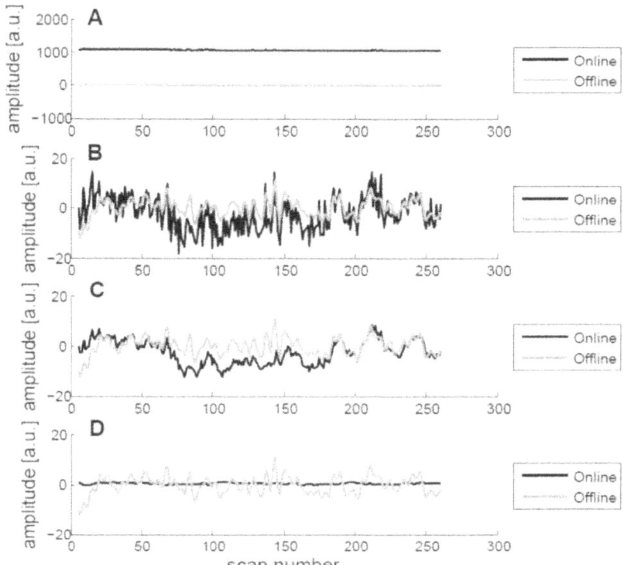

Figure 2: Online process step by step. (A) Scanner data (B) after EMA filtering (C) after Kalman filter (D) after normalization

The scanner data come directly from the fMRI scanner and are not edited yet. The EMA filter sets the baseline of the data to zero so that the graphics are comparable now. Additionally, the EMA filter removes fluctuations of the baseline. One can see that the online signal is very noisy and the wanted signal is not really seen.

The Kalman filter removes the high-frequency noise and the spikes. After this the signals look very similar. Just the baseline is a little different but in the normalization step another EMA filter will compensate this error. The last step is the normalization where the signal is scaled into the interval [0,1] to get the signal onto the display.

Table 1: GLM parameter for each online processing step. The parameter for offline data for comparison is 2.4692

Online processing step	GLM parameter
Scanner data	3.5002
1. EMA filter	3.4781
Kalmanfilter	2.4545
2. EMA filter	2.6262

Table 1 shows the GLM parameter for each online processing step and demonstrates that the beta values approach to the offline parameter with the value 2.4692 with each step. The second EMA, which belongs to the normaliza-

tion, worsened the parameter again. This could be because the Kalman filter removes errors and spikes and the second EMA tries to adapt the baseline again to the signal.
To show how important every filter is for the process every filter has been turned off one time to see how the finished data changes. The other filters were all used normally and on the same position as normal. Only the normalization step is not done because the offline data is not normalized either. However, the second EMA filter is used although.

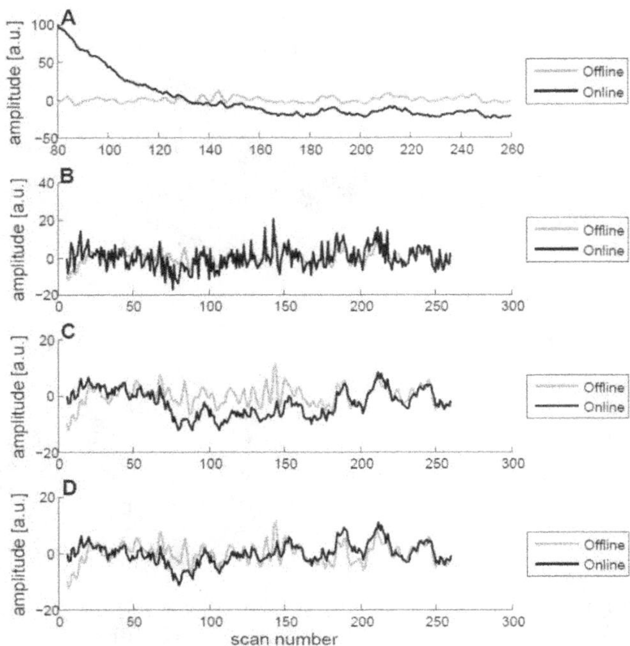

Figure 3: Online processing, when each filter has been turned off one time (A) without EMA-filter (B) without Kalman filter (C) without EMA filter in Normalization step (D) data with all named filter

The EMA filter sets the baseline of the data to zero and removes fluctuations of this baseline. Without this filter the signal would not have a clear baseline and is not very comparable to other signals. One can see that graphic A in Fig. 3 begins at scan number 80 because the maximum of the amplitude before is up to 800 a.u. (arbitrary units). This way the signal could not be present on a practical scale. If the GLM parameter is calculated for this result it deviates greatly from the parameter when all filters are used. The value of the parameter without the EMA filter is -19.248 and the normal value is 2.6262.
The Kalman filter removes spikes and noise from the signal. Without the Kalman filter the signal, which is important for the neurofeedback, cannot be detected. Fig. 3 graphic B shows how much noise is filtered with help from the Kalman filter. The GLM parameter without the Kalman filter is 3.4728 so that one can see that the signal is changed a lot, too.
Finally, the second EMA filter from the normalization step has been turned off. The result is shown in Fig. 3 graphic C and one can see that the difference is not significant without this filter. This underlines the GLM parameter with the value 2.6967, which is very similar to the value of the normal processing parameter 2.6262.

4 Conclusion

All in all the online processing matches the offline processing very well and the offline processing is considered as a gold standard. Every step in the processing is important for a special task and if this step is not used the feedback is not as good as it can be. The EMA filter has to correct the baseline of the signal so that the signal can be scaled on a practical axis. Without the Kalman filter the signal would be too noisy to detect each single value for the feedback. So it looks that the Kalman filter is the most important filter in this case. The normalization is only important if the signal has to be shown on a display since a special interval has to be chosen. Generally the feedback with this online processing method is good to help subjects to train their brain activity with neurofeedback.

Acknowledgement

The work has been carried out at the University hospital Aachen in the clinic for Psychiatry, Psychotherapy and Psychosomatic Disorders.

5 References

[1] Y. Koush, M. Zvyagintsev, M. Dyck, K. A. Mathiak, K. Mathiak, *Signal quality and Bayesian signal processing in neurofeedback based on real-time fMRI*. Elsevier, 2011.

[2] H. Devlin, *What is Functional Magnetic Resonance Imaging (fMRI)?*. Available: http://psychcentral.com/lib/what-is-functional-magnetic-resonance-imaging-fmri/0001056 [last accessed on 29.01.2015]

[3] D. Schetler (HAW-Hamburg), *Kalman Filter zur Rekonstruktion von Messsignalen*. Faculty of Engineering and Computer Science, Hamburg, 2007

[4] Brainvoyager, *BrainVoyager QX User's Guide*. Available:http://www.brainvoyager.com/bvqx/doc/UsersGuide/BrainVoyagerQXUsersGuide.html [last accessed on 29.01.2015]

[5] W. M. K. Trochim, *General Linear Model*. Available: http://www.socialresearchmethods.net/kb/genlin.php [last accessed on 29.01.2015]

Different k-Space Sampling Sequences for MR Image Reconstruction with Blind Sparse Motion Estimation

C. Clauß [1], A. Möller [2], and A. Mertins [2]
[1] Medizinische Ingenieurwissenschaft, Universität zu Lübeck, clauss@miw.uni-luebeck.de
[2] Institute for Signal Processing, Universität zu Lübeck, {moeller, mertins}@isip.uni-luebeck.de

Abstract

Sudden movements during MRI lead to ghost artifacts in the recorded images. A first approach, where such images were improved without any additional information has been shown in [1] and [2]. This method is extended to a linear translational motion. To integrate a noise reduction step and examine dependencies between sampling sequences and reconstruction results, different k-space sampling sequences are tested on different translational movements of the brainweb data [3]. Results are shown as motion corrected images while using the linear subpixel interpolation approach. Images with motion up to one third of *field of view* (FOV) will be reconstructed. A Poisson disk sampling method is presented to reconstruct those images with a non-fully sampled k-space, additionally.

1 Introduction

If a patient moves during an MR scan, there will be artifacts in the recorded images. Those artifacts are mostly ghost artifacts [4]. The intensity of the artifacts will largely depend on the strength of the motion. It is noted that not only active movement, but also inner body motion like breathing or heart beating can cause such artifacts. Obviously, a physician cannot give a clear diagnosis with such images. Diverse groups are dealing with this matter in different ways. Mostly additional information is used to perform a triggered [5] and/or faster sampling to reduce unwanted image effects. In [1], it is shown that no additional information is needed to reconstruct images with artifacts produced by translational movements. The enhancement to reconstruct subpixel movement is shown in [2].

In this work, we study the dependence between reconstruction results and sampling sequences without any additional information. It is an advantage to use a random sample line approach for *compressed sensing* (CS) [6], which will be used in further reconstruction algorithms. Anyway, it is useful to collect low-frequency information as soon and fast as possible because the energy is higher in this part of the k-space. This implies more information in the part of lowest frequencies.

We introduce a method where k-space lines out of different intervals are sampled in random order. The number of randomly picked sample lines increases for intervals with lower frequencies. In addition, we present a Poisson disk distributed sample line selection which will result in an undersampled k-space. The advantage of this approach is that a single MR slice scan could be done faster than usual. For example, this has the consequence that patients do not need to hold breath for a longer time during a thorax slice scan.

2 Material and Methods

The MR scan of one slice results in a discretely recorded k-space $\mathcal{K} \in \mathbb{C}^{O \times N}$. In our approach, we work on a k-space matrix $K \in \mathbb{C}^{M \times N}$, $M = \frac{O}{2}$, because we deal with real valued images. In K, the low frequencies are in the first lines. The highest frequencies are in the last lines. With knowledge about the spatial encoding [4], we assume that one k-space line $\boldsymbol{m}_i \in \mathbb{R}^{1 \times N}$, $i = 1, ..., M$, is recorded without any motion. Therefore, each k-space line needs to be frequency encoded. Accordingly, the phase encoding will be in k_y direction. Due to the fact that phase encoding takes longer time, motion will appear between different k_y lines.

Let $\mathcal{M}$ be the set of all lines $\boldsymbol{m}_i$ (cf. Fig. 1) with

$$\mathcal{M} = \{\boldsymbol{m}_i \mid i = 1, ..., M\}. \tag{1}$$

$\mathcal{M}$ will be needed to describe the total random sample line approach and the method of random lines out of splitted intervals, which we introduce in the following. After this, the dart-throwing Poisson disk sampling is shown.

2.1 Total Random Sample Sequence

Due to the fact that we want to use CS to reconstruct the image, we sample the complete k-space randomly line wise. Therefore, $\mathsf{rnd}[\mathcal{M}]$ is an operator which randomly chooses one index i of one element $\boldsymbol{m}_i$ of set $\mathcal{M}$ with respect to the uniform distribution on the interval $[0, 1]$ and no replacement. After using this operator, the number of elements in set $\mathcal{M}$ decreases by one. Now, we can construct each k-space line $K(i, 1...N)$ as

$$K(i, 1...N) = \mathcal{F}_2(I(t))(i, 1...N) \tag{2}$$

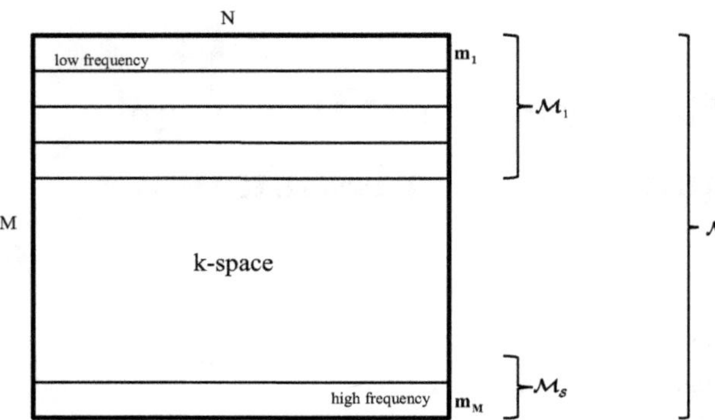

Figure 1: Scheme of k-space with set $\mathcal{M}$ and subsets $\mathcal{M}_s$.

with the two-dimensional Fourier transform $\mathcal{F}_2$, the actual image $I(t)$ of the focused body slice at discrete time t and $i = \mathsf{rnd}[\mathcal{M}]$. Motion will occur between two time points t_1 and t_2. The decreasing of the cardinality of $\mathcal{M}$ can be denoted by $\mathcal{M}^{t+1} = \mathcal{M}^t \setminus \{\boldsymbol{m}_i\}$ with $\mathcal{M}^0 = \mathcal{M}$, t being an index.

2.2 Splitted Interval Sampling Order

To achieve better results than the method in 2.1, it is necessary to sample low frequencies with low motion. Moreover, it is important to retain the random approach to be able to use CS [7]. A fusion of both aspects is the method of random sample lines out of splitted intervals.

For this purpose, we divide the set $\mathcal{M}$ into S strict subsets $\mathcal{M}_s \subset \mathcal{M}$ and $\mathcal{M}_s \bigcap \mathcal{M}_r = \varnothing$ for $s, r \in 1, ..., S$ (Fig. 1). Note that $S \leq M$. Thus, the lowest frequency line is in $\mathcal{M}_1$ and the highest one is in $\mathcal{M}_S$.

The sequence of random line selections depends on the cardinality of the subsets. So, it makes more sense to have more elements e_s in the lowest subset $\mathcal{M}_1$.

We propose an algorithm to choose random lines from each subset proportionally distributed to the cardinalities of $\mathcal{M}_1$ to $\mathcal{M}_S$. The algorithm chooses subsets $\mathfrak{M}_1, ..., \mathfrak{M}_S$ of the sets $\mathcal{M}_1, ..., \mathcal{M}_S$ respectively with the condition that the ratios of the subsets' cardinalities are nearly equal to the ratios of the cardinalities of the sets $\mathcal{M}_1, ..., \mathcal{M}_S$. This can be formulated as

$$\frac{|\mathfrak{M}_s|}{|\mathfrak{M}_r|} \approx \frac{|\mathcal{M}_s|}{|\mathcal{M}_r|} \tag{3}$$

with

$$\mathfrak{M}_s \subset \mathcal{M}_s.$$

This method is iterated until no elements are left in the sets $\mathcal{M}_1, ..., \mathcal{M}_S$. If a set is empty before others, this set will be skipped. This can only happen in the last iteration of the algorithm. For a better generality, the number and size of sets are given by a vector $\boldsymbol{v}$ with length S. The entries v_s of the vector $\boldsymbol{v}$ specify the ratio of the cardinality of the corresponding set $\mathcal{M}_s$ to the one of $\mathcal{M}$. The sum of all elements of $\boldsymbol{v}$ needs to be one, accordingly. We determine $\boldsymbol{v} = [0.6, 0.1, 0.1, 0.1, 0.1]$ empirically.

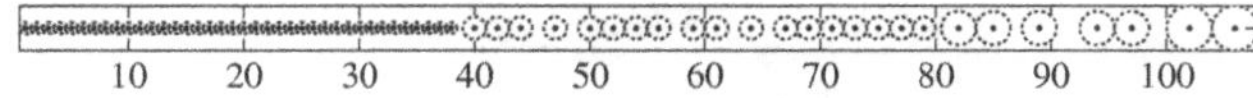

Figure 2: Distribution of indices (index vector $\boldsymbol{i}$) with dart-throwing Poisson disk approach and variable density ($\lambda = 0.7$).

2.3 Poisson Disk Distributed Sample Sequence

To extend the reconstruction method in [2] to work with an undersampled k-space, we introduce a Poisson disk distribution with variable density [8]. For this, we use a basic dart-throwing algorithm [9] to generate a Poisson disk distributed index vector $\boldsymbol{i}$ (Fig. 2). To restrict variable areas around each point, a vector $\boldsymbol{d}$ of length M is generated as

$$\boldsymbol{d} = \begin{bmatrix} d_1 \\ \vdots \\ d_M \end{bmatrix}, \quad d_i \in \mathbb{N}_0, \quad i = 1, ..., M. \tag{4}$$

The entries d_i of $\boldsymbol{d}$ describe the restriction radius for corresponding points (cf. circles in Fig. 2). This restriction radius gives the possibility to reduce the density of higher frequencies, while the lowest frequencies are fully sampled. In this work, we use

$$d_i = \begin{cases} 0, & i \in [1, 40[\\ 1, & i \in [40, 80] \\ 2, & i \in]80, 100] \\ 3 & \text{otherwise.} \end{cases} \tag{5}$$

The index vector $\boldsymbol{i}$ is created with the algorithm in Alg. 1. To adjust the undersampling intensity, we denote L as the maximal desired number of sample lines. Therefore, the computed rate of k-space lines is described by $\lambda = \frac{L}{M}$. To abort the algorithm if no index is found, the variable $thresh$ sets a maximum number of iterations. This point could be reached when all available indices are restricted by already chosen neighboring indices. For adjustments, a function handle fch gives the possibility to get the next index randomly proportional to a self modulated distribution. In our case, we choose an empirical distribution generated from k-spaces of adjacent slices [8]. This distribution is shown in Fig. 3.

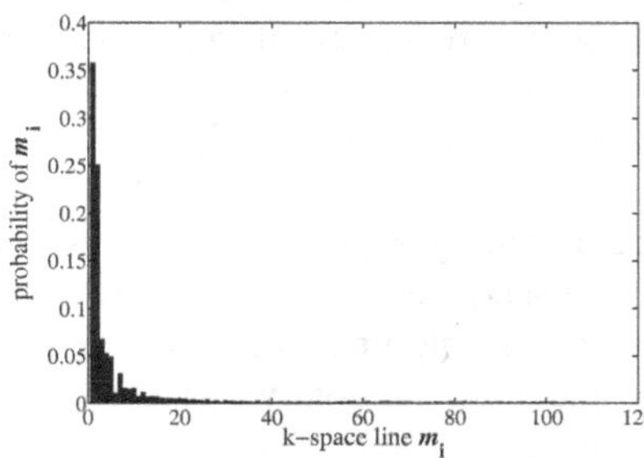

Figure 3: Self-modulated distribution to adjust random process.

Algorithm 1 Poisson disk with variable density

```
procedure GETPOISSONIND(L, fch, thresh, d)
    counter ← 0
    foundL ← 0
    run ← 1
    while run ≠ 0 do
        counter ← counter + 1
        actualIndex ← getRandomIndex(fch)
        isGood ← checkArea(actualIndex,d)
        if isGood = 1 then
            foundL ← foundL + 1
            counter ← 0
            setToVec(actualIndex)
        if counter > thresh then
            run ← 0
        if foundL = L then
            run ← 0
    ï ← getIndexVec()
    return ï
```

3 Results

The different algorithms are examined for a circular translation of 15 px to 120 px. The selected brainweb data [3] has a size of 217 $px \times 181$ px.
In the following, we only present the results for 30 px (Fig. 4), 70 px (Fig. 5) and 100 px (Fig. 6). We chose the split vector $\boldsymbol{v}$ for all results as defined before. Furthermore, we set a rate of $\lambda = 0.7$ while using Poisson disk sampling together with the index vector shown in Fig. 2.
As expected, more movement will result in more artifacts. It is clearly recognizable while comparing the images (a) in Fig. 4, 5 and 6. Additional to ghost artifacts, some deformation occurs. It is possible to reconstruct images with a motion up to 70 px (cf. Fig. 5). The deformation intensifies (cf. Fig. 6) for larger pixel shifts.
Between the total random sample lines and splitted interval algorithms, only inconclusive differences exist. It seems to be a better contrast while using the method of splitted intervals.
In Fig. 7 the results of Poisson disk sampling of a movement over 50 px for different rates $\lambda = 0.7$ down to $\lambda = 0.3$ are shown. While only a few ghost artifacts are left in the image Fig. 7(b), no fine structure is visible in a half sampled k-space (Fig. 7 (c)). A 30% sampled k-space (cf. Fig. 7 (d)) results in more unusable reconstruction. No edge information is left here.
In comparison to the fully sampled approaches, the 70% sampled k-space of Poisson disk sampling results in reconstructions with equivalent quality.

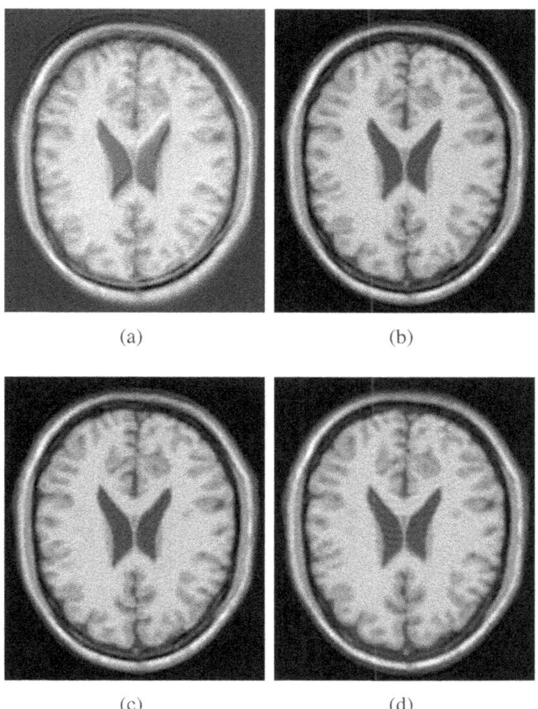

Figure 4: Linear shift of 30 px: (a) original moved image, (b) total random sampling, (c) splitted interval sampling, (d) Poisson disk sampling.

4 Conclusions

Different k-space sampling sequences were introduced in this work. A Poisson disk sampling approach was presented to reconstruct images without ghost artifacts from an undersampled k-space gained from an corrupted image.

The results showed that all approaches are useful to reconstruct artifact free images. Translational motion up to 70 px could be reconstructed sufficiently. Furthermore, an undersampling of the k-space is possible. The quality of reconstructed images is good enough for better clinical diagnostic.
In the future, it will be necessary to find an objective measure to compare reconstructed images to the original ones. The advantages of each method should be used in reconstruction. Moreover, information about sampling sequences should be used in the motion estimation method.
Especially for Poisson disk sampling, the best restriction areas and different self-modulated distributions need to be evaluated. Using Poisson disk sampling with an iterative reduction of the restriction areas could lead to an "online" reconstruction method.
Furthermore, it will be useful to test the algorithms with real data. In addition, the reconstruction algorithm should be expanded to other kinds of motion like rotation, scaling, and non-affine movement.

5 Acknowledgement

This work has been carried out at Institute for Signal Processing, Universität zu Lübeck.

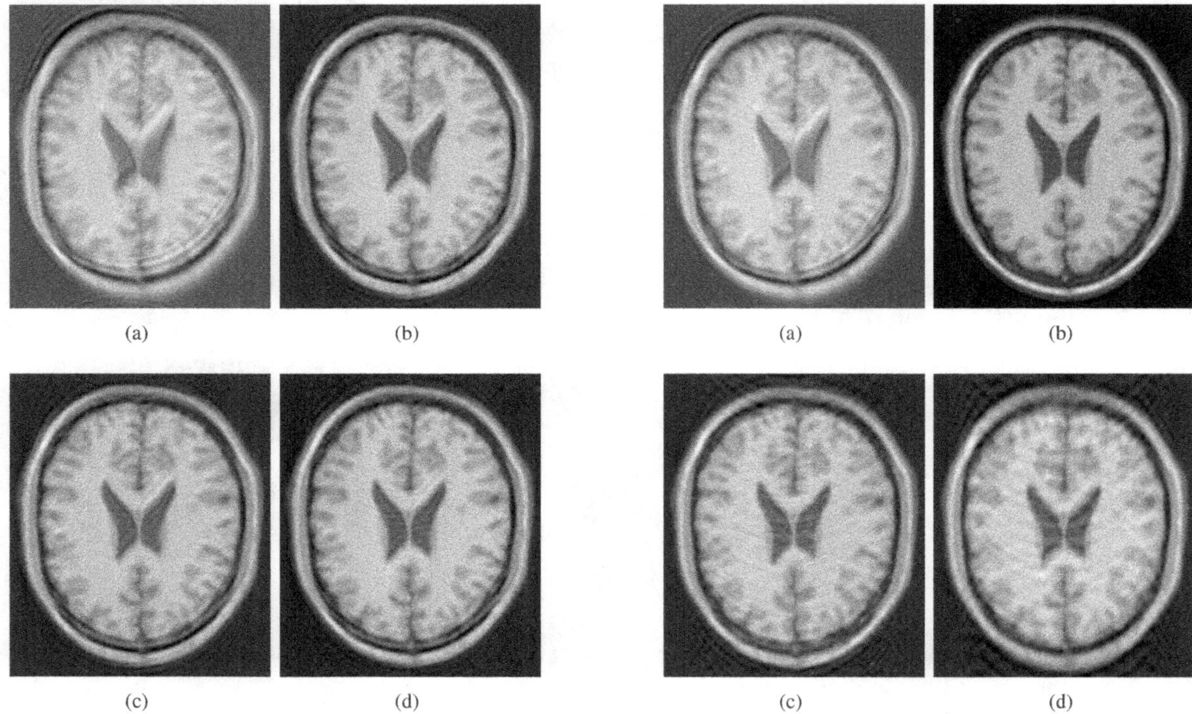

Figure 5: Linear shift of 70 px: (a) original moved image, (b) total random sampling, (c) splitted interval sampling, (d) Poisson disk sampling.

Figure 7: Different reconstructions depending on the rates of Poisson disk sampling: (a) original 50 px moved image, (b) $\lambda = 0.7$, (c) $\lambda = 0.5$, (d) $\lambda = 0.3$.

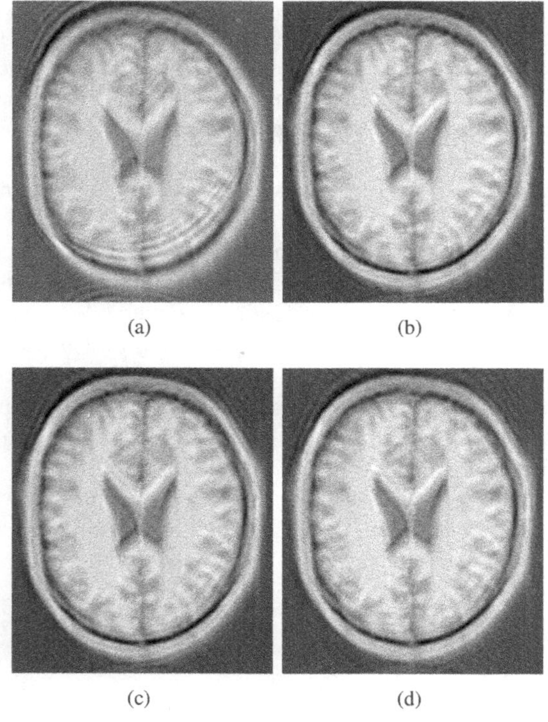

Figure 6: Linear shift of 100 px: (a) original moved image, (b) total random sampling, (c) splitted interval sampling, (d) Poisson disk sampling.

6 References

[1] Z. Yang, C. Zhang, and L. Xie, "Sparse MRI for motion correction," in *IEEE 10th International Symposium on Biomedical Imaging (ISBI)*, pp. 962–965, 2013.

[2] A. Möller, M. Maaß, and A. Mertins, "Blind sparse motion MRI with linear subpixel interpolation," in *Proc. Bildverarbeitung für die Medizin (BVM)(accepted)*, March 2015.

[3] C. A. Cocosco, V. Kollokian, R. K.-S. Kwan, G. B. Pike, and A. C. Evans, "Brainweb: Online interface to a 3d MRI simulated brain database," in *NeuroImage*, 1997.

[4] R. E. Hendrick, *Breast MRI: Fundamentals and Technical Aspects*, vol. 1. New York: Springer, 2008.

[5] Y. Wang, P. J. Rossman, R. C. Grimm, S. J. Riederer, and R. L. Ehman, "Navigator-echo-based real-time respiratory gating and triggering for reduction of respiration effects in three-dimensional coronary MR angiography," *Radiology*, vol. 198, no. 1, pp. 55–60, 1996.

[6] D. L. Donoho, "Compressed sensing," *IEEE Transactions on Information Theory*, vol. 52, no. 4, pp. 1289–1306, 2006.

[7] M. Lustig, D. Donoho, and J. M. Pauly, "Sparse MRI: The application of compressed sensing for rapid MR imaging," *Magnetic resonance in medicine*, vol. 58, no. 6, pp. 1182–1195, 2007.

[8] N. Gdaniec, *Robust breath-held abdominal magnetic resonance imaging based on compressed sensing*. PhD thesis, Lübeck, Univ., 2014.

[9] R. L. Cook, "Stochastic sampling in computer graphics," *ACM Transactions on Graphics (TOG)*, vol. 5, no. 1, pp. 51–72, 1986.

Exploiting Sparse Representations of the Plenacoustic Function for Compressive Sensing

F. Katzberg [1], R. Mazur [2], J. O. Jungmann [2], and A. Mertins [2]
[1] Medizinische Ingenieurwissenschaft, Universität zu Lübeck, katzberg@miw.uni-luebeck.de
[2] Institute for Signal Processing, Universität zu Lübeck, {mazur, jungmann, mertins}@isip.uni-luebeck.de

Abstract

The knowledge about the entire sound pressure field of a room can be used for acoustic scenarios in virtual reality and for listening room compensation [1]. In conventional signal processing the measurement of a signal is subjected to the Nyquist–Shannon sampling theorem. Therefore, sampling of a sound pressure field requires a huge number of measurements. For reducing this effort, methods of compressed sensing can be used exploiting sparsity in some representation of the signal. Here, we will show that sound fields are sparse in frequency domain. We propose an algebraic reconstruction approach using the basic spatial properties of the sound pressure field. Additionally, this method will be compared to the physically motivated plane wave approximation.

1 Introduction

Imagine you are walking up and down a room, listening to fixed positioned music speakers. Which is your most convenient location in space to enjoy the music with the best experience of sound? To acquire this knowledge, you must find a way to constitute information about the space and time dependent sound pressure field.
Measuring the sound pressure field is basically a sampling problem. A finite number of points, uniformly sampled in space and time, allows us to compute a reconstruction of the entire acoustic wavefield. According to the Nyquist–Shannon sampling theorem and considering a bandlimited signal with cutoff frequency f_c, the sampling frequency f_s has to fulfill the condition $f_s > 2f_c$, in order to avoid aliasing. In our setup, where we consider sampling in time and space, this implies

$$\Delta d < \frac{c_0}{2f_c} \tag{1}$$

where c_0 is the speed of sound and Δd denotes the spatial sampling intervall. This is the requirement for gathering the minimal spatial wavelength

$$\lambda_{\min} = \frac{c_0}{f_c}. \tag{2}$$

For example, to reconstruct the sound pressure field inside a cube of $1\,\mathrm{m}^3$ with $f_c = 8\,\mathrm{kHz}$, about $12 \cdot 10^3$ spatial measuring points for microphones are needed. In order to reduce this infeasible number, the technique of compressed sensing can be used. For that purpose, two compressive-sensing based approaches will be described and applied.

2 Material and Methods

In this section, we follow the approach [2] and model an acoustic environment as a linear transmission system. A sound source emits an auditory event which stimulates the surroundings to give an acoustic feedback. The relation between an input sound signal and the corresponding behaviour of the acoustic environment is described by the room impulse response (RIR). In the continuous case, for a certain listener position, the specific RIR $h(t)$ characterises the time t dependent sequence of the received sound waves, which result from a sound impulse effected at a particular source location. Usually, the received signal $x(t)$ is a succession of the first incoming direct sound, the early reflections, and the diffuse late-field reverberation. The temporal connection between the emitted and the received signal is stated by the convolution integral

$$x(t) = s(t) * h(t) = \int_{-\infty}^{\infty} s(\tau)h(t-\tau)d\tau. \tag{3}$$

2.1 The Plenacoustic Function

The introduced motivation to describe the whole spatio-temporal sound pressure field in a room leads to the concept of the *plenacoustic function* (PAF) [2]. Consider a single point source which emits the signal $s(t)$ at a fixed position. Then, the PAF $p(\mathbf{r}, t)$ depends on the listener location $\mathbf{r} = (x, y, z)^{\mathrm{T}}$ as well as on time t, and it is composed by the convolution integral

$$p(\mathbf{r}, t) = \int_{-\infty}^{\infty} s(\tau)h(\mathbf{r}, t-\tau)d\tau. \tag{4}$$

In case of an emitted Dirac pulse, the PAF is simply a set of time and space dependent RIRs. Postulating that the acoustic environment embodies an LTI system, the impact of multiple sources can be modeled as the superposition of single sources. Then, the sound pressure field is assembled by the sum of all source signals, each of them previously convolved with their spatio-temporal RIR as in (4). Without loss of generality, the PAF will be regarded as a depiction of the spatio-temporal sound pressure field, given one fixed positioned source that emits a Dirac impulse at $t = 0$, so $p(\mathbf{r}, t) = h(\mathbf{r}, t)$. To study the properties of the PAF inside a concluded rectangular room we simulated RIRs on a uniformly sampled grid within a confined space regarding (1) at discrete time n. Here, we use the image method from [3]. This shoe-box model allows for simulation of sound reflections in closed rooms by mirroring the acoustic scenario along the room walls. The sound source and the microphones are considered to be omnidirectional in our simulations.

2.2 The Principle of Compressed Sensing

By use of *compressed sensing* (CS), reconstructing an unknown signal is possible even in the case where the Shannon-Nyquist requirements are not met [4]. The underlying idea is to represent an unknown vector $\mathbf{g}$ of length N as a linear combination of basis vectors in matrix $\mathbf{T}$ as

$$\mathbf{g} = \mathbf{T}\mathbf{c} \tag{5}$$

with vector $\mathbf{c}$ containing the weighting coefficients. The principle of CS requires that $\mathbf{g}$ can be approximated by a linear combination of only few basis vectors. This translates to the requirement of $\mathbf{c}$ being sparse, which means that most of the elements are zero. That can be exploited to reconstruct $\mathbf{g}$ using just a few measurements. For this purpose, the measuring process is modeled as

$$\mathbf{b} = \mathbf{S}\mathbf{g} \tag{6}$$

with vector $\mathbf{b}$ containing M measurements and $\mathbf{S}$ being an interpolation matrix, which serves as sampling operator. It interrelates the measurements with the unknowns in $\mathbf{g}$. Inserting (5) into (6) and defining $\mathbf{A} = \mathbf{S}\mathbf{T}$ yields the underdetermined linear system of equations

$$\mathbf{b} = \mathbf{A}\mathbf{c} \tag{7}$$

with less measurements in $\mathbf{b}$ than unknowns in $\mathbf{c}$ ($M < N$). For obtaining a unique solution, we need to impose the sparsity on $\mathbf{c}$. This can be reformulated as a convex linear programming problem with quadratic contraints

$$\min \|\mathbf{c}\|_1 \text{ subject to } \|\mathbf{b} - \mathbf{A}\mathbf{c}\|_2 \leq \varepsilon \tag{8}$$

which can be solved via standard interior point methods [5]. Here, the tradeoff between sparsity and fineness of reconstruction is defined by ε. However, a solution $\mathbf{c}_s$ of the underdeterminded system (7) with ℓ_1-norm regularization approximates the wanted signal $\mathbf{g}$ as

$$\mathbf{g} \approx \mathbf{T}\mathbf{c}_s. \tag{9}$$

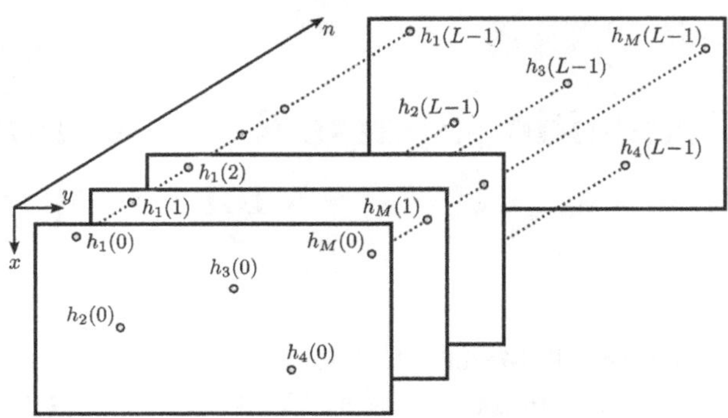

Figure 1: Partition of M measured RIRs at random positions $[x, y]^{\mathrm{T}}$ into time layers n.

2.3 Approach I: Thresholding in Layers

For the purpose of illustration and without loss of generality, we will consider the PAF for the two-dimensional case by setting z to some constant. The task is simplified to reconstruct the PAF on a plane with spatial coordinates x and y and discrete time n. More specifically, we want to recontruct a uniform grid on a plane satisfying the sampling theorem (1) using only a small set of M RIRs with length L, each of them measured at a random position on the plane. The spatial property of the RIRs is calculated by examining the progress of each time tap n in space separately. This procedure is shown in Fig. 1. Iterating over all L slices we reconstruct the spatial variation of each tap position $n \in \{0, \ldots, L-1\}$ by applying CS. Imagine a uniform sampled grid in each layer satisfying (1). At the corresponding grid positions are the unknown RIRs $g_{x_i,y_i}(n)$ on the plane we need to reconstruct using M measurements. The discrete indices $x_d \in \{0, \ldots, k-1\}$ and $y_d \in \{0, \ldots, l-1\}$ span the two-dimensional grid of size $k \times l$. For layer n, the matrix

$$\mathbf{G}_n = \begin{bmatrix} g_{0,0}(n) & g_{0,1}(n) & \cdots & g_{0,l-1}(n) \\ g_{1,0}(n) & g_{1,1}(n) & \cdots & g_{1,l-1}(n) \\ \vdots & \vdots & \ddots & \vdots \\ g_{k-1,0}(n) & g_{k-1,1}(n) & \cdots & g_{k-1,l-1}(n) \end{bmatrix}$$

contains the unknown values for the grid indices at time n. These can be represented as a two-dimensional transformation

$$\mathbf{G}_n = \mathbf{T}\mathbf{C}_n\mathbf{T}^{\mathrm{H}} \tag{10}$$

with the $k \times l$ coefficient matrix $\mathbf{C}_n$. Concatenating all columns of $\mathbf{G}_n$ to one vector $\mathbf{g}_n$ and defining $\mathbf{b}_n = [h_1(n), h_2(n), \ldots, h_M(n)]^{\mathrm{T}}$, the measuring process is modeled by

$$\mathbf{b}_n = \mathbf{S}\mathbf{g}_n \tag{11}$$

where $\mathbf{S}$ interrelates $\mathbf{b}_n$ with the unknowns $\mathbf{g}_n$ on the grid by the bias of bilinear interpolation. For solving this underdetermined system of linear equations we apply a kind of iterative hard thresholding algorithm similar to [6] and minimize

$$\|\mathbf{b}_n - \mathbf{S}\mathbf{g}_n\|_2^2 \tag{12}$$

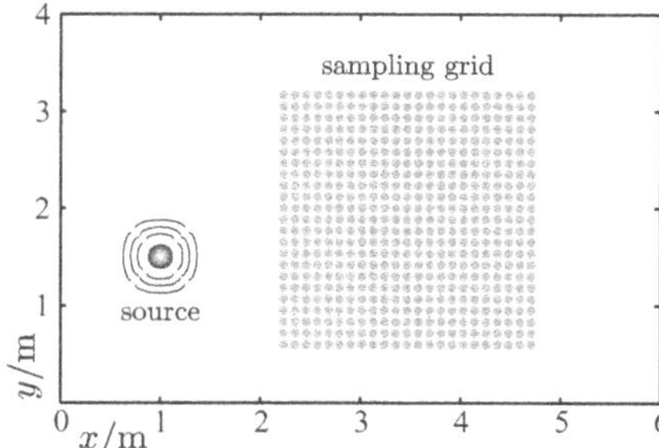

Figure 2: Plane x-y-perspective of the simulated three-dimensional room.

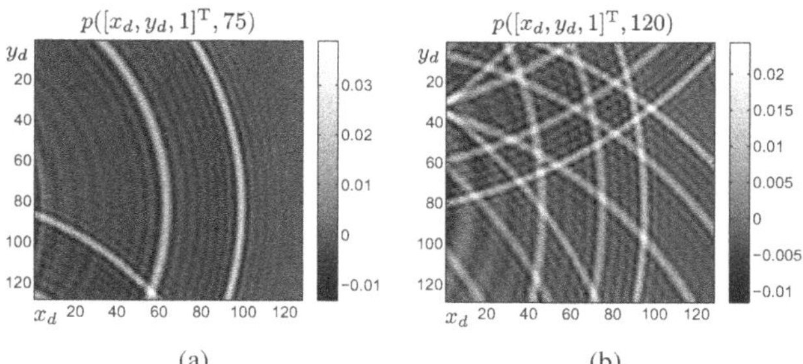

Figure 3: Spatial representation of the PAF on the plane. (a) Time index $n = 75$. (b) Time index $n = 120$. Note the different scaling of the gray values.

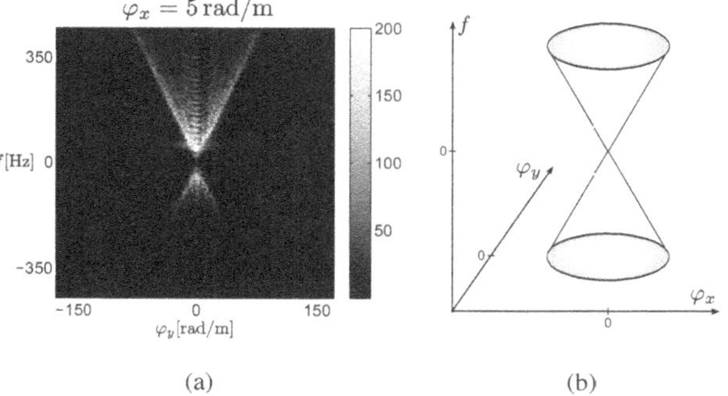

Figure 4: Spectrum of the PAF on the plane. (a) Fixed spatial frequency $\varphi_x = 5\,\mathrm{rad/m}$. (b) Entire spectrum outlined.

with nonlinear regularization. In each iteration i, after inverse transform of the current estimate $\tilde{\mathbf{G}}_n$, we get the estimated coefficient matrix $\tilde{\mathbf{C}}_n$. Then, the sparsity is enforced by retaining only the K most dominant coefficients. By transforming this K-sparse matrix back using (10) we obtain a new approximation $\tilde{\mathbf{G}}_n$, respectively $\tilde{\mathbf{g}}_n$. Finally, that one is updated applying the gradient descent

$$\tilde{\mathbf{g}}_n^{i+1} = \tilde{\mathbf{g}}_n^i - a\left(-2\mathbf{S}^{\mathrm{H}}\left(\mathbf{b}_n - \mathbf{S}\tilde{\mathbf{g}}_n^i\right)\right) \tag{13}$$

with a small step size a.

2.4 Approach II: Modal Analysis

In [7] a physically based approach is presented exploiting the modal properties of any star-shaped room. Assuming a structured sparsity of the sound pressure field at low temporal frequencies, the PAF is estimated as the discrete sum of complex harmonics q, each of them approximated with R wavevectors $\mathbf{k}_{q,r}$. After finding Q room modes using a few measured RIRs employed on SOMP [8], the PAF is reconstructed as

$$p(\mathbf{r}, t) \approx \sum_{q=1}^{2Q} \sum_{r=1}^{R} a_{q,r} e^{j\mathbf{k}_{q,r}^{\mathrm{T}}\mathbf{r}} e^{-\mu_q t} e^{j\omega_q t} \tag{14}$$

with complex amplitudes $a_{q,r}$, positive time damping coefficients μ_q, and angular frequencies ω_q.

3 Results and Discussion

To discuss the properties of the PAF on a plane, a room of length 6 m (x coordinate), width 4 m (y coordinate) and height 2.5 m (z coordinate) was modeled. The position of the sound source was set to $[1, 1.5, 1]^{\mathrm{T}}$ concerning a coordinate system with unit 1 m. Then, beginning from position $[2.2, 0.6, 1]^{\mathrm{T}}$ RIRs of length $L = 1000$ were simulated on a uniform sampling grid of size 128×128 at constant height $z = 1\,\mathrm{m}$. This was accomplished by applying the spatial sampling step $\Delta d = 0.02\,\mathrm{m}$ at temporal sampling frequency $f_s = 8\,\mathrm{kHz}$. The x-y-perspective of the simulated room including the positions of the sound source as well as the sampling grid is outlined in Fig. 2. Regarding this scenario, the spatial variation of different fixed time indices is illustrated in Fig. 3. In these images one pixel represents one sample on the grid in Fig. 2 at fixed time. The gray values represent the values of the PAF at the appropriate positions. In Fig. 3(a) one can see the wave front of the direct sound with most energy at the right-hand side coming from the left. Furthermore, there are the delayed and attenuated first reflections from the left und lower wall. With proceeding time, more and more reflections occur (Fig. 3(b)), and finally the PAF results in diffuse late-field reverberation. So, the spatio-temporal RIRs of the PAF have a wave structured sparsity in space, especially at early time taps. Transforming the whole simulated PAF considering one discrete time dimension n and two discrete space dimensions x_d, y_d into Fourier domain, yields even a stronger sparsity. The spectrum of the three-dimensional discrete Fourier transform for one fixed space frequency $\varphi_x = 5\,\mathrm{rad/m}$ is shown in Fig. 4(a). The entire three-dimensional frequency spectrum is outlined in Fig. 4(b). The most information lives inside a cone along the temporal frequency axis f. This is an excellent prerequisite for CS-based sound-field reconstruction.

3.1 Quality of Reconstruction

To compare the quality of reconstruction between both approaches, the same acoustic scenario as modeled in [7] is considered. Beginning from position $[0.95, 1.95, 1]^{\mathrm{T}}$ RIRs of length $L = 500$ were simulated on a uniform sampling grid of size 20×20 at constant height $z = 1\,\mathrm{m}$. This was accomplished by applying the spatial sampling step $\Delta d = 0.02\,\mathrm{m}$ at temporal sampling frequency $f_s = 750\,\mathrm{Hz}$. So, the simulated PAF involves 400 spatio-temporal RIRs to be

Table 1: Mean NSM in dB for approach I using M measurements and retaining K coefficients of the 2D-DCT

M \ K	10	20	30	100	200
5	-0.41	-0.42	-0.42	-0.33	-0.31
10	-1.94	-2.11	-1.88	-1.12	-0.90
20	-4.60	-3.56	-3.25	-2.13	-1.76
30	-5.45	-3.51	-3.28	-2.65	-2.18
50	-10.28	-10.44	-8.11	-4.35	-3.57
100	-12.70	-15.02	-15.15	-8.54	-7.05
150	-13.13	-15.64	-16.34	-12.70	-9.64
200	-14.55	-17.18	-18.24	-16.08	-12.01

Table 2: Mean NSM in dB for approach I using M measurements and retaining K coefficient pairs of the 2D-DFT

M \ K	10	20	30	100	200
5	-1.15	-0.75	-0.64	-0.40	-0.31
10	-2.27	-2.17	-1.74	-1.00	-0.76
20	-6.01	-3.36	-2.81	-1.76	-1.49
30	-7.09	-4.48	-3.84	-2.24	-2.03
50	-12.41	-8.47	-5.92	-3.76	-3.25
100	-15.91	-16.36	-13.65	-6.96	-6.52
150	-17.08	-18.65	-18.30	-9.87	-9.12
200	-18.76	-20.09	-20.30	-12.67	-10.78

recontructed. The quality of the reconstruction of an RIR on the sampling grid is evaluated using the normalized system misalignment (NSM) in dB

$$\mathrm{NSM}_{\mathrm{dB}} = 20\log_{10}\left(\frac{\|\mathbf{g}_{x_d,y_d} - \tilde{\mathbf{g}}_{x_i,y_i}\|_2}{\|\mathbf{g}_{x_d,y_d}\|_2}\right) \quad (15)$$

where $\mathbf{g}_{x_d,y_d} = [g_{x_d,y_d}(0), \dots, g_{x_d,y_d}(L-1)]^{\mathrm{T}}$ contains the simulated RIR and $\tilde{\mathbf{g}}_{x_d,y_d} = [\tilde{g}_{x_d,y_d}(0), \dots, \tilde{g}_{x_d,y_d}(L-1)]^{\mathrm{T}}$ contains the reconstructed RIR at the subscripted discrete grid position. For reconstructing via thresholding in layers (approach I), the 2D discrete cosine transform (2D-DCT) and the 2D discrete Fourier transform (2D-DFT) was tested. Using M random located measuring points, the mean NSM in dB over all grid positions is listed in Tab. 1 (2D-DCT) for retaining K coefficients, respectively in Tab. 2 (2D-DFT) for retaining $2K$ Fourier coefficients. In comparison to that, the results for reconstructing via modal analysis (approach II) are shown in Tab. 3. Here, on the basis of the same M measuring points, $Q = 100$ joint damped harmonic plane waves (modes) were estimated, each of them approximated with R directions in space.

4 Conclusion

For $M < 100$, the modal analysis delivers the best results. But, concerning a higher number of measurements the quality of reconstruction does not improve significantly anymore . In contrast to that, the reconstruction via thresholding in layers gets steadily better with increasing M. Regarding both approaches, an excessive order of approximation impairs the quality of reconstruction, especially for little M. Then, the reconstructed PAF is overfitted to the sampling positions, so that areas being far away from the measuring points are approximated poorly.

Table 3: Mean NSM in dB for approach II using M measurements and R-order approximation for each mode

M \ R	10	20	30	50	100
5	-10.87	-10.89	-10.88	-10.87	-10.87
10	-3.59	-2.00	-3.49	-3.49	-3.54
20	-10.80	2.73	11.70	8.49	8.50
30	-12.79	-12.05	2.83	-2.88	-3.66
50	-12.62	-12.38	-10.73	4.64	9.33
100	-12.78	-12.88	-12.63	-11.62	-9.33
150	-12.98	-13.05	-12.96	-12.58	-11.81
200	-12.00	-13.07	-13.03	-12.78	-12.33

Acknowledgement

This work has been carried out at the Institute for Signal Processing (ISIP), Universität zu Lübeck.

5 References

[1] J. O. Jungmann, R. Mazur, and A. Mertins, "Perturbation of room impulse responses and its application in robust listening room compensation," *Proc. IEEE Int. Conf. Acoust., Speech, and Signal Process. (ICASSP 2013)*, pp. 433–437, May 2013.

[2] T. Ajdler, L. Sbaiz, and M. Vetterli, "The plenacoustic function and its sampling," *IEEE Trans. Signal Process.*, vol. 54, no. 10, pp. 3790–3804, October 2006.

[3] J. B. Allen and D. A. Berkley, "Image method for efficiently simulating small-room acoustics," *Journal Acoustic Society of America*, vol. 65/4, pp. 943–950, April 1979.

[4] E. Candès and M. Wakin, "An introduction to compressive sampling," *IEEE Signal Process. Magazine*, vol. 25, no. 2, pp. 21–30, March 2008.

[5] S.-J. Kim, K. Koh, M. Lustig, S. Boyd, and D. Gorinevsky, "An interior-point method for large-scaled ℓ_1-regularized least squares," *IEEE Journal of Selected Topics in Signal Process.*, vol. 1, no. 4, pp. 606–617, December 2007.

[6] T. Blumensath and M. E. Davies, "Iterative thresholding for sparse approximations," *The Journal of Fourier Analysis and Applications*, vol. 14, pp. 629–654, December 2008.

[7] R. Mignot, G. Chardon, and L. Daudet, "Low frequency interpolation of room impulse responses using compressed sensing," *IEEE Trans. Audio, Speech, and Language Process.*, vol. 22, pp. 205–216, January 2014.

[8] G. Chardon and L. Daudet, "Optimal subsampling of multichannel damped sinusoids," *IEEE Sensor Array Multichannel Signal Process. Workshop*, pp. 25–28, October 2010.

9
Signal Processing II

Robust Pattern Recognition of Hand Movement with Multi-Channel Surface EMG Using Random Forest

V. Haase [1], P. Koch [1], L. Hertel [2], and A. Mertins [2]
[1] Medizinische Ingenieurwissenschaft, Universität zu Lübeck, {haase, kochp}@miw.uni-luebeck.de
[2] Institute for Signal Processing, Universität zu Lübeck, {hertel, mertins}@isip.uni-luebeck.de

Abstract

For the control system of a neuroprosthetic hand, a robust classification of the desired hand movement is necessary. The temporary loss of an electrode contact is one of the problems a robust recognition based on sEMG has to deal with. In contrast to hardware-based approaches, this work is trying to overcome these difficulties by adapting a learning algorithm on selected features. The considered time-domain features are extracted from a given data set, containing multi-channel sEMG signals of eight different hand movements, recorded from three able-bodied subjects. The recognition of movement is realized by the Random Forest algorithm. The results show that the training of a classifier with dropout related data is useful to moderate the effects of missing signals. Particularly suitable features for this problem are not found. These findings cannot replace the complex hardware solutions, but they can complement them to reduce the dropout disturbances.

1 Introduction

Modern prosthetic systems for the upper limb are based on human-machine interfaces. A neuroprosthetic hand is an example of the direct interaction of the user's thoughts and the control system of an artificial limb. The intended hand movement can be determined by the changes of the electrical potential inside the muscles, located in the forearm. The technique for evaluating this electrical activity is called *electromyography*. The non-invasive alternative, where electrodes are placed on the skin, is named *surface electromyography* (sEMG).

Current commercial neuroprosthesis hands are working with a maximum of two bipolar electrodes to detect the requested movement. To achieve a more natural control of the prosthesis, without sequentially executing complex hand movements, multi-channel sEMG signals are necessary. Because of diverse disturbances of the sEMG signal source, there is still no clinical application for this kind of intuitive controlled prosthetic hand. A robust recognition has to deal with changes in electrode location, variability of muscle contraction effort, and muscle fatigue [1]. This work considers the problem of temporarily missing contacts between sEMG electrodes and the user's skin, which is required to record the electrical activity. These *dropouts* can appear e.g. when too much weight is put on one side of an artificial limb and so the socket electrodes on the opposite side are lifted from the skin.

To prevent dropouts, different solutions are explored by enhancing parts of the used hardware [2]. Considering a software-based approach to minimize the effects of dropouts for the recognition of hand movements, this work examines a specific classification algorithm called *Random Forest* (RF) [3]. T. Friedrich has shown that RF is a useful method to overcome shift variances of sEMG electrodes for controlling a prosthetic system [4]. To extend the previous work the same data set is used. This specific set of sEMG signals is provided by Ottobock Healthcare GmbH[1]. It was recorded for the research project AMYO (Advanced Myoelectric Control of Prosthetic Systems) of the Department of Neurorehabilitation Engineering at the University Medical Center Göttingen[2].

2 Material and Methods

In the following section the given data set, the applied feature extraction, and the used classification algorithm are described.

2.1 Data Set

To gain more generalized information, the AMYO data set contains the sEMG recordings of three able-bodied subjects with no neuromuscular disorders. Eight electrodes are placed equidistantly around the forearm of each subject. They provide an eight-channel sEMG signal of a specific hand movement. The recordings are repeated on five consecutive days with five iterations for every hand movement on each day. An example of a typical signal sequence is shown in Fig. 1. The eight hand movements, which define the different classes for the classifier are wrist supination,

[1] http://www.ottobock.com.
[2] http://www.nre.bccn.uni-goettingen.de/?id=22.

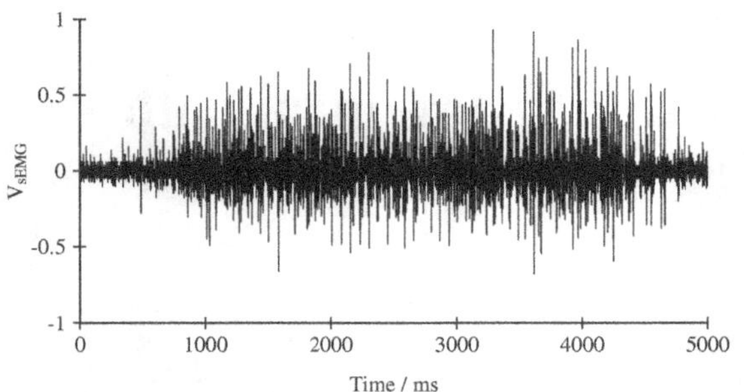

Figure 1: Typical normalized sEMG signal of a wrist pronation of subject 1, recorded as first repetition on day 1. For simplicity, only sEMG channel no. 3 is plotted.

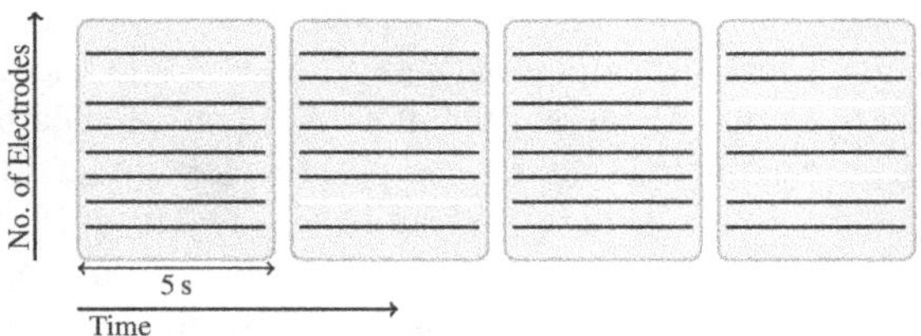

Figure 2: Scheme of the implementation of dropouts. The black stripes symbolize sEMG signals from working electrodes, whereas the white strides represent the dropout of the electrode. A dropout probability of 12.5 % is applied exemplarily.

wrist pronation, wrist flexion, wrist extension, hand open, lateral pinch, disk grip, and no movement of the hand as a relaxed posture. The used data only includes a muscle contraction effort of 60 % of the maximal voluntary contraction (MVC) and no intended shifts of the electrodes.

Every sEMG sample of a recorded hand movement has a duration of 5 s and a sampling rate of 1 kHz. For the following calculations only the central 2 s of the sample are used because of a non-immediate start and a too early ending of the movement noticed in a few samples. This parameter is determined empirically.

2.2 Simulated Dropouts

To simulate a missing contact between electrode and skin, the signal of an electrode is set to zero for the whole recording of the hand's movement. The adaptable probability of dropouts is based on a uniform probability distribution. An example of this procedure can be seen in Fig. 2.

2.3 Feature Extraction

The features are extracted from an analysis window of size N =128 ms. This frame is shifted with a step size of 50 ms, resulting in an overlap of 78 ms (Fig. 3). Therefore, a 2 s sample of the recorded movement provides 38 feature vectors for a framewise classification. For the feature extraction, only time-domain features are used due to the low

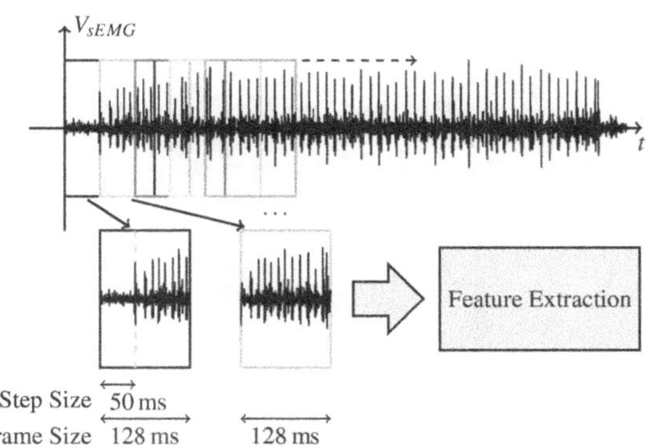

Figure 3: Scheme of the applied feature extraction. The features are calculated with single, overlapping parts of the original sEMG signal.

computational complexity, explained in [1]. The following eight features are calculated for the mean free sEMG signal $\vec{x} = [x_{1501}, \ldots, x_{3500}]$, which are also used in the AMYO project. More detailed information about these features can be found in [1], [5], and [6].

Root mean square (RMS) describes the constant force and non-fatiguing contraction of a muscle when the signal is modelled as a Gaussian random process. This feature relates to the standard deviation and is calculated over the analysis window of size N by

$$x_{RMS} = \sqrt{\frac{1}{N}\sum_{i=1}^{N} x_i^2}. \tag{1}$$

Mean absolute value (MAV) is used for a signal modeled as a Laplacian random process to detect different levels of a muscle contraction. It is defined as

$$x_{MAV} = \frac{1}{N}\sum_{i=1}^{N} |x_i|. \tag{2}$$

Zero crossings (ZC) is defined as the number of times, the signal passes the zero amplitude axes and is associated with the frequency of a signal. It is given by

$$x_{ZC} = \sum_{i=1}^{N-1} f(x_i \cdot x_{i+1}), \tag{3}$$

where $f(x)$ is the Heaviside step function.

Slope sign changes (SSC) is another way to represent the frequency information of a signal. With $f(x)$ as Heaviside step function it is formulated as

$$x_{SSC} = \sum_{i=2}^{N-2} f((x_i - x_{i-1}) \cdot (x_i - x_{i+1})). \tag{4}$$

Waveform length (WL) is the cumulative length of the waveform over a time segment and measures the complexity of the signal. The definition is as

$$x_{WL} = \sum_{i=1}^{N-1} |x_{i+1} - x_i|. \tag{5}$$

Autoregressive model coefficients (ARC) describes each sample of the signal $\hat{x}_i$ as a linear combination of the p previous samples with an additional white noise s_k:

$$\hat{x}_i = \sum_{k=1}^{p} a_k x_{i-k} + s_k. \quad (6)$$

In this work the ARC a_k are calculated using the Burg method [7]. Considering [8], the order is set to $p = 6$, which results in the only multidimensional feature that is analyzed.
The *energy* (POW) of an sEMG signal is defined as

$$x_{POW} = \frac{1}{N} \sum_{i=1}^{N} x_i^2. \quad (7)$$

Also the *logarithmic energy* (LOGPOW) of the signal is calculated by taking the logarithm of (7).
When all eight features are calculated for the sEMG signal of each electrode, the feature vector contains 104 features for every frame that is classified. To find a significant subset of features, a backward search as a wrapper approach [9] is implemented.

2.4 Random Forest

In 2001 Leo Breiman developed the Random Forest algorithm for classification [3]. RF is an extension of normal decision or classification trees. To receive a RF, an ensemble of classification trees is built, using random bootstrap samples of the given data. This process of randomly choosing subsets of data is called bootstrap aggregating, also known as bagging, and allows to examine a large amount of data in a short time. In addition to this, the candidate set of features at each node of one tree is a random subset of the available features. There is no pruning step performed, meaning all trees of the forest are fully grown. Due to this special way of constructing a RF the individual trees have a low correlation to each other. Other advantages of the RF algorithm are the non-overfitting characteristic and a good predictive performance even with noise-impaired data.
The most important parameters of a RF are the number of trees ($ntree$), which are built and the number of features ($mtry$) at each split of the tree. These parameters have to be adapted to the particular classification problem.
When a trained RF is tested, each feature vector, extracted from the data, is running simultaneously through every tree from the root to its allocated leaf. The class-dependent probability distributions in these leaves are then used to calculate the most likely class over all trees.
In this work, the MATLAB package for RF[3] is used to classify the calculated sEMG features. The classification performance is quantified by the classification error (CE) over all frames of every hand movement sample:

$$CE = \frac{\text{Number of wrong classifications}}{\text{Total number of classifications}}. \quad (8)$$

[3]Random Forest (regression, classification and clustering) implementation for MATLAB provided by Abhishek Jaiantilal, http://code.google.com/p/randomforest-matlab.

Table 1: Classification error of RF for different dropout probabilities in train and test data

Test	Train				
	0 %	5 %	10 %	25 %	50 %
0 %	0.066 ±0.007	0.079 ±0.008	0.096 ±0.012	0.122 ±0.024	0.228 ±0.046
5 %	0.113 ±0.014	0.118 ±0.020	0.104 ±0.011	0.129 ±0.022	0.232 ±0.034
10 %	0.175 ±0.022	0.148 ±0.020	0.1486 ±0.010	0.1568 ±0.024	0.275 ±0.022
25 %	0.394 ±0.045	0.270 ±0.037	0.256 ±0.021	0.245 ±0.008	0.304 ±0.041
50 %	0.699 ±0.039	0.554 ±0.041	0.475 ±0.014	0.441 ±0.030	0.461 ±0.038

The RF is trained with the described data of all three subjects recorded in the first two days without any shift variances and a contraction effort of 60 MVC. After the training procedure, the classifier is tested with the data of the same specification of the third recording day.

3 Results and Discussion

Due to the special characteristic of the RF, the classification result varies, depending on the random sequences of the learning procedure. To enable a convincing outcome, the training and testing of the classifier are repeated ten times for every experiment. The listed error rates are the mean value and the standard deviation of these repetition. All of the eight time-domain features mentioned above are calculated during the feature extraction.
As a first reference value for the described data set, the classification error rate of $6.6\,\% \pm 0.7\,\%$ is achieved, when no dropouts are interfering. In this case, the number of trees and the number of variables at each node is set to the default setting of $ntree = 100$ and $mtry = 2$.
Table 1 shows how the RF reacts to different dropout probabilities in the train and test data. When the classifier is trained without any defective signals but is tested with it, the error rate increases steeply up to $69.9\,\%$ for $50\,\%$ of dropouts. If the classifier is trained with dropout containing signals, this ascending behavior is reduced: only $22.8\,\%$ of the data is classified incorrectly for $50\,\%$ of missing signals. However, the classifier loses its effectiveness, if it is trained with a lot of dropouts in the data but is tested with faultless signals.
The experiments, listed in Table 2, with a varying number of trees that are growing during the learning procedure of a RF, confirm the default setting of 100 trees. With more than 100 trees the classification error can not be reduced. Note that the calculation effort has to be taken into account: an approximately linear correlation between the needed time to train the classifier and number of trees can be noticed.
A further improvement of the classifier, depending on the correct choice of the second parameter $mtry$, is shown in

Table 2: CE for dropout (D) and non-dropout (ND) impaired data with different numbers of trees in the RF

	ntree				
	10	50	75	100	200
D	0.224	0.153	0.148	0.129	0.133
	±0.018	±0.020	±0.024	±0.022	±0.024
ND	0.116	0.073	0.068	0.067	0.065
	±0.011	±0.008	±0.007	±0.006	±0.007

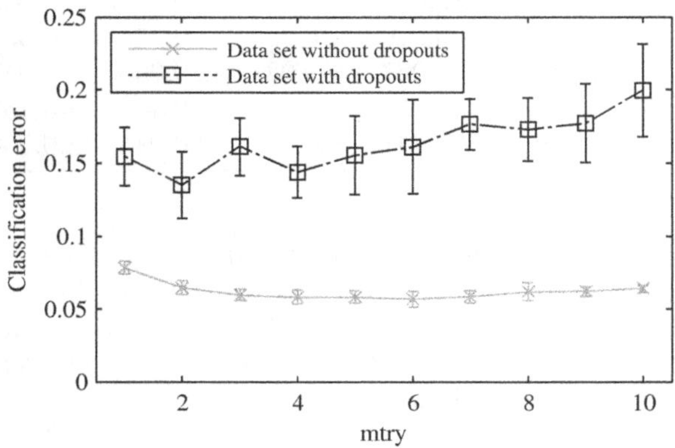

Figure 4: The classification error depends on the correct number of features taken as candidates at each node of a decision tree.

Fig. 4. The optimal value for this specific train and test set related with dropouts is $mtry = 2$. For faultless data the determination of $mtry$ is less decisive. The smallest classification error is achieved with $mtry$ between 4 and 6. For both of the different data sets $mtry$ should not be larger than 10.

The feature selection applied to the data set without any dropouts as well as on a data set with different settings for the dropout probability on test and train data does not improve the number of right classifications. Furthermore, there is no clear tendency in the chosen subsets of features recognizable. Due to the high standard deviation that appears for calculations with dropout related data, the backward search with the classification error as decision criterion can not be recommended.

4 Conclusion

The purpose of this work is a robust recognition of hand movement despite dropout related sEMG signals. The implemented experiments and its results show that learning a Random Forest with missing sEMG signals is favorable for the correct classification if dropouts appear in the test sequence. This improvement is not possible without the trade-off against the optimal classification of faultless signals. The respective classification results can be improved by choosing the correct settings for the RF parameters. A significant subset of the provided sEMG features that either reduces the calculation effort or improves the classification result on data with a specific dropout probability is not identified.

For further research, a more complex system of multiple Random Forests can be implemented: Every RF has to diverge from each other by the dropout probability of the trained data set. An early event detector is needed to recognize the amount of dropouts in the test data as soon as possible. This observation decides which special trained RF is used to classify the upcoming sequence of sEMG features.

Acknowledgement

The work has been carried out at the Institute for Signal Processing, Universität zu Lübeck.

5 References

[1] D. Tkach, H. Huang, and T. A. Kuiken, "Research study of stability of time-domain features for electromyographic pattern recognition," *Journal of Neuroengineering and Rehabilitation*, vol. 7, p. 21, 2010.

[2] S. H. Roy, G. De Luca, M. Cheng, A. Johansson, L. D. Gilmore, and C. J. De Luca, "Electro-mechanical stability of surface emg sensors," *Medical & biological engineering & computing*, vol. 45, no. 5, pp. 447–457, 2007.

[3] L. Breiman, "Random forests," *Machine learning*, vol. 45, no. 1, pp. 5–32, 2001.

[4] T. Friedrich and A. Mertins, "Overcoming electrodes shift variances in multi-channel surface emg recordings for prosthetic controlling," in *Student Conference Medical Engineering Science 2014: Proceedings*, vol. 3, p. 127, GRIN Verlag, 2014.

[5] A. Phinyomark, C. Limsakul, and P. Phukpattaranont, "A novel feature extraction for robust emg pattern recognition," *Journal of Computing*, vol. 1, pp. 71–80, December 2009.

[6] R. Boostani and M. H. Moradi, "Evaluation of the forearm emg signal features for the control of a prosthetic hand," *Physiological measurement*, vol. 24, no. 2, p. 309, 2003.

[7] J. P. Burg, "A new analysis technique for time series data," *NATO Advanced Study Institute on Signal Processing with Emphasis on Underwater Acoustics*, vol. 1, 1968.

[8] D. Farina and R. Merletti, "Comparison of algorithms for estimation of emg variables during voluntary isometric contractions," *Journal of Electromyography and Kinesiology*, vol. 10, no. 5, pp. 337–349, 2000.

[9] R. Kohavi and G. H. John, "Wrappers for feature subset selection," *Artificial intelligence*, vol. 97, no. 1, pp. 273–324, 1997.

Noise Cancellation using Room Equalization Filters

T. Parbs [1] and A. Mertins[2]
[1] Medizinische Ingenieurwissenschaft, Universität zu Lübeck, parbs@miw.uni-luebeck.de
[2] Institute for Signal Processing, Universität zu Lübeck, mertins@isip.uni-luebeck.de

Abstract

Mechanical noise is a problem in many applications, as well as in cars as in magnetic resonance imaging. Active noise cancellation has been implemented together with passive insulation methods to suppress undesired noise. In this paper, a stationary prefilter is developed to cancel out a known noise signal, thus creating a silence zone. A filter design based on the Wiener-Hopf equations is compared with a recently proposed p-norm optimizing filter including a spectral flatness criterion in respect to performance and speaker displacement. A significant reduction in noise amplitude is achieved with both filters, with the Wiener-Hopf filter offering better performance than the p-norm optimizing filter while introducing more spectral distortion.

1 Introduction

Active noise cancellation (ANC) systems received a lot of attention lately. While traditional, passive approaches, which aim at insulating the acoustic source with foams and barriers, offer good attenuation at high frequencies, they are generally bulky and expensive. Modern ANC systems are typically more effective at low-frequency noise associated with mechanical systems and can be realized with few electromechanical components, often making them smaller and more versatile. ANC systems aim to introduce additional sound into the system by means of a speaker or exciter, which is tailored to cancel out the unwanted noise via destructive interference. Since the propagation paths of the noise source and the speaker of the ANC system necessarily differ, the noise cancelling system needs to compensate for the differences in the impulse response. Therefore, measurement or approximation of the room impulse responses (RIRs) of both channels is required. The signal created by the ANC system is a measurement of the unwanted noise processed by a digital filter which aims to mitigate these differences. Therefore, ANC systems perform best for unchanging RIRs and non-moving listeners. In the last two decades, advancements in available digital processing systems has driven progress towards highly adaptive noise cancelling systems which are able to cope with changes in both noise and RIRs [1]. Today, the most wide-spread application of ANC systems are noise-cancelling headphones, in which they are used alongside passive insulation materials to attenuate outside sounds.
Here, we try to find a stationary solution for a single channel ANC system using impulse response equalization techniques normally used in listening room compensation. We assume that the unwanted noise is periodic, as it is in most mechanical applications. We construct prefilters using the well-established Wiener-Hopf approach and compare their performance with filters created using a more recently developed approach using p-norm optimization with joint frequency-domain regularization.
In this paper, the following notation will be used: bold face lower-case letters are used for vectors, bold face capital letters for matrices. Series and scalar values are denoted by regular letters. The superscript ^{T} is used for transposition. E represents the expectation operator, $\Re$ the real part of a value.

2 Material and Methods

Our measurements used two identical exciters as sound sources. One was used as a acoustic source producing unwanted noise (the *noise source*), the other as output for the ANC system (the *antinoise exciter*). A wooden panel was used as a mounting surface for the two sources as metallic surfaces proved to introduce strong resonance oscillations in the measurements. The two exciters were positioned on opposing sites of the panel. In the following notation, $\mathbf{h_1}$ and $\mathbf{h_2}$ will denote the RIRs of length L_h from the noise output exciter and the noise cancelling output exciter to an arbitrary listener position, respectively. Furthermore, let $c(n)$ be the finite impulse response of the prefilter designed for the noise cancelling system of length L_c. The resulting residual signal at the listener position for a noise signal x(n) then equals

$$e(n) = \mathbf{H_1}x(n) + \mathbf{CH_2}x(n) \quad (1)$$

in which $\mathbf{C}$ is the L_c by $L_h + L_c - 1$ convolution matrix of $\mathbf{c}$ while $\mathbf{H_1}$ and $\mathbf{H_2}$ are the appropriately sized convolution matrices of the RIRs. By setting $e(n)$ to zero and and rearranging the formula, one can see that perfect noise cancellation can be achieved if the convolution of $h_2(n)$ and $\mathbf{c}$

equals the negative of $\mathbf{h_1}$. This formulation is very similar to listening room compensation, in which a prefilter is designed to reshape a specific RIR to resemble to some target function to remove reverberation effects as in this case, $\mathbf{h_2}$ is reshaped in respect to $\mathbf{h_1}$. The prefilter $\mathbf{c}$ can then be described by setting the residual to zero.

$$\begin{aligned} \mathbf{0} &= \mathbf{h_1} + \mathbf{H_2c} \\ \mathbf{c} &= -\mathbf{H_2}^{-1}\mathbf{h_1}. \end{aligned} \tag{2}$$

However, since room impulse responses are generally non-minimum phase [2], the exact inverse $\mathbf{H_2}^{-1}$ does not exist and has to be approximated. Generally, gradient descent least squares (LS) approaches are used in the filter design because of their robustness and simple implementation. In this paper, a closed-form expression of the LS filter as well as a gradient descent p-norm optimization approach are used.

2.1 Wiener-Hopf Filter

Our first approach was based on a finite impulse response filter based on the well-known Wiener-Hopf equations as described in [3] which is often used in similar studies. The Wiener filter minimizes the mean square error between the input signal and some desired signal. As mentioned, $\mathbf{h_2}$ should be reshaped to match $\mathbf{h_1}$, therefore the problem can be reformulated as

$$\min_{\mathbf{c}} E\{\|\mathbf{e}\|^2\} = E\{\|\mathbf{h_1} + \mathbf{H_2c}\|^2\} \tag{3}$$

$$= E\{\mathbf{h_1}^2\} + 2E\{\mathbf{h_1H_2}\}\mathbf{c} + \mathbf{c}^T E\{\mathbf{H_2}^T\mathbf{H_2}\}\mathbf{c}. \tag{4}$$

Using these equations and assuming $\mathbf{h_1}$ and $\mathbf{h_2}$ to be stationary, the cross-correlation column vector $\mathbf{p_{h_1h_2}}$ and the symmetric autocorrelation matrix $\mathbf{R_{h_2h_2}}$ can be defined as

$$\mathbf{p_{h_1h_2}} = E\{\mathbf{h_1H_2}\} \tag{5}$$

$$\mathbf{R_{h_2h_2}} = E\{\mathbf{H_2}^T\mathbf{H_2}\}. \tag{6}$$

By differentiating (4) for c and setting the gradient to zero, one arrives at the minimum mean square error solution

$$\mathbf{0} = 2\mathbf{R_{h_2h_2}c} + 2\mathbf{p_{h_1h_2}} \tag{7}$$

$$\mathbf{c} = -\mathbf{R_{h_2h_2}}^{-1}\mathbf{p_{h_1h_2}} \tag{8}$$

from which the filter coefficients can be derived. Except for some special cases, $\mathbf{R_{h_2h_2}}$ is not singular and therefore invertible [4]. In linear time-invariant systems, LS designs should converge to the solution of the Wiener-Hopf equation. Therefore, the Wiener-Hopf filter represents a closed-form solution for the LS-problem.

2.2 Iterative P-Norm Optimization Filter

The Wiener-Hopf filter in the previous section solves the LS-problem, but its impulse response generally contains high spectral peaks, which introduced very noticeable distortion during noise cancellation. To mitigate this, an alternative filter design was used in comparison. The p-norm optimization criterion has been shown to be superior to traditional LS approaches [5] for RIR equalization purposes. Furthermore, a spectral flatness measure can easily be added to the gradient descent equation [6].
The basic p-norm optimization problem is defined as

$$\min_{\mathbf{c}} f(\mathbf{c}) = \|h_1(n) - g(n)\|_p \tag{9}$$

$$= \left(\sum_{n=0}^{L_h} |h_1(n) - g(n)|^p\right)^{\frac{1}{p}} \tag{10}$$

using $\mathbf{g} = \mathbf{H_2c}$ and p as some integer value greater than two. Furthermore, the spectral flatness criterion is similarly defined as

$$\min_{\mathbf{c}} y(\mathbf{c}) = \|\mathbf{a}\|_p \tag{11}$$

$$= \left(\sum_{k=0}^{L_a} |a(k)|^p\right)^{\frac{1}{p}} \tag{12}$$

in which $\mathbf{a} = \mathbf{Fc}$ is the L_a-component Fourier transform, and $\mathbf{F}$ is the $L_a \times L_h$ discrete Fourier transform matrix. The gradients of (10) and (12) with respect to $\mathbf{c}$ then read

$$\nabla_{\mathbf{c}} f(\mathbf{c}) = \left(\sum_{n=0}^{L_h} |h_1(n) - g(n)|^p\right)^{\frac{1}{p}-1} \mathbf{C}^T b(\mathbf{g}) \tag{13}$$

$$\nabla_{\mathbf{c}} y(\mathbf{c}) = \Re\left(\sum_{k=0}^{L_a} |a(k)|^p\right)^{\frac{1}{p}-1} \mathbf{F}^T b(\mathbf{a}) \tag{14}$$

with

$$b(\mathbf{m}) = diag(sign(\mathbf{m}))|\mathbf{m}|^{p-1}. \tag{15}$$

The iterative filter update then simply reads

$$\mathbf{c}^{l+1} = \mathbf{c}^l - \mu(\nabla_{\mathbf{c}} f(\mathbf{c}^l) + \alpha\nabla_{\mathbf{c}} y(\mathbf{c}^l)) \tag{16}$$

where l is the current iteration, μ is the step size of the algorithm and α denotes the weighting of the spectral constraint. A more detailed explanation of the gradients and the p-norm optimization scheme is given in [5] and [6].

2.3 Data acquisition and signal processing

In these measurements, two identical, proprietary surface exciters driven by two identical amplifiers (Thomann t.amp PM40C) were used. All acoustic signals were measured using measuring microphones (Beyerdynamic MM1). SoundMexPro (Hörteck gGmbH) was utilized for playback and recording, filter design and signal processing was done using MATLAB 2014.
We assumed the noise to be cancelled to be band-limited to below 500 Hz. For every measurement, room impulse responses for both paths were recorded using exponential sine sweeps [7]. To reduce the computational load and improve

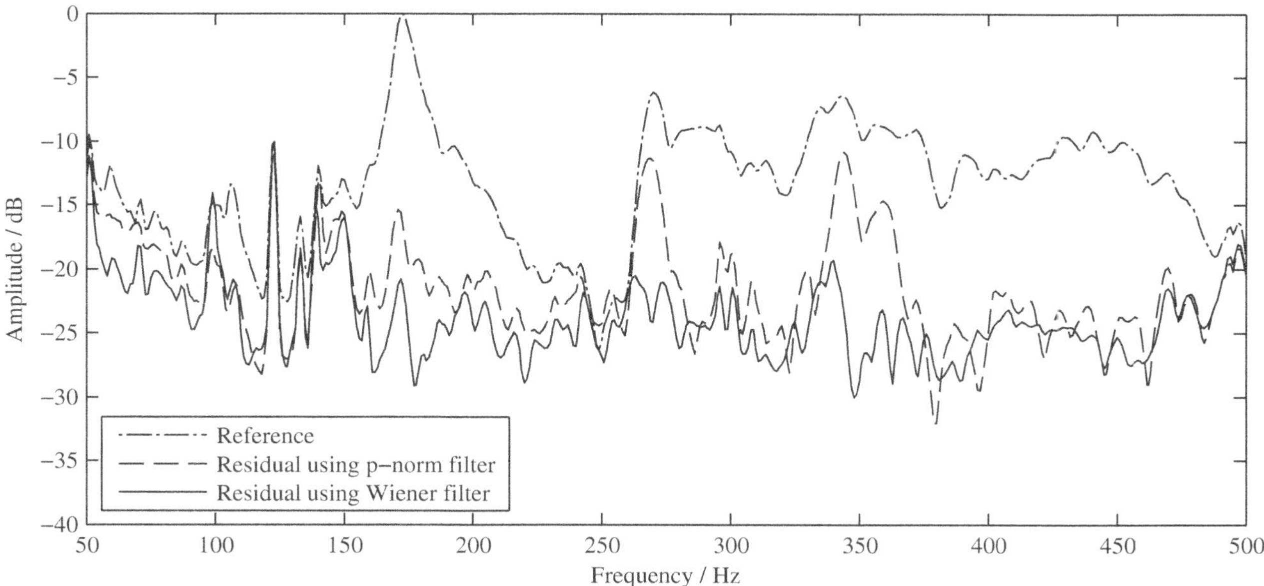

Figure 1: Amplitude levels of reference signal and residual signal when using Wiener filter and p-norm filter at 8 cm exciter displacement over a frequency range of 50 to 500 Hz

stability of the algorithms, the calculated RIRs were resampled to 1000 Hz. Furthermore, a relatively short reverberation time of 0.25 seconds was assumed. This resulted in impulse responses of $L_g = 250$ taps.

The frequency-dependent signal distortion of the whole system was approximated together with the background noise from several three second signals using the 'total harmonic distortion + noise' (THD+N) measure for 10 to 500 Hz. A signal containing a sine wave of a single frequency was played back, the recorded signal was filtered with a narrowbanded notch filter which removed the testing signal. The signal energy was calculated for the filtered and the unfiltered recorded signal, the quotient equals the THD+N measure. Smaller values thus correspond to less influence of distortion and noise towards the signal amplitude.

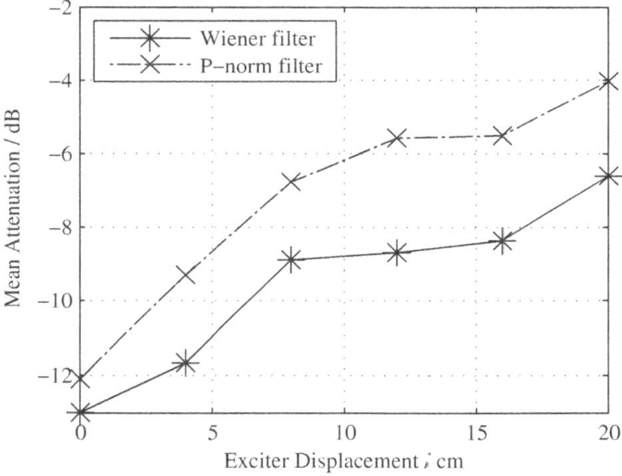

Figure 2: Mean attenuation quotient over exciter displacement for both filter designs

3 Results and Discussion

To compare the performance of the different filters for various positions of the exciters, a linear sine sweep was used that covered the range of 0 to 500 Hz. The sweep was then filtered by the constructed prefilter and both the unfiltered and the filtered signal were played back simultaneously from the noise source and antinoise exciter, respectively. For each measurement a reference signal was recorded, in which a sweep was played solely through the noise source. Then, the Fourier transform was taken of both recordings. The attenuation can then be calculated as the quotient between the two spectra. The performance of the ANC system was measured for multiple positions of the antinoise exciter. As a starting position, the exciters were placed directly opposite of each other on the wooden panel. The antinoise exciter was then displaced in four centimeter increments to up to 20 centimeter from the noise source. Figure 1 shows such a measurement at a exciter displacement of 8 cm. All values are relative to the maximum amplitude of the reference measurement, which was set to 0 dB. The frequency response of the exciters is noticeably non-linear, as seen in various peaks and troughs throughout the spectrum of the reference signal. Nevertheless, good cancellation was achieved in the range of 150 to 450 Hz, with the Wiener-Hopf filter providing all around better attenuation than the p-norm optimizing filter. It has to be noted however, that the p-norm optimizing filter provided better subjective quality, as the Wiener-Hopf filter introduced more audible distortion. Additionally, the performance of the system using either filter deteriorated when tested with higher frequencies than 500 Hz.

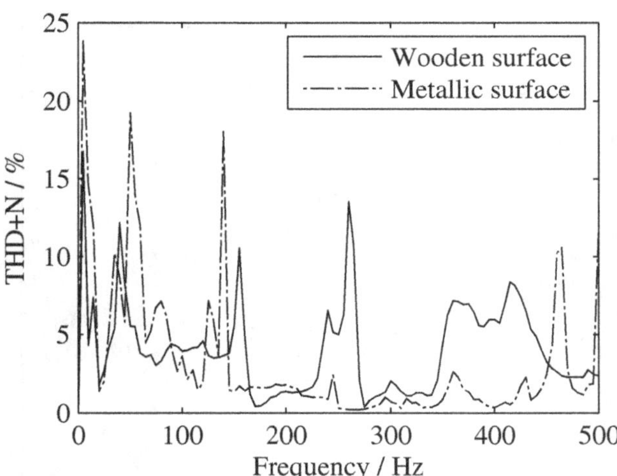

Figure 3: Total harmonic distortion + noise over the relevant frequencies for two mounting surfaces

Figure 2 shows the mean attenuation coefficient as a function of exciter displacement. One can see that the system performance deteriorates with rising exciter distance as expected. Additionally, the divergence in filter performance increases with rising distance, while they provide very similar results for low distances.This not only underlines the importance of filter design, but of speaker placement. Still, even for large displacements a mean noise cancellation of -6.5 dB was achieved using the Wiener filter while for optimal placement, a mean attenuation of more than -12 dB was possible for either filter.
Figure 3 shows the THD+N of the whole system for two different mounting surfaces. There are several high peaks which indicate very poor performance of the exciters for these frequencies. For this reason, both the amplitude of the reference measurement and the performance of the ANC system drop for some frequencies, as seen in Fig. 1. The position and shape of the distortion peaks vary between surfaces, with the metallic surface showing more discrete peaks. Therefore, the surface used by the exciter system has to be carefully chosen in respect to the properties of the unwanted noise.

3.1 Outlook

In these experiments, it is assumed that the noise we try to cancel is known in advance. This simplifies the system, but is generally not true for real-life applications. We plan to use a vibration sensor for noise measurement, whose signal will be used for the noise cancelling system. Furthermore, the influence of the surroundings on the stability of the system will be estimated and an adaptive RIR estimation will be implemented if deemed necessary.

4 Conclusion

In this paper, an ANC system based on room impulse response equalization was presented. Two methods of filter design were implemented and evaluated for noise cancelling performance, especially in respect to speaker placement. Though the p-norm filter generally provided inferior attenuation when compared to the Wiener-Hopf filter, both provided robust cancellation in the low frequency band and could be used together with insulating materials to attenuate unwanted noise. It is shown that the performance of the system is dependent of the mounting surface of the exciter, which indicates that the surface material has to be chosen based on the characteristics of the unwanted noise.

Acknowledgement

The work has been carried out at the Institute for Signal Processing at the University of Lübeck with the friendly cooperation of the Kendrion Kuhnke Automation GmbH.

5 References

[1] S. M. Kuo and D.R. Morgan, *Active Noise Control.* Springer Handbook of Speech Processing, pp. 1001–1018, 2008.

[2] S. T. Neely, *Invertibility of a Room Impulse Response.* in: The Journal of the Acoustical Society of America, vol. 66, no. 1, pp. 165–169, 1979

[3] B. Widrow and S. D. Stearns, *Adaptive signal processing.* John Wiley & Sons, 1985.

[4] M. H. Hayes, *Statistical Digital Signal Processing and Modeling.* John Wiley & Sons, 1996.

[5] A. Mertins and T. Mei and M. Kallinger, *Room impulse Response Shortening / Reshaping with Infinity- and p -Norm Optimization.* in: IEEE Transactions on Audio, Speech and Language Processing, vol. 18, no. 2, pp. 249–259, 2010.

[6] J. O. Jungmann and T. Mei and S. Goetze and A. Mertins, *Room Impulse Response Reshaping by Joint Optimization of Multiple p-Norm Based Criteria.* in: Proc. European Signal Processing Conference 2011, pp. 1658–1662, 2011.

[7] A. Farina, *Advancements in Impulse Response Measurements by Sine Sweeps.* in: 122nd AES Convention, 2007

Receive Chain Noise Matching For Magnetic Particle Imaging

M. Melchger [1], M. Graeser [2], and T. M. Buzug [2]

[1] Institute of Medical Engineering, Universität zu Lübeck, melchger@miw.uni-luebeck.de

[2] Institute of Medical Engineering, Universität zu Lübeck, {graeser, buzug}@imt.uni-luebeck.de

Abstract

In *Magnetic Particle Imaging* (MPI) the signal quality strongly depends on the properties of the components used in the receive chain. The main sources of noise are the receive coil, the parts used in the analog filter circuit and the electronics of the *Low Noise Amplifier* (LNA). In the receive coil peak voltages of 200 mV are commonly recorded in the band between 5 kHz and 2 MHz [1]. These signals are then filtered by an analog circuit and fed into an LNA in preparation for further processing. Operating at *radio frequency* (RF) with small signals, any noise affects the *Signal-to-Noise Ratio* (SNR) of the measurement significantly and reduces the spatial resolution of the measured data. This paper examines noise matching between the combined output noise of both receive coil and filter, and the LNA as an approach and possible solution for SNR improvement.

1 Introduction

Magnetic Particle Imaging (MPI) is a new imaging modality proposed in 2005 by Weizenecker and Gleich [1] based on the nonlinear response of *Superparamagnetic Iron Oxid* (SPIO) nanoparticles. The SPIO nanoparticles are very responsive to magnetic fields and can be used for in vivo imaging and medical applications [2], [1].
The SPIO nanoparticles are injected into a patient who then is placed inside the MPI scanner. The spatial distribution of the nanoparticles can be reconstructed from distortions caused by their nonlinear magnetization. These distortions are measured with a *Receive Coil* (R_X), filtered with an electric circuit to attenuate the direct feedthrough and finally amplified by a *Low Noise Amplifier* (LNA) for further processing. Fig. 1 shows the current receive chain setup as described, refer to Fig. 2 for details of the receive coil . Relevant technical details of each component in the receive chain are listed in Table 2.

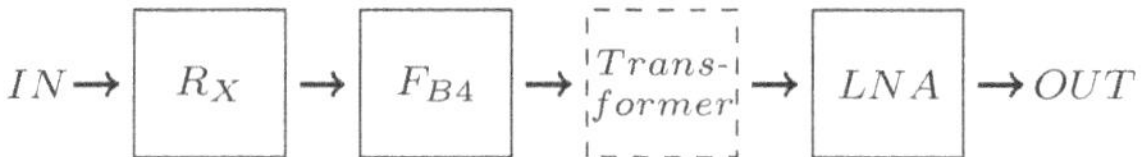

Figure 1: Receive chain setup: R_X receive coil, F_{B4} filter circuit (4th order Butterworth), LNA *Low Noise Amplifier*.

1.1 Receive Chain Noise

The measured distortions of the nonlinear magnetization are composed of frequencies between 5 kHz and 2 MHz [1] with very small signal amplitudes ranging down to a few mV. The relevant band for our current measurements however ranges from 5 kHz to 1 MHz [3]. To preserve the high sensitivity of the system, analog pre-processing by the filter and the LNA is required as digital pre-processing would not sufficiently resolve the incoming signal amplitudes and frequencies. Analog circuits allow faster processing but at the same time generate noise by the parts used in the components. Electronic parts and semiconductors are commonly affected by a multitude of external and internal factors that inherently cause noise such as *Johnson–Nyquist noise* [5]. All of the variables used in the following calculations are either explained explicitly, explained in the corresponding figure or listed in Tab.2 with their corresponding properties and values. The noise voltage is calculated as:

$$V_N = \sqrt{4k_bTR}. \tag{1}$$

Fig. 2 shows the equivalent, non-ideal RF circuit of a coil with capacitive, inductive and parasitic properties [9]. Similar to the coil any other part used in the system is non-ideal and generates noise in accordance with 1.

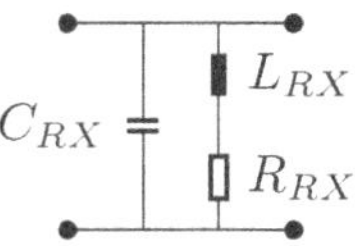

Figure 2: *Radio Frequency* (RF) equivalent circuit of the receive coil. Measured properties are listed in Table 2 under *Receive Coil*.

In order to reduce the impact of noise on the signal quality and to maintain a high spatial resolution throughout the receive chain it is therefore required to either significantly reduce the noise generation by greatly reducing or eliminating most of the noise sources. Alternatively the signal-to-noise ratio can be improved by matching the combined

output noise figures of the filter circuit with the input noise of the LNA. Since it is very hard to reduce or eliminate noise as most sources are intrinsic, noise matching poses a far more feasible approach for resolution enhancement.
A significant part of the measured signal in the receive coil is very small and below the noise level of the amplifier. Through noise matching the noise of the incoming signal is adjusted to the noise of the amplifier, therefore effectively amplifying both the signal and the noise. Since the noise level of the LNA is the dominant noise source (Tab. 2, [3]) the noise matching as the measurement sensitivity for signals below the noise voltage of the LNA is increased significantly. The feasibility of noise matching with a transformer is examined for the application in MPI in the following sections.

2 Material and Methods

In order to design a suitable transformer it is necessary to determine the noise of the receive coil. With the ratio of the receive coil noise and the LNA noise it is then possible to calculate the turn ratio required for the noise matching.

2.1 Receive Coil Noise

The measured resistance and (1) can be used to calculate the noise figure (k_b: Boltzmann constant):

$$V_N = \sqrt{4k_b \cdot 300\,K \cdot 0.8\,\Omega} \approx 115\,pV/\sqrt{Hz}. \quad (2)$$

This result coincides with the simulation and the findings of Biederer [3], [4]. With the simulated noise of the LNA from Tab. 2 it is now possible to determine the turn ratio required for the noise matching:

$$a = \frac{115\,pV\sqrt{Hz}}{440\,pV\sqrt{Hz}} = \frac{N_P}{N_S} = \sqrt{\frac{L_P}{L_S}} \approx \frac{1}{3.826}. \quad (3)$$

2.2 Radio Frequency Transformer Layout

A transformer consists of two or more windings, often separated by a core, between which energy is transferred through electromagnetic induction. Ideal transformers can be modeled as coupled coils [6][7] with a transfer ratio equivalent to (2), however capacitive and parasitic effects in radio frequency transformers require a modified, non-ideal equivalent circuit. Fig. 3 shows a non-ideal 2 winding transformer with capacities between turns, the core and in-between windings such as used for the following analysis.

With the equivalent circuit of a coil such as shown in Fig. 2 the windings of the non-ideal transformer can be modeled [7][8]. For an accurate description of the capacitive and inductive effects as well as the parasitic properties, such as core and iron losses, it is necessary to introduce additional parts for the RF analysis. Fig. 4 shows the equivalent circuit of non-ideal RF transformer. For further analysis and readability the circuit can be transformed into a circuit with an ideal transformer such as displayed in Fig. 5.

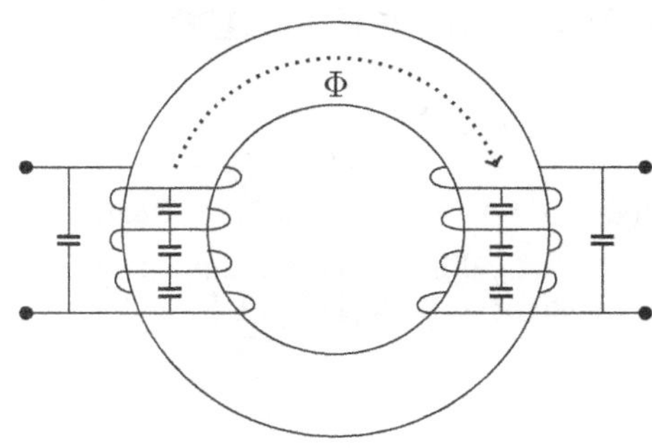

Figure 3: Parasitic properties in a RF transformer are prevalent in-between any conductive material due to the non-ideal nature of materials and coupling. Copper, iron and core losses additionally reduce the efficacy, capacities cause lower resonance frequencies. This requires additional modeling for the correct description and analysis of a RF transformer.

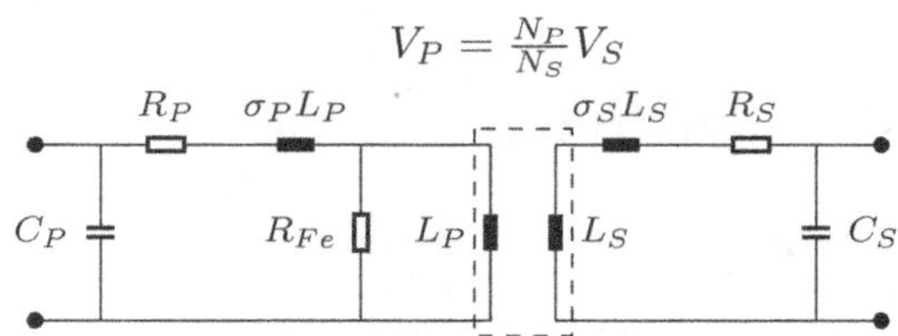

Figure 4: Radio frequency transformer, ($L_{P,S}$: inductance, $N_{P,S}$: turns of the winding, $C_{P,S}$: winding capacitance, $\sigma_{P,S}$: scattering factor, calculated from the coupling factor of the winding $k_{P,S}$: $\sigma_{P,S} = 1 - k^2_{P,S}$, $R_{P,S}$: copper losses, $V_{P,S}$: voltage over $L_{P,S}$)

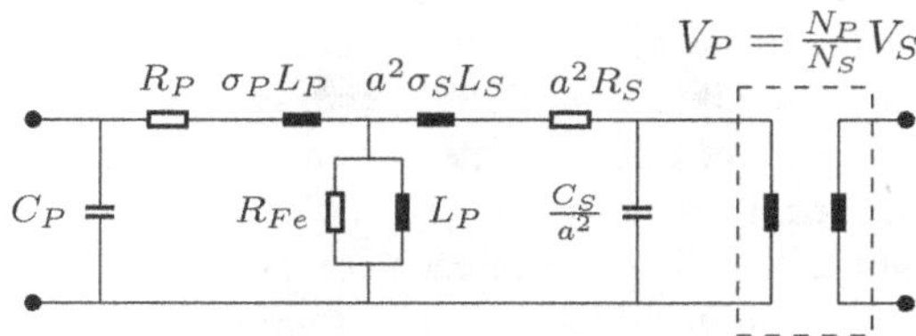

Figure 5: Radio frequency transformer equivalent circuit with all elements on the primary side and an ideal transformer, ($L_{P,S}$: inductance, $N_{P,S}$: turns of the winding, $C_{P,S}$: winding capacitance, $\sigma_{P,S}$: scattering factor, calculated from the coupling factor of the winding $k_{P,S}$: $\sigma_{P,S} = 1 - k^2_{P,S}$, $R_{P,S}$: copper losses, a: $\frac{N_P}{N_S}$, $V_{P,S}$: voltage over $L_{P,S}$)

2.2.1 Windings

The inductance of the primary transformer winding should be at least equal to the inductance of the receive coil in order to minimize losses and maximize the effect of the transformer. With the turn ratio from (3) and the induction of the receive coil (Tab. 2) it is now possible to calculate the required induction of the secondary winding:

$$L_S = \frac{300\ \mu H}{a^2} = 300\ \mu H \cdot 3.826^2 \approx 4.39\ mH. \tag{4}$$

The permeability of a material largely affects, amongst other, the inductance per turn which is commonly called the A_L value:

$$A_L = \frac{\mu_0\ \mu_r h}{2\pi} ln\left(\frac{R}{r}\right). \tag{5}$$

In (5), μ_0 is the vacuum permeability, μ_r the core material permeability, h the height, R and r the outer respectively the inner radius of the toroid core. With A_L and a given number of turns N it is possible to calculate the overall inductance of a winding:

$$L = A_L \cdot N^2. \tag{6}$$

Too keep the resistance of the primary and secondary winding at a minimum it is furthermore necessary to find a material with a high permeability and small dimensions to reduce the total amount of copper wire used. For the primary winding a maximum of 10 turns is desirable which in return results in 40 turns for the secondary winding.
The experimental setup does not permit a transformer size larger than $(15\ cm)^3$ Due to these requirements and the spatial limitations, the solution to this problem was the stacking of multiple cores of lower permeability to retrieve a high A_L value. A suitable core for 10 turns on the primary side has to have an AL-value roughly equal to:

$$A_{L,P} = \frac{300\ \mu H}{10^2} = 3\ \mu H/N^2. \tag{7}$$

The selected core material is listed in Tab. 2 under *Toroid Core*. The theoretic A_L value of 3 stacked cores of this material is $3.9\ \mu H/N^2$, the measured value however is far closer to $3.05\ \mu H/N^2$ due to the isolating finish of the individual cores and coupling. The resulting details of the wired transformer are listed in Tab. 1.

Table 1: TRANSFORMER DETAILS

Element	Property	Value
General	Turn ratio	a = 0.25
	Gain	$V_P = \frac{1}{4}\ V_S$
	Resonance frequency	f_0 = 1.43 MHz
1st *winding*	Turns	N = 10
	Inductance	$L_P = 305\ \mu H$
2nd *winding*	Turns	N = 40
	Inductance	$L_S = 4.88\ mH$

2.3 Experimental Verification of the Transformer

The correct amplification respectively turn ratio of the transformer can be confirmed experimentally by manipulating the resonance frequency of the transformer with a capacitor. Under the assumption that the coupling and iron losses are ideal ($k = 1$, $R_F \to \infty$) the equivalent circuit from Fig. 5 can be simplified for the calculation of the altered resonance frequency as shown in Fig. 6. According to (8) as well as Fig. 6 adding a parallel capacitor with a sufficiently high capacitance at the output of the secondary winding lowers the resonance frequency of the transformer and can be calculated as

$$f_0 = \frac{1}{2\pi\sqrt{L_P \cdot C_S \cdot a^{-2}}} \tag{8}$$

which shows that the resonance frequency is proportional to the capacitance of the secondary winding:

$$f_0 \propto \frac{a}{C_S}. \tag{9}$$

Table 2: SYSTEM PARAMETERS

Element	Property	Value
Receive Coil	Resistance	$R_{RX} = 800\ m\Omega$
	Inductance	$L_{RX} = 30\ \mu H$
	Capacity	$C_{RX} = 8.7\ pF$
	Noise sim.	$V_{N,RX} = 115\ pVHz^{-2}$
	Noise calc.	$V_{N,RX} = 115\ pVHz^{-2}$
	Noise meas.	$V_{N,RX} \approx 115\ pVHz^{-2}$
LNA	Noise sim.	$V_{N,LNA} = 440\ pVHz^{-2}$
	Turn ratio req.	$a \approx 3.9 \to 4$
Toroid core Fair-Rite 5943011101	A_L	$1.3\ \mu H/N \pm 25\%$
	$A_{L,3stack,calc}$	$3.9\ \mu H/N^2$
	$A_{L,3,stack,meas}$	$3.05\ \mu H/N^2$
	Permeability	10
Other	Temperature	$T = 300\ K$
	Boltzmann Const.	$k_b \approx 1.38064 \cdot 10^{-3}\ JK^{-1}$

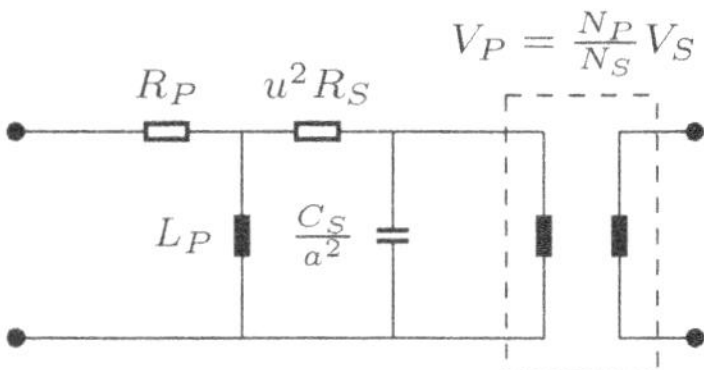

Figure 6: Simplified radio frequency transformer equivalent circuit. (L_P: winding inductance, C_S: winding capacitance, $R_{P,S}$: copper resistivity, a: transfer ratio)

The capacitor C_S was selected with a sufficiently high capacity of $C_S = 1\ nF$ that the other capacities in the transformer would be negligible for the calculation and returns a frequency of

$$f_0 = \frac{1}{2\pi\sqrt{300\ \mu H \cdot 1\ nF}} \approx 128.7581\ kHz. \tag{10}$$

This coincides with the measured resonance frequency of 129 kHz and verifies the correct turn ratio within measurement accuracy. The properties of the manufactured transformer are listed in Tab.1.

3 Results and Discussion

The final transformer has a very stable gain of about 12 dB for frequencies up to 0.5 MHz as shown in Fig. 7. After the implementation of a shielding box it was possible to shift the resonance frequency from 1.13 MHz up to 1.43 MHz, with a peak gain of 39 dB at the resonance frequency. The nonlinear gain increases from 12 dB up to 39 dB for frequencies between 0.5 MHz and 1.43 MHz. For measurements at frequencies higher than the resonance frequency the signal will be largely affected by the capacitive load behaviour (Fig. 7) as it effectively short-circuits the secondary side of the transformer. The measured load behaviour of the transformer is displayed in the phase plot of Fig. 7 and shows the inductive load up to 1.43 MHz as well as the capacitive load for frequencies higher than 1.43 MHz.
Unlike most MPI scanners the current measurement setup operates in the band between 5 kHz and 1 MHz and therefore is not affected by the resonance frequency. The nonlinearity of the gain can be compensated by a modification of the filter circuit of by digital post-processing of the MPI scanner's system transfer function. Contrary to the aquisition process, digital post-processing of already aquired data does not affect the spatial resolution.

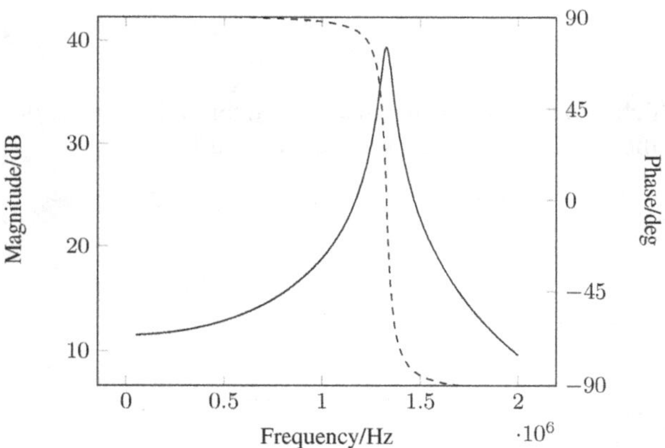

Figure 7: Magnitude and phase plot of the transformer with the resonance frequency at 1.43 MHz.

4 Conclusion

The implementation of this transformer theoretically improves the measurement sensitivity through noise matching and therefore is a very effective component for the improvement of MPI measurement sensitivity. Further research of the effects of noise matching on MPI measurement sensitivity improvement is expected to verify the theoretic results. Any additional improvement of sensitivity does require a significantly lower noise of the LNA because a higher turn ratio inherently introduces more capacitance and therefore lower resonance frequencies. Additionally the receive coil can be modified to include more windings raising both signal and noise level.

Acknowledgement

The work has been carried out at the Institute of Medical Engineering at the University of Lübeck, Germany. Dirk Steinhagen helped with the construction of the shielding box.

5 References

[1] Gleich, Weizenecker, *Tomographic imaging using the nonlinear response of magnetic particles*. Nature 435, pp 1214-1217,2005.

[2] Weizenecker, Gleich, *Three-dimensional real-time in vivo magnetic particle imaging*. Phys. Med. Biol. 54 L1, 2009.

[3] S. Biederer, *Magnet-Partikel-Spektrometer: Entwicklung Eines Spektrometers zur Analyse Superparamagnetischer Eisenoxid-Nanopartikel für Magnetic-Particle-Imaging*. Vieweg+Teubner Verlag, 2012.

[4] Biederer, S., Sattel, T., Knopp, T., Erbe, M., Lüdtke-Buzug, K., Vogt, F., Barkhausen, J., and Buzug, T., *A Spectrometer to Measure the Usability of Nanoparticles for Magnetic Particle Imaging. Magnetic Nanoparticles*. Particle Science, Imaging Technology, and Clinical Applications, World Scientific Publishing Company, vol. 1, pp. 60-65, 2010.

[5] J. B. Johnson, *Thermal Agitation of Electricity in Conductors*. Phys. Rev. 32, 97 – Published 1 July 1928.

[6] Seidel, Wagner, *Allgemeine Elektrotechnik Band 1*. Carl Hanser Verlag, München/Wien, 1992.

[7] Seidel, Wagner, *Allgemeine Elektrotechnik Band 2*. Carl Hanser Verlag, München/Wien, 1993.

[8] Fischer, *Elektrische Maschinen*. Carl Hanser Verlag, München/Wien, 1995.

[9] Würth Elektronik GmbH & Co KG, *Trilogy of Magnetics*. Siwiridoff, 2009.

[10] *Fair-Rite transformer core, part number 5943011101, material mix 43*. http://www.fair-rite.com/catalog_pdfs/5943011101.pdf, last checked 27/01/2015.

Experimental Evaluation of Different Weighting Schemes in Magnetic Particle Imaging Reconstruction

P. Szwargulski [1], J. Rahmer [2], M. Ahlborg [3], C. Kaethner [3], and T. M. Buzug [3]

[1] Medizinische Ingenieurwissenschaft, Universität zu Lübeck, szwargul@miw.uni-luebeck.de

[2] Philips GmbH Innovative Technologies, Research Laboratories Hamburg, juergen.rahmer@philips.com

[3] Institute of Medical Engineering, Universität zu Lübeck, {ahlborg, kaethner, buzug}@imt.uni-luebeck.de

Abstract

Magnetic Particle Imaging (MPI) is a new imaging technique with an outstanding sensitivity, a high temporal and spatial resolution. MPI is based on the excitation and detection of magnetic tracer material by using magnetic fields. The spatial resolution strongly depends on the reconstruction parameters and on the selection and weighting of the system function frequency components. Currently, no fundamental strategy to weight the system function for the reconstruction is given. In this contribution, the influence on the spatial resolution of different selection and weighting methods is analyzed. Thereby, a new strategy is proposed to select and weight the components with respect to their mixing order. As a result, it is confirmed that a weighted system function provides better results of image reconstruction than a non-weighted one. In addition to this, it is shown that the usage of the mixing order in combination with established weightings improves the resolution.

1 Introduction

Magnetic Particle Imaging (MPI) is a novel imaging technique based on the detection of superparamagnetic iron oxide particles [1]. The generation of a detectable signal is based on the non-linear magnetization of those particles. This signal is the induced voltage generated by the excitation of the particles. This excitation is realized with orthogonal sinusoidal drive fields generated by orthogonal sets of coils [2]. Currently, two reconstruction methods are established to obtain the image of the particle distribution, the time-domain reconstruction, known as the x-space approach [3, 4], and the frequency-domain reconstruction [2, 5].

In frequency space, typically a system matrix is used to calibrate the system. Therefore, a system function (SF) for every position in the field of view (FOV) is acquired. It has been shown in [6] that the image reconstruction can be improved with an additional weighting of individual SF frequency components.

In this contribution, the mixing orders of measured SFs, as described in [5], are analyzed. In order to evaluate those mixing orders with respect to their influence on the reconstruction results, different regularization, selection, and weighting schemes are used.

2 Material and Methods

The measurements used in this work are performed with the MPI preclinical demonstrator from the Philips research laboratories, Hamburg, Germany [7]. These measurements are performed with a 16 mT drive field amplitude on all three axes and a gradient strength of $G_x = G_y = 1.25\,\text{T/m}/\mu_0$ and accordingly $G_z = 2.5\,\text{T/m}/\mu_0$. The frequencies to generate a Lissajous measurement cycle with a repetition time T_R are $f_x = 528\Delta f$, $f_y = 561\Delta f$, and $f_z = 544\Delta f$ [5]. Thereby, Δf is given by $1/T_R = 46.42\,\text{Hz}$. The FOV is sampled at $20 \times 36 \times 36 = 25920$ positions with a voxel and a delta probe size of $1\,\text{mm}^3$. The phantom consists of seven tubes centered in the volume and filled with a tracer similar to Resovist with a concentration of 0.03 mol(Fe)/l. Each tube has a diameter of 2 mm and a distance of 2 mm to the next tube. In the following, a characterization of the SF is given followed by the description of the reconstruction. With respect to the reconstruction, the regularization, the selection, and the weighting of the frequency components are represented in relation to the mixing order.

2.1 System Function

The SF is a complex valued matrix, which includes all information about the system and the particle behavior in every sampled position of the FOV. Typically, the SF is determined by a robot-based method, which is very time consuming [1]. Alternative acquisition methods are already presented in [8] and [9], but currently not established, because of the uncertainty of the particle behavior.

In [5], the characteristics of a 3D SF have been presented.

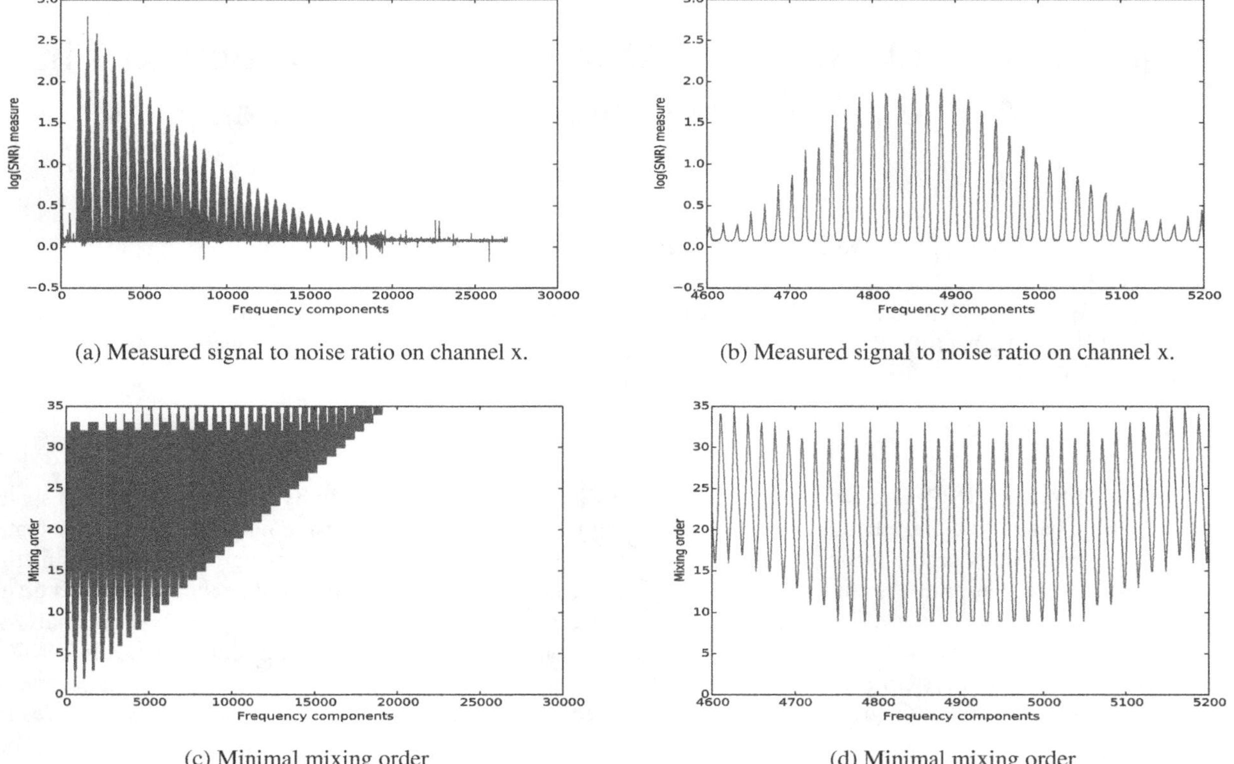

(a) Measured signal to noise ratio on channel x.

(b) Measured signal to noise ratio on channel x.

(c) Minimal mixing order

(d) Minimal mixing order

Figure 1: Logarithmic visualisation of the measured x channel SNR in comparison with the minimal mixing order. Thereby, in (a) and (c), all measured components are presented. In (b) and (d), a closer look to the components 4600 until 5200 is given, which equals the band around the 9th harmonic.

The system matrix of one receive channel G is defined as

$$G = \begin{pmatrix} \tilde{s}(f_1, p_1) & \tilde{s}(f_1, p_2) & \cdots & \tilde{s}(f_1, p_n) \\ \tilde{s}(f_2, p_1) & \tilde{s}(f_2, p_2) & \cdots & \tilde{s}(f_2, p_n) \\ \vdots & \vdots & \ddots & \vdots \\ \tilde{s}(f_m, p_1) & \tilde{s}(f_m, p_2) & \cdots & \tilde{s}(f_m, p_n) \end{pmatrix}, \quad (1)$$

with $\tilde{s}$ as the signal in Fourier space, the rows M_{freq}, representing the number of stored frequencies f_i, and the columns N_{samp}, the number of sampled positions in the FOV p_j. In this work, $\tilde{s}$ is given with $M_{\text{freq}} = 26929$ frequencies per channel.

Every frequency component can be described by a linear combination of the excitation frequencies for each drive field channel and positive/negative integers n_x, n_y and n_z like

$$f = |n_x f_x + n_y f_y + n_z f_z| \quad (2)$$

[5]. The mixing order n_{mo} of the frequencies is defined as

$$n_{\text{mo}} = |n_x| + |n_y| + |n_z|. \quad (3)$$

An example visualization of the minimal mixing order n_{mo} over all frequencies for one channel is presented in Fig. 1c. Furthermore, the measured signal-to-noise ratio (SNR) for the same channel is visualized in Fig. 1a. It can be seen that there is a direct link between a high SNR and a low mixing order. As proposed in [10], this correlation can be used to choose frequencies with high SNR via the mixing order.

2.2 Image Reconstruction

Image reconstruction in MPI decodes the particle distribution from the measured signal in the sampled FOV. The previously described SF is necessary for the system matrix based frequency-domain reconstruction. For this reconstruction, a discrete system of equations can be established, which in the matrix vector notation is given as

$$Gc = \hat{u}, \quad (4)$$

with c being the desired particle concentration and $\hat{u}$ being the Fourier transformed voltage signal. Due to the dimension of the system matrix, this inverse problem is ill-posed, so that a regularization is needed. Furthermore, it has been shown in [6] that a weighting matrix can be used to improve the solution of the problem. The reconstruction can be expressed as a weighted regularized least-squares problem

$$||W(G_S c - \hat{u})||^2 + \lambda ||c||^2 \rightarrow \min \quad (5)$$

with W as the weighting matrix, G_S as the system matrix with selected components and λ as the regularization parameter. In the practical realization, a reconstruction kernel $\kappa = W \cdot G_S$ including information about the selected, weighted frequency components is generated.

Further, as described in [6], a non-negativity and non-complexity constraint justified by the particle physics can be applied to refine the reconstructions. The reconstruction,

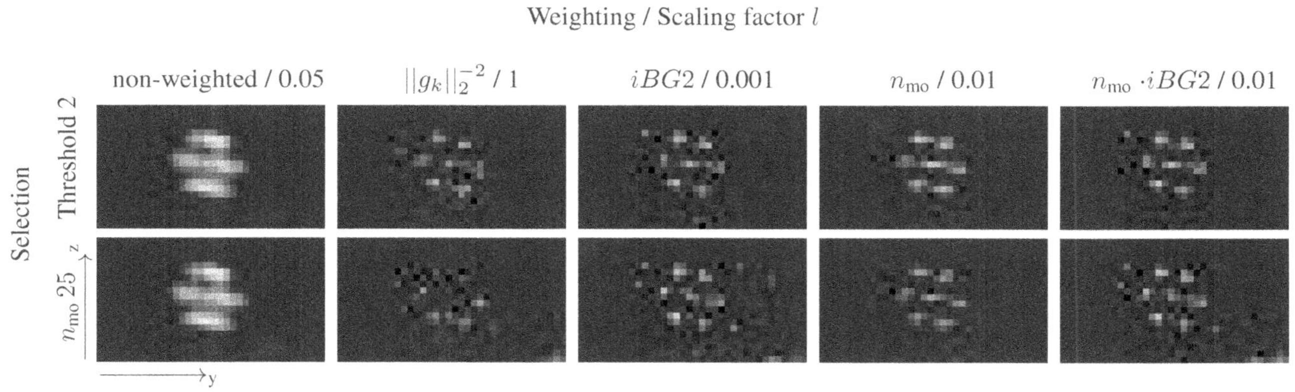

Weighting / Scaling factor l

	non-weighted / 0.05	$\|\|g_k\|\|_2^{-2}$ / 1	$iBG2$ / 0.001	n_{mo} / 0.01	$n_{\text{mo}} \cdot iBG2$ / 0.01
Selection: Threshold 2					
Selection: n_{mo} 25					

Figure 2: Comparison of the yz-plane of the reconstruction results achieved with different weighting schemes. In the rows, the selection strategies based on the SNR threshold and the minimal mixing order threshold are presented. In the columns, the new investigated weightings in comparison with the non-weighted and the energy weighted results are shown. Additionally, the scaling factor l is given, which represents the regularization.

which is used in this work, follows the approach presented in [11].

2.2.1 Selection of individual frequency components

Many of the components of the SF are highly noisy and therefore should not be used for the reconstruction. A possible way to improve the reconstruction is to introduce a preprocessing step, where only specific components are selected. This aspect suggests to choose the components based on an SNR threshold [6]. This means, only the components with an SNR above the threshold are used for the reconstruction.

The correlation between the SNR and the mixing order, which is visualized in Fig. 1, is presented in [5]. Based on that relation, the selection of the frequency components using the mixing order is determined in this work. The idea is to select only those frequency components that can be generated by a given minimal mixing order threshold.

2.2.2 Weighting of the system function

In [6], it has been proven that an additional weighting of the system of equations as defined in (5) does not change the mathematical correctness. A weighting has the effect to raise or decrease the rows of the matrix and therefore the corresponding frequencies in every position. It has been proposed in [6] to use a weighting, that adjusts the energy of the system matrix rows. The representation for the k-th row of G is g_k, so that the weighting can be written as

$$\tilde{w_k} = ||g_k||_2^{-2} \tag{6}$$

where $W = \text{diag}((\tilde{w_k})_{k=1}^{M_{\text{freq}}})$ and $||\cdot||_2^{-2}$ denote the squared inverse Euclidean norm.

An additional approach is to weight the system matrix with the squared inverse background norm $iBG2$, which includes information about the sensitivity of the receive coils. The background information can be obtained by empty measurements g_{empty} during the acquisition of the SF.

A new strategy, presented in this work, is to use the mixing order for the weighting, like $\tilde{w_k} = n_{\text{mo}}$. The idea is to increase the influence of the components with a high mixing order and hence a low SNR, to achieve a homogeneous distribution of the SNR over all components.

Additionally, the mixing order weighting is extended to integrate system properties by a multiplication with $iBG2$, like

$$\tilde{w_k} = n_{\text{mo}} \cdot iBG2. \tag{7}$$

2.2.3 Regularization

The main idea of regularization is to establish a balance between the discrepancy of $||Gc - \hat{u}||^2$ and the energy of the solution $||c||^2$. Possible approaches to determine the mathematically optimal regularization parameter λ are presented in [6]. In this work, the regularization parameter λ is defined as

$$\lambda = l \cdot \lambda_0 = l \frac{||\kappa||_F^2}{r}, \tag{8}$$

with l being a scaling factor of the measurement dependent λ_0, $||\kappa||_F^2$ is the squared Frobenius norm of the kernel κ, and r the number of voxels. In (8) it is shown that the regularization is directly linked to the weighting and selection of the SF. Therefore, the following regularization will be described via the scaling factor l, independent of the used weighting and selection.

3 Results and Discussion

In this work, several weighting and selection aspects are investigated. The achieved reconstruction results are presented in Fig. 2 for both investigated selection methods, i.e. the SNR threshold and the mixing order threshold. Further, the different weighting types are shown: the non-weighted, the energy based, the $iBG2$, the mixing order, and the product of mixing order and $iBG2$. In addition to this, the scaling factor for all reconstructions is given.

The results of the $iBG2$ weighting demonstrate a better resolution in comparison with the non-weighted and energy-based weighting. However, some noise patterns are visible, what could be explained by the very low regularization.
The reconstruction results of the weighting with the mixing order are satisfactory. This is very significant, because the information used for the weighting and selecting are independent of the measured SNR.
In addition to the aforementioned approaches, reconstructions are presented, where the mixing order is combined with the $iBG2$. The idea is to integrate system information and especially information about the receive channels. It is visible that this approach improves the reconstruction in comparison to the non-weighted and energy based method, so that a resolution of almost 2 mm also in the low gradient direction y is achieved. Furthermore, the noise in the background is at an acceptable level.
All results include some minor artifacts, which can be explained by the fact that the images are not post processed and that the areas where the artifacts occur are not sampled by the Lissajous trajectory.
In the reconstructions shown in Fig. 2, only minor differences between the selection methods are visible, which could be explained by the selection of nearly the same frequency components. This emphasizes the importance of the mixing order, not only for the weighting, but also for the selection of the frequency components carrying the important information for image reconstruction.

4 Conclusion

In this work, different weighting and selection methods for the frequency components of the MPI system function are analyzed. It has been shown that the idea presented in [5], where the system is characterized with the mixing order, can be used for the weighting as well as for the selection of the frequency components.
Furthermore, it has been shown that a combination of the theoretical mixing order and system information improves the reconstruction results in comparison to the presented weighting schemes.
Summarized, it could be shown that a weighting and selection of the system function components based on the mixing order of the excitation frequencies improves the image reconstruction.
In the future, the theoretical aspects of the SF should be investigated further. Through this, it might be possible to improve the resolution even further.

Acknowledgments

This work has been carried out in the Philips Research Laboratories, Hamburg, Germany in cooperation with the Institute of Medical Engineering, Universität zu Lübeck, Lübeck, Germany.

5 References

[1] B. Gleich and J. Weizenecker, "Tomographic imaging using the nonlinear response of magnetic particles," *Nature*, vol. 435, no. 7046, pp. 1214–1217, 2005.

[2] J. Rahmer, J. Weizenecker, B. Gleich, and J. Borgert, "Signal Encoding in Magnetic Particle Imaging: Properties of the System Function," *BMC Medical Imaging*, vol. 9, no. 1, p. 4, 2009.

[3] P. W. Goodwill and S. M. Conolly, "The X-Space Formulation of the Magnetic Particle Imaging Process: 1-D Signal, Resolution, Bandwidth, SNR, SAR, and Magnetostimulation," *IEEE Transactions on Medical Imaging*, vol. 29, no. 11, pp. 1851–1859, 2010.

[4] P. W. Goodwill and S. M. Conolly, "Multidimensional X-Space Magnetic Particle Imaging," *IEEE Transactions on Medical Imaging*, vol. 30, no. 9, pp. 1581–1590, 2011.

[5] J. Rahmer, J. Weizenecker, B. Gleich, and J. Borgert, "Analysis of a 3-d system function measured for magnetic particle imaging," *IEEE Transactions on Medical Imaging*, vol. 31, no. 6, pp. 1289–1299, 2012.

[6] T. Knopp, J. Rahmer, T. F. Sattel, S. Biederer, J. Weizenecker, B. Gleich, J. Borgert, and T. M. Buzug, "Weighted Iterative Reconstruction for Magnetic Particle Imaging," *Physics in Medicine and Biology*, vol. 55, no. 6, pp. 1577–1589, 2010.

[7] B. Gleich, J. Weizenecker, H. Timminger, C. Bontus, I. Schmale, J. Rahmer, J. Schmidt, J. Kanzenbach, and J. Borgert, "Fast mpi demonstrator with enlarged field of view," in *Proceedings of the International Society for Magnetic Resonance in Medicine*, vol. 18, p. 218, 2010.

[8] T. Knopp, T. F. Sattel, S. Biederer, J. Rahmer, J. Weizenecker, B. Gleich, J. Borgert, and T. M. Buzug, "Model-Based Reconstruction for Magnetic Particle Imaging," *IEEE Transactions on Medical Imaging*, vol. 29, no. 1, pp. 12–18, 2010.

[9] M. Grüttner, T. Knopp, J. Franke, M. Heidenreich, J. Rahmer, A. Halkola, C. Kaethner, J. Borgert, and T. M. Buzug, "On the formulation of the image reconstruction problem in magnetic particle imaging," *Biomedizinische Technik/Biomedical Engineering*, vol. 58, no. 6, pp. 583–591, 2013.

[10] T. Knopp, *Effiziente Rekonstruktion und alternative Spulentopologien für Magnetic-Particle-Imaging*. Vieweg und Teubner, Wiesbaden, 2011.

[11] A. Dax, "On row relaxation methods for large constrained least squares problems," *SIAM Journal on Scientific Computing*, vol. 14, no. 3, pp. 570–584, 1993.

10
Image Processing I

Comparison and Performance Evaluation of Indoor Localization Algorithms based on an Error Model for an Optical System

Lifang Zhao[1], Mathias Pelka[2], C. Bollmeyer[2], and H. Hellbrück[2]

[1]Applied Mathematics, East China University of Science and Technology (e-mail:030130131@mail.ecust.edu.cn).
[2]Center of Excellence CoSA, Lübeck University of Applied Sciences, Germany (e-mail: mathias.pelka, christian.bollmeyer, hellbrueck@fh-luebeck.de).

Abstract

Recently indoor localization has gained attention in current research and emergent applications. Especially design and development of a low budget optical indoor localization system requires preliminary simulations and performance evaluation. Efficient and robust algorithms to determine a position from distance measurement are crucial for indoor localization. Distance measurements are noisy and affect performance of algorithms to calculate the position of a tag. Current evaluation of indoor localization algorithm do not consider error models systematically. In this work, we present an error model for the Microsoft Kinect for deterministic and random errors of distance measurements. We evaluate the mean square error and computational cost with a selection of localization algorithms. Based on simulations we identify suited algorithms for a low budget optical indoor localization system.

1 Introduction

Indoor localization enables new applications within medical environments e.g. tracking of medical equipment or reference points related to the patient [4]. Optical systems are beneficial for medical applications since they provide accurate localization based on colored objects and are robust against hygienic procedures. However, distance based systems are influenced by measurements error influencing the calculated position of a tag. Therefore, indoor localization based on distance measurement is still a challenge for inexpensive optical systems. An indoor localization system consists of anchors and tags. Anchors are fixed and serve as infrastructure for an application. Tags are mobile objects with a position of interest.

Indoor localization algorithms are subject to research for years e.g. [1]-[3]. In [5], Lui et al. provided a broad survey of indoor positioning approaches, including Time of Arrival (ToA) and Time Difference of Arrival (TDoA), to retrieve the position of a tag. In our work, we focus solely on ToA. Shen et al. provided algorithms but he did not present a Quasi-Newton algorithm or the Levenberg-Marquardt algorithm. In his presentation, Shen did not provide an error model [1]. To the best of our knowledge this is the first suggestion to use an error model to study the effects of localization errors yet.

In this paper we study the influence of a noise model and its affect to localization algorithms for calculation of the position of a tag. We evaluate each algorithm in terms of mean squared error (MSE), maximum error and computational cost. Maximum error allows comparison of areas, where the algorithm violate a certain minimum localization requirement.

The contribution of this paper is an evaluation of an error model for distance estimation and evaluation of indoor localization algorithms based on noisy distance measurements.

This paper is organized as follows: Section II explains our error model for the Microsoft Kinect. In section III, we present the details of our algorithms. In Section IV we evaluate the algorithms. Finally, we draw our conclusion in section V and provide an outlook to future research.

2 Error Model

Each measurement contains uncertainty in form of a deterministic error and a random error. To describe the deterministic error, we use the mean error, which is the Euclidian distance between real value and the measured value. We describe the random errors as variance of distance measurements. Mean and variance can be a function of the distance.

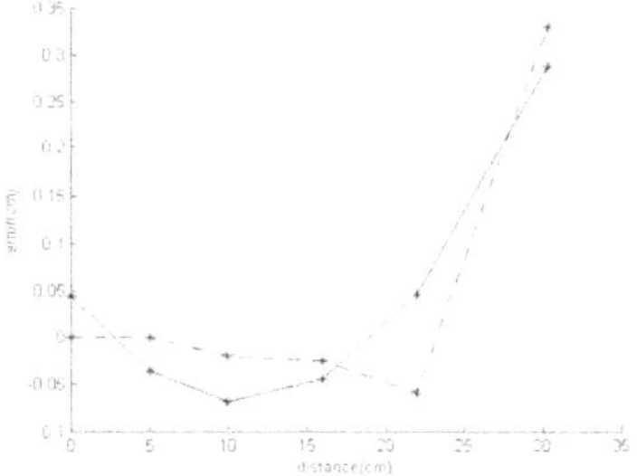

Figure 1: Mean error for Microsoft Kinect (dotted line) and third order polynomial approximation (solid line)

In previous work, we evaluated the Microsoft Kinect for a medical application in terms of accuracy and precision [8]. We found, that the mean error increases with distance which is shown in the left part of Figure 1. It presents the relationship between real distances and mean error. The error is smaller than 2 cm for distances below 250 cm. If distance increases above 2 m, the error increases linearly. Variance σ^2 of the Microsoft Kinect is $\sigma^2 = 5.29\ \text{cm}^2$ ($\sigma = 2.30$ cm) [4]. We employ a third order polynomial approximation of the data with a sum squared error (SSE) of 0.45 cm². The polynomial is shown in the right part of Figure 1 along with the drawn sample points. Such approximation is useful to extrapolate missing data. With increasing degree, the sum squared error decreases as the curve fits better. The higher the order of the polynomial, the more it will oscillate. Further, the function grows with maximum order in areas where no data is available, in this case for distances larger than 3.5 m.

3 Algorithms

In this section we present briefly the four different algorithms: Least Square (LS) as the only analytical solution, Taylor Series (TS) as an historical solution [7], Quasi-Newton-Davidon–Fletcher–Powell (QN-DFP) and the Levenberg-Marquardt (LM) algorithm for nowadays solutions. Each algorithm can be used to determine the position of a tag. We implement and present LS and TS algorithms according to [1]. We highlight the important details in our paper as they share several similarities with QN-DFP and LM.

A. Least Square

The following equation establishes a relationship between distances d_i between tag and anchors and the coordinates $\boldsymbol{r} = [x \quad y \quad z]^T$ of the tag

$$(x_i - x)^2 + (y_i - y)^2 + (z_i - z)^2 = d_i^2. \tag{1}$$

In (1), x_i, y_i, z_i are the coordinates of anchors. We use $i = 1,2,\dots,n$ equations given for n anchors.

We retrieve the following matrix by subtracting $i = 1$ from the rest of the equations, (here only for two dimensions)

$$2\underbrace{\begin{bmatrix} x_2 - x_1 & y_2 - y_1 \\ \vdots & \vdots \\ x_n - x_1 & y_n - y_1 \end{bmatrix}}_{\mathbf{A}} \underbrace{\begin{bmatrix} x \\ y \end{bmatrix}}_{\boldsymbol{r}} = \underbrace{\begin{bmatrix} d_1^2 - d_2^2 + k_2 - k_1 \\ d_1^2 - d_3^2 + k_3 - k_1 \\ \vdots \\ d_1^2 - d_n^2 + k_n - k_1 \end{bmatrix}}_{\mathbf{b}} \tag{2}$$

We write $k_i = x_i^2 + y_i^2 + z_i^2$, and we write (2) as $2\mathbf{A}\boldsymbol{r} = \boldsymbol{b}$. We obtain the position of the tag with respect to anchors according to Least Square as follow,

$$\boldsymbol{r} = \frac{1}{2}(\mathbf{A}^T\mathbf{A})^{-1}\mathbf{A}^T\boldsymbol{b}. \tag{3}$$

B. Taylor Series

We rewrite (1), as a function of $f(\boldsymbol{r})$ and arrange it as a vector:

$$f(\boldsymbol{r}) = \begin{bmatrix} \sqrt{(x_1 - x)^2 + (y_1 - y)^2 + (z_1 - z)^2} - d_1 \\ \vdots \\ \sqrt{(x_n - x)^2 + (y_n - y)^2 + (z_n - z)^2} - d_n \end{bmatrix} = \begin{bmatrix} d_1 + \varepsilon_1 \\ \vdots \\ d_n + \varepsilon_n \end{bmatrix} \tag{4}$$

We denote ε_n as range estimation error. Given an initial estimation as $\boldsymbol{r_0} = [x_0\, y_0\, z_0]^T$ we find $\boldsymbol{r} = \boldsymbol{r_0} + \boldsymbol{\delta}$. Let $\boldsymbol{\delta} = [\delta_x \quad \delta_y \quad \delta_z]^T$ denote the location estimation error vector which is to be determined. Expanding $f(\boldsymbol{r})$ into a Taylor series and retain the linear elements: $f(\boldsymbol{r}) \approx f_{i,0} + j_{i,1}\delta_x + j_{i,2}\delta_y + j_{i,3}\delta_z \approx d_i + \varepsilon_i$ where $j_{i,l}$ is defined as the Jacobian

$$\mathbf{J} = \begin{bmatrix} \frac{\partial f_1}{\partial x} & \dots & \frac{\partial f_1}{\partial z} \\ \vdots & \ddots & \vdots \\ \frac{\partial f_n}{\partial x} & \dots & \frac{\partial f_n}{\partial z} \end{bmatrix} = \begin{bmatrix} j_{1,1} & j_{1,2} & j_{1,3} \\ j_{2,1} & j_{2,2} & j_{2,3} \\ \vdots & \vdots & \vdots \\ j_{n,1} & j_{n,2} & j_{n,3} \end{bmatrix}. \tag{5}$$

We solve $\mathbf{J}\boldsymbol{\delta} = \boldsymbol{D} + \boldsymbol{e}$, $\boldsymbol{D} = [d_1 - f_{1,0} \quad \cdots \quad d_n - f_{n,0}]^T$ and $\boldsymbol{e} = [\varepsilon_1 \quad \cdots \quad \varepsilon_n]$. With Least Square we retrieve

$$\boldsymbol{\delta} = (\mathbf{J}^T\mathbf{J})^{-1}\mathbf{J}\boldsymbol{D}. \tag{6}$$

From the initial guess, we can update the location estimation. By iterating, one continually get a better solution. To find a suitable stop criterion for the iteration, choose ε in the magnitude of the desired accuracy.

C. Quasi-Newton-Davidon–Fletcher–Powell

One can also consider (4) as an optimization problem. To find a solution, we interpret each column of (4) as an error which is squared and summed up. To find the minimum of the function we apply Newton-iteration, which requires finding the Jacobian and Hessian of this equation. We approximate both matrices with the Davidon-Fletcher-Powell formulas, and thus become a Quasi-Newton approach.

$$f(\boldsymbol{r}) = \sum_{i=1}^{n} \left(\sqrt{(x_i - x)^2 + (y_i - y)^2 + (z_i - z)^2} - d_i\right)^2$$

We estimate $f(\boldsymbol{r})$ with a second order Taylor series around a point $\boldsymbol{r}_0$ and find

$$f(\boldsymbol{r_0} + \boldsymbol{h}) \cong f(\boldsymbol{r_k}) + \boldsymbol{h}^T\boldsymbol{g}_k + \frac{1}{2}\boldsymbol{h}^T\boldsymbol{B}_k\boldsymbol{h}. \tag{7}$$

In this equation we denote $\boldsymbol{g}_k = \nabla f(\boldsymbol{r_k})$ and $\boldsymbol{h}_k = -\boldsymbol{B}_k^{-1}\boldsymbol{g}_k$, $\boldsymbol{B}_0$ is the Hessian matrix of $f(\boldsymbol{r})$ and positive definite. We provide pseudo-code for the implementation.

begin
$k := 0; \boldsymbol{r} := \boldsymbol{r_0}; \boldsymbol{H_0} = \boldsymbol{B}_0\,;\ \varepsilon;$
$\boldsymbol{g}_0 := J(\boldsymbol{r_0})^T f(\boldsymbol{r_0})$
while($\|\boldsymbol{g}_k\| \geq \varepsilon$)
$\boldsymbol{g}_k := \boldsymbol{J}_k^T f_k$
$\boldsymbol{h}_k = -\boldsymbol{H}_k\boldsymbol{g}_k$
$\alpha_k = \arg\min_{\alpha} f(\boldsymbol{r_k} + \alpha\boldsymbol{h}_k)$
$\boldsymbol{r_{k+1}} := \boldsymbol{r_k} + \alpha_k\boldsymbol{h}_k$
$\boldsymbol{s_k} = \boldsymbol{r_{k+1}} - \boldsymbol{r_k}$
$\boldsymbol{y_k} = \boldsymbol{g_{k+1}} - \boldsymbol{g_k}$
$\boldsymbol{H}_{k+1} = \boldsymbol{H}_k - \frac{\boldsymbol{H}_k\boldsymbol{y}_k\boldsymbol{y}_k^T\boldsymbol{H}_k}{\boldsymbol{y}_k^T\boldsymbol{H}_k\boldsymbol{y}_k} + \frac{\boldsymbol{s}_k\boldsymbol{s}_k^T}{\boldsymbol{y}_k^T\boldsymbol{s}_k}$
$k := k + 1;$
end
end

We update $\boldsymbol{H}_k$ according to the Davidon–Fletcher–Powell formula as follow,

$$\boldsymbol{H}_{k+1} = \boldsymbol{H}_k - \frac{\boldsymbol{H}_k\boldsymbol{y}_k\boldsymbol{y}_k^T\boldsymbol{H}_k}{\boldsymbol{y}_k^T\boldsymbol{H}_k\boldsymbol{y}_k} + \frac{\boldsymbol{s}_k\boldsymbol{s}_k^T}{\boldsymbol{y}_k^T\boldsymbol{s}_k} \tag{8}$$

The iteration continues until $\|\boldsymbol{g}_k\| \leq \varepsilon$ with $0 \leq \varepsilon < 1$. With smallerε, the accuracy increases, but requires more computational effort since more iterations are required.

D. Levenberg-Marquardt

The last algorithm to retrieve a tag position from distances is the Levenberg-Marquardt algorithm [6]. We use the same function as in (4).

We aim to minimize $\|f(\boldsymbol{r})\|_2$, or equivalently to find $r^* = arg\,\min_{r}\{F(\boldsymbol{r})\}$, where

$$F(\mathbf{r}) = \frac{1}{2}\sum_{i=1}^{n}(f_i(\mathbf{r}))^2 = \frac{1}{2}\|f(\mathbf{r})\|^2 = \frac{1}{2}f(\mathbf{r})^T f(\mathbf{r}) \quad (9)$$

We write the Taylor expansion of $f(\boldsymbol{r})$ as follow with first order partial derivatives:

$$f(\boldsymbol{r}+\boldsymbol{h}) \cong f(\boldsymbol{r}) + \boldsymbol{J}(r)\boldsymbol{h} \quad (10)$$

$$F(\boldsymbol{r}+\boldsymbol{h}) \cong F(\boldsymbol{r}) + \boldsymbol{h}^T\boldsymbol{J}^T f + \frac{1}{2}\boldsymbol{h}^T\boldsymbol{J}^T\boldsymbol{J}\boldsymbol{h} \quad (11)$$

According to LM, the step $\boldsymbol{h}$ is defined by the following:

$$(\boldsymbol{J}^T\boldsymbol{J} + \mu\boldsymbol{I})\boldsymbol{h} = -\boldsymbol{g} \text{ with } \boldsymbol{g} = \boldsymbol{J}^T f \text{ and } \mu \geq 0$$

The initial value of μ should be related to the size of elements in $\mathbf{A} := \boldsymbol{J}(\boldsymbol{r})^T\boldsymbol{J}(\boldsymbol{r})$ [2].We provide the pseudo-code here.

```
begin
  k := 0; r := r_0
  A_0 := J_0^T J_0; g_0 := J_0^T f_0
  % τ is used to control the initial step size.
  μ := τ * max{a_ii}
  while(||g|| ≥ ε_1)
     h_k = (A + μI)\g_k
   if F(r_0 + h_0) < F(r_0)
        r_{k+1} := r_k + h_k
        A_{k+1} := J_{k+1}^T J_{k+1}
        g_{k+1} := J_{k+1}^T f_{k+1}
        k = k + 1
     else
        set μ larger
  end
end
```

4 Evaluation

In this part, we evaluate performance of our proposed algorithms. The assumed scenario is an over determined system in a 2D square space under Line of Sight (LOS) conditions. To provide results which are typical for a Microsoft Kinect, we limit the size of each dimension by $r = 3.5$ m and divide each dimension in 100 steps, resulting in a step size of 0.035 cm, which is in the magnitude of the standard deviation of the Microsoft Kinect [4]. The largest distance is given as $d_{\max} = \sqrt{2r^2} \approx 5$ m. We aim for an accuracy $\varepsilon < 10$ cm which is sufficient for many applications. We place four anchors in the four corners of this target space. We iterate through each tag position in the target space and calculate the distance to each anchor. Based on our error model, we add a deterministic and random Gaussian noise with variance $\sigma^2 = 5.29\ \text{cm}^2$ to the distance estimation. Last, we compute the position with one of our algorithms. We determine the accuracy of an algorithm by the MSE between true position and noisy position for every possible tag position.

First, each algorithm is evaluated with no noise to test the computational runtime of the algorithms. Runtime depends on actual implementation and desired accuracy of the algorithms. Based on the simulation we calculate the time required to determine one position. The results of the simulation are in Table 1.

We notice that LS takes the least time per position calculation, followed by TS. LM algorithm takes approximately three times more computational effort than LS or TS. QN-DFP takes seven times longer than LS or TS and even two times more than LM.

Table 1: Computational Efforts

	LS	TS	QN-DFP	LM
Total Runtime [s]	10.92	11.9	71.08	27.67
Per Calc. [ms]	1.07	1.16	6.97	2.71

Additionally we add the deterministic error and finally the random error. To measure the performance, we calculate the MSE for all tag positions. We further use the maximum error between true position and calculated position as an evaluation criteria. In Figure 2 we show typical results for every algorithm. Fig 2. Shows a heat map where dark areas indicate zero MSE and bright areas indicate an error of 20 cm. Anchors are indicated as dots. Error increases as the tag becomes closer to one anchor. MSE for LS in the target space is 8.3 cm which is the worst of all four algorithms. Maximum error for LS is 31.7 cm, which is the worst for all algorithms – compared to the other algorithms, TS (upper right part, 6.67 cm MSE), QN-DFP (lower left part, 5.36 cm MSE) and LM (lower right part, 6.67 cm MSE). QN-DFP performs best in terms of MSE. When the maximum error is used as a metric, then TS, QN-DFP and LM outperforms LS. Each algorithm provides best results, then the tag is in the center of the target space. The results are in Table 2.

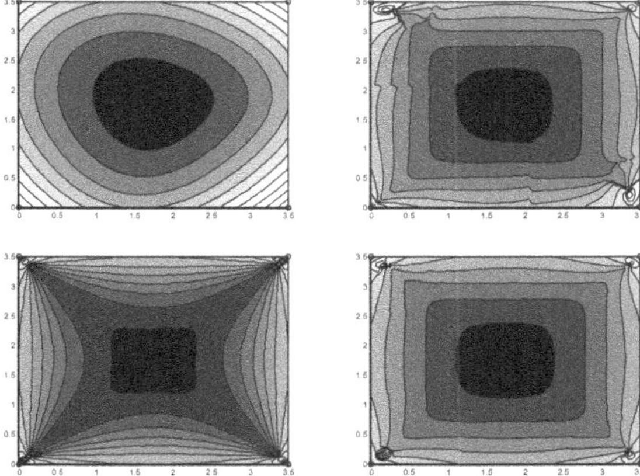

Figure 2: Results for deterministic error for LS (upper left), TS (upper right), QN-DFP (bottom left) and LM (bottom right)

We also evaluate the direction of the error vector. This is shown in the left part of Figure 3. The direction of the error tends to point to the center.

Table 2: Algorithm comparisons for deterministic error

	LS	TS	QN-DFP	LM
MSE [cm]	8,30	6,67	5,36	6,67
Max error [cm]	31,8	19,6	21,4	20,0

In the next test, we will add a random error to the simulation. To provide the same test environment, we manipulate the random number generator to provide the same random numbers for each algorithm. The results are

shown in Figure 4. We use the same scaling and the same alignment as in the previous test.
We notice that the principle shape of the heat maps looks the same, only with increased noise. The MSE did not increase by the same value of the standard deviation of the Microsoft Kinect. The impact was marginal as shown by Table 03. The LM algorithm shows the least impact of the random error and LS shows the most impact to the evaluation criteria.

Table 3: Algorithm comparisons for random error

	LS	TS	QN-DFP	LM
MSE [cm]	8,30	6,67	5,36	6,67
Max error [cm]	34,4	21,5	21,2	21,5

Figure 3: Error vectors for LM algorithm.

The error vectors point in the middle randomly and at the outer parts of the figure to the center of the figure. This is shown in the right part of Figure 3. We conclude that the random error dominates in areas, where the deterministic error is small compared to the standard deviation of the random error.

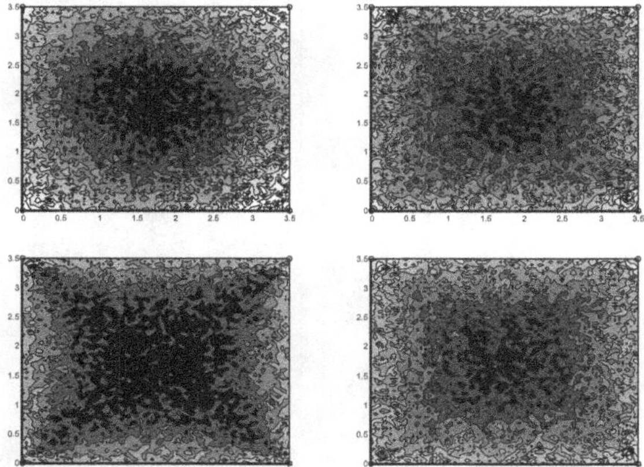

Figure 4: Results for non-systematic noise for the four different algorithms

QN performs best in terms of MSE. This however comes at the price of high computational costs. LS has the highest MSE error for both test scenarios.
LM performs worse than QN-DFP but is considerable faster than QN-DFP but still slower than TS and LS.
The introduction of an error model influences the outcome of a simulation. The influence of the random error is neglectable for large distances, as long as the systematic error is dominant. Based on this evaluation we can choose an algorithm for our desired low budget optical reference system.

5 Conclusion and Future Work

QN-DFP is the best algorithm to calculate the position of tags in terms of mean squared error (MSE). Least Square is the fastest algorithm to retrieve the position of a tag. The best trade-off in terms of MSE and computational cost is the Levenberg-Marquardt algorithm. We find that the random error has no influence to the MSE.
Future work will consider room geometry and we optimize the anchor locations based on a given metric. We want to determine the optimal number of anchors for a given room. Based on our results in this paper, we aim to build a low budget optical system.

Acknowledgement

This publication is a result of the research within the Center of Excellence CoSA in the m:flo project, which is funded by German Federal Ministry for Economic Affairs and Energy (BMWi, FKZ KF3177201ED3). This publication is also a result of the ongoing research within the LUMEN research group, which is funded by the German Federal Ministry of Education and Research (BMBF, FKZ 13EZ1140A/B).
LUMEN is a joint research project of Lübeck University of Applied Sciences and University of Lübeck and represents a branch of the Graduate School for Computing in Medicine and Life Sciences of University of Lübeck.

6 References

[1] Guowei Shen, Rudolf Zetik, and Reiner S. Thoma. *Performance Comparison of TOA and TDOA Based Location Estimation Algorithm in LOS Environment.* Proceeding of the 5th workshop on positioning, Navigation and communication 2008.

[2] K.Madsen, H.B.Nielsen, O.Tingleff. *Methods for non-linear least squares problems.* 2nd Edition, April 2004.

[3] Amitangshu Pal, *Localization Algorithms in Wireless Sensor Networks: Current Approaches and Future Challenges.* Network Protocols and Algorithms, ISSN 1943-3581, 2010, Vol. 2, No. 1.

[4] Q. Ma, C. Bollmeyer, Y. Zhu, H. Hellbrück, *Localization of Heart Reference Point of a Lying Patient with Microsoft Kinect Sensor.* GRIN (T. M. Buzug et. al., ed.), 2014.

[5] Liu Hui,Houshang Darabi,Pat Banerjee,and Jing Liu, *Survey of wireless indoor positioning techniques and systems.* Systems. Man, and Cybernetics, Part C: Applications and Reviews, IEEE Transactions on 37.6 (2007): 1067-1080.

[6] Marquardt, Donald W. *An algorithm for least-squares estimation of nonlinear parameters.* Journal of the Society for Industrial & Applied Mathematics 11.2 (1963): 431-441.

[7] W. H. Foy, *Position-location solutions by Taylor-series estimation.* IEEE Trans. Aerosp. Elecctron. Syst., vol. 12, pp. 187–194, Mar. 1976.

A machine learning approach for planning valve-sparing aortic root reconstruction

J. Hagenah [1], M. Scharfschwerdt [2], Z. Zhang [3], and C. Metzner [4]

[1] Medizinische Ingenieurwissenschaft, Universität zu Lübeck, jannis.hagenah@miw.uni-luebeck.de
[2] Department of Cardiac Surgery, University Hospital Schleswig-Holstein, Lübeck, michael.scharfschwerdt@web.de
[3] Institute of Biomedical Analytical Technology and Instrumentation, Xi'an Jiaotong University, zxzhang@mail.xjtu.edu.cn
[4] Institute for Robotic and Cognitive Systems, Universität zu Lübeck, metzner@rob.uni-luebeck.de

Abstract

Choosing the optimal prosthesis size and shape is a difficult task during surgical valve-sparing aortic root reconstruction. Hence, there is a need for surgery planning tools. Common surgery planning approaches try to model the mechanical behaviour of the aortic valve and its leaflets. However, these approaches suffer from inaccuracies due to unknown biomechanical properties and from a high computational complexity. In this paper, we present a new approach based on machine learning that avoids these problems. The valve geometry is described by geometrical features obtained from ultrasound images. We interpret the surgery planning as a learning problem, in which the features of the healthy valve are predicted from these of the dilated valve using support vector regression (SVR). Our first results indicate that a machine learning based surgery planing can be possible.

1 Introduction

The aortic valve is an important structure located in the aortic root to provide the right direction of the blood flow in the human body. However, the functionality of the valve can be restricted, which can finally lead to a heart insufficiency. One reason for such a restriction is the dilatation of the aortic root wall. In this case, the geometry of the valve is distorted while the shape of the valve leaflets stays unchanged [1]. This distortion causes a valve insufficiency, which happens especially in patients with the Marfan-syndrome [2].
For these patients, the valve-sparing aortic root reconstruction is an alternative to valve replacement. The basic idea of this technique is to remodel the healthy shape of the aortic root using a prosthesis [4]. The patients leaflets are attached to this prosthesis. The advantages of this method are the natural valve leaflets much better mechanical properties and the longer durability compared to artificial valve prosthesis'. Fig. 1 shows the aortic root in the healthy, the dilated and the reconstructed state.

However, the estimation of the actual valve geometry and the determination of the optimal prosthesis size and shape are difficult tasks. During surgery, the heart is not pressurized, which limits the possibilities of detecting the actual root geometry. One further problem is that one can only obtain the root geometry in the dilated state, so the optimal prosthesis shape can only be estimated based on this distorted geometry. Performing this estimation before the treatment could improve the method significantly.
Previous approaches are aiming at finite element based simulation to evaluate the individual valves mechanics as well as the bloodflow through the valve with different prosthesis sizes virtually [5], [6]. One problem of these approaches are the complex, non-isotropic biomechanical properties of the valve leaflets, which are not yet completely understood [7], so it's hard to find biologically reasonable model parameters. Furthermore, three-dimensional image acquisition of the valve leaflets can be quite intricate [8] and the models are computational expansive. The simulation of the blood flow raises additionally raises the complexity.
In this paper, we want to present a new machine learning

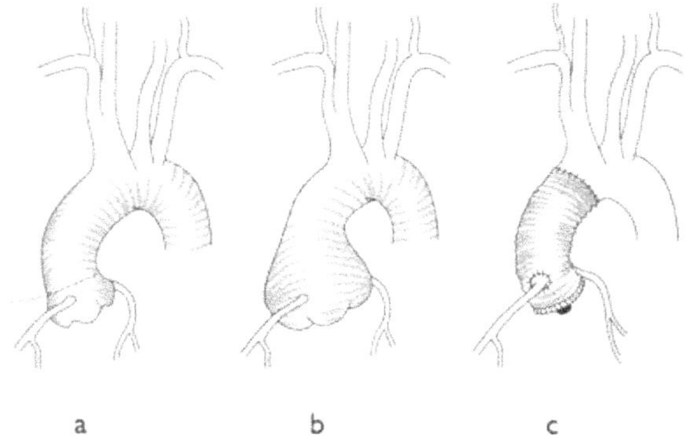

Figure 1: The aortic root. a) healthy state b) dilated state c) reconstructed state [3].

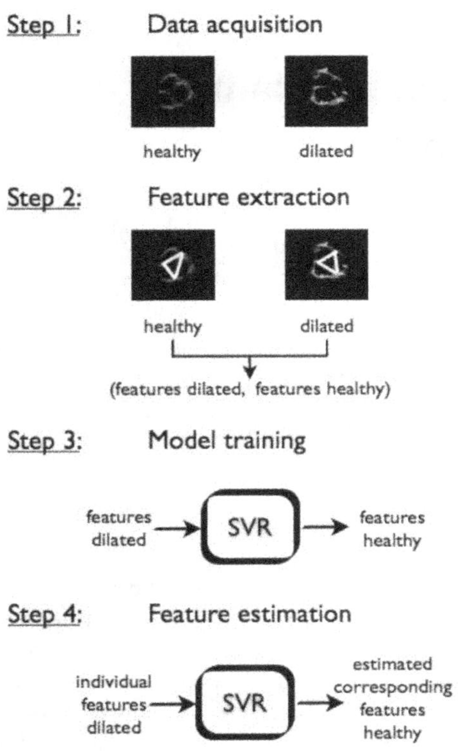

Figure 2: The main steps of the presented method. At first, ultrasound images are acquired. Then, geometrical features are extracted to get tupels of features in the healthy and dilated state. With these tupels, an SVR-model is trained. This model allows feature estimation.

based approach to solve this problem avoiding biomechanical uncertainties.

2 Material and Methods

The basic idea of the approach is to describe the valve geometry by geometric parameters called *features*. We assume the dilatation to be a mapping from the features of the healthy valve to the features of the dilated valve. Hence, the aim of the surgery planning is to estimate the mapping from the dilated to the healthy features.

In our experiments, we obtained healthy and dilated features of porcine aortic roots, which results in a *(features dilated, features healthy)* tupel for each examined valve. Accordingly, the problem of finding the optimal prosthesis can be described as a learning problem: the aim is to calculate the features in the healthy state based on the individual features in the dilated state. This problem can be solved using *Support Vector Regression* (SVR) where the obtained tupels *(features dilated, features healthy)* serve as training data.

The presented method can be separated into four steps: the experimental data acquisition, the feature extraction, the model training and the feature prediction. These steps are visualized in Fig. 2 and are described in the following paragraphs.

2.1 Data Acquisition

To obtain features of an aortic root, a suitable imaging modality is needed. Due to their fine structure and their fast movement during the cardiac cycle, the detailed leaflet geometry is hard to extract from typical volumetric images like CT or MRI. Because of this reason, we previously proposed the usage of transesophageal ultrasound (TEE) [9]. The benefits of this modality are the high temporal resolution, low examination costs and the availability in clinical practice.

We designed a setup to simulate a TEE-examination on ex-vivo porcine aortic roots [9]. In this setup, a porcine aortic root is pressurized by a constant diastolic pressure created by a water head. The ultrasound images are taken sequentially while the imaging plane is rotating. After that, a three-dimensional reconstruction is done by transforming the image data to a Cartesian coordinate representation. The result is a volumetric image frame of the aortic root.

As mentioned above, we examined ex-vivo porcine aortic roots. To get information about the root geometry before and after the pathological dilatation, we studied each aortic root in two different states: the *healthy* state and the *dilated* state. To examine the healthy state, we took volumetric ultrasound images of the unchanged root. To simulate the dilated state, the root wall was manually enlarged by adding additional aortic tissue into cuts in the root wall. After that, we acquired three-dimensional image data of the dilated root. The result are three-dimensional images of the root in both states.

2.2 Feature extraction

The aim of this step is to generate tupels of features that describe the geometry of the valve in the healthy and the dilated state. The extracted features are the three commissure distances k_1, k_2 and k_3, the effective height h_{eff} and the leaflet-specific characteristic parameters F and α. The effective height is defined as the height difference between the commissure plane, where the leaflets are attached to the root wall, and the coaptation plane, where the three leaflets meet each other. It has a high influence on the functionality of the valve [5]. The leaflet-specific parameter F describes the area of the triangle formed by the two commissure points of the leaflet and the coaptation point (cf. Fig. 3). Hence, F measures the size of the leaflet. α is one of the angles of the same triangle and describes the leaflets sheering. Both F and α affect the performance of the valve [10]. The commissure distances are defined as the distances between the three commissure points, respectively (cf. Fig. 3). The features were manually obtained from the ultrasound images using the open-source image analysis tool *3dSlicer* (Harvard Medical School, Boston, USA).

At the moment, the prostheses used in clinical practice is shaped as a tube, so we aim to estimate the optimal prosthesis diameter. This diameter can be calculated based on the three commissure distances as the diameter of the circumcircle of the triangle formed by the commissure points.

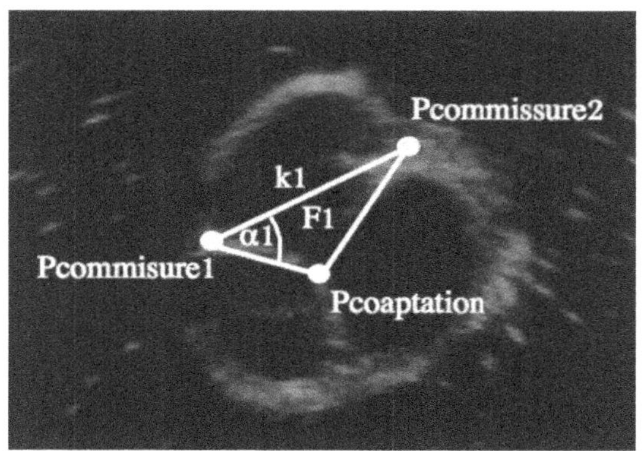

Figure 3: Ultrasound image of a porcine aortic root. For one leaflet, the commissure points $P_{commissure1}$ and $P_{commissure2}$, the coaptation point $P_{coaptation}$ and the geometrical features k_1, F_1 and α_1 are shown.

Hence, the commissure distances k_1, k_2 and k_3 are very important and the focus of this paper lies on the good estimation of them.

2.3 Model Training

The surgery planning method aims at estimating the healthy features only based on the knowledge of the dilated features. In the previous steps we have obtained tupels *(features dilated, features healthy)*. Using this data set we train a support vector regression (SVR) algorithm to learn the mapping between the dilated and the healthy states. The SVR is a machine learning method that performs regression without initial knowledge of the underlying model [11]. In this paper, we used the so called ϵ-SVR with a *Gaussian radial basis function* kernel (RBF) using the *MATLAB*-implementation of the open-source library *libsvm* [12].
As mentioned above, the focus of this paper lies on a good estimation of the commissure distances. To find the best parameter combination for reaching this goal, we implemented a nonlinear simplex optimization method that minimizes the sum of absolute differences between the healthy commissure distances and the estimated commissure distances.
With this parameter set, we can train our SVR-model with the *(features dilated, features healthy)* tupels, which serve as *support vectors*.

2.4 Feature estimation

After the training, the model is ready to reconstruct the healthy features of a valve from the individual dilated features. We obtained tupels of the healthy and dilated features of six aortic roots using the method previously described. We trained the SVM-model with five of the tupels and estimated the healthy features of the sixth valve with it. To evaluate the accuracy we compared all estimated features to the reference by calculating relative distances. Additionally, we calculated the root diameter based on the estimated features and the reference.

This evaluation was performed six times, each time estimating the healthy features of another valve while the other five valves where used for training (leave-one-out).

3 Results and Discussion

In the following paragraphs, the results of the feature estimation are shown and discussed.

Table 1: Relative differences in percentage between the estimated features and the reference for the six examined valves.

Feature	Valve 1	Valve 2	Valve 3	Valve 4
k_1	23,07	14,10	3,76	1,38
k_2	21,00	16,89	1,81	9,02
k_3	10,96	24,68	77,64	27,63
h_{eff}	50,901	69,77	9,30	38,65
α_1	8,81	47,18	54,85	6,31
α_2	16,24	26,18	4,48	2,18
α_3	0,87	3,41	1,24	16,76
F_1	38,22	50,70	17,64	27,40
F_2	26,64	85,92	110,83	33,21
F_3	38,77	39,02	100,82	18,00

Feature	Valve 5	Valve 6	Analysis:	Mean
k_1	18,61	2,73		10,61
k_2	7,42	17,18		10,72
k_3	4,52	4,94		25,06
h_{eff}	29,93	10,13		34,78
α_1	45,82	5,25		28,04
α_2	3,04	12,20		10,72
α_3	41,00	48,68		18,60
F_1	51,06	18,06		33,85
F_2	27,44	23,81		51,31
F_3	80,71	27,72		50,84

3.1 Results

We examined six porcine aortic valves using the method describes in chapter 2. Accordingly, we estimated the healthy features of each of the six valves using an SVR-model trained with the other five valves' features, respectively. Table 1 shows the relative distances between the estimated features and the reference as well as the mean difference for each feature. As mentioned in section 2.2, our aim is to calculate the optimal prosthesis diameter based on the commissure distances. For this purpose, this diameter was calculated for the estimated healthy features as well as the reference features. The resulting prosthesis sizes are presented in Table 2. As the commonly used prostheses are produced with even-numbered diameters, we rounded our results adequate.

Table 2: Estimated and reference prosthesis diameters in mm.

Valve	Reference	Estimated
1	24	26
2	18	20
3	16	20
4	28	28
5	20	20
6	22	24

3.2 Discussion

Table 1 shows particular differences between the estimated and the reference features. Some parameters for some valves are estimated good, others depict a high discrepancy. This is mainly due to the fact that the regression was performed with only five training samples. This is obviously not enough information to produce reliable feature estimations.

However, Table 2 depicts that in two cases, the calculated prosthesis diameter fits to the diameter of the healthy valve. In three other cases, the difference is one prosthesis size step. Hence, even with this small data set, an estimation of the best prosthesis diameter is possible.

Further work should aim for the enlargement of the training data set. This enhances the accuracy of the SVR-model. Additionally, a greater number of support vectors allows a higher dimensional regression, i.e. the estimation of one feature can be based on all other features.

Another interesting point is the further processing of the estimated features. If the features could be translated to a geometric model of the aortic root, it would be possible to produce patient individual prosthesis' with the specific shape of that patients aortic root in the healthy state. Estimating the prosthesis diameter could be just the beginning of individualization of cardiovascular implants.

4 Conclusion

We presented a new machine learning based approach for planning valve-sparing aortic root reconstruction. The advantage is that no biomechanical modeling of the valve leaflets or the surrounding blood is needed. Our first results indicate that a planning for valve-sparing aortic root reconstruction based on a simple machine learning could be possible.

Acknowledgement

The work has been carried out at the Institute of Biomedical Analytical Technology and Instrumentation, Xi'an Jiaotong University, and the Institute for Robotics and Cognitive Systems, Universität zu Lübeck. This publication is a result of the ongoing research within the LUMEN research group, which is funded by the German Bundesministerium für Bildung und Forschung (BMBF) (FKZ 13EZ1140A/B). LUMEN is a joint research project of Lübeck University of Applied Sciences and University of Lübeck and represents an own branch of the Graduate School for Computing in Medicine and Life Sciences of University of Lübeck.

5 References

[1] M. Scharfschwerdt, HH. Sievers, A. Hussein, ED. Kraatz and M. Misfeld, *Impact of progressive sinotubular junction dilatation on valve competence of the 3F Aortic and Sorin Solo stentless bioprosthetic heart valves.* Eur J Cardiothorac Surg, 37:631-634, 2010.

[2] A. Schuerhaus, *Aortale Eingriffe bei Patienten mit Marfan-Syndrom.* PhD thesis, Universität zu Lübeck, 2008.

[3] P. Nataf and E. Lansac, *Dilation thoracic aorta: medical surgical management.* Heart 92(9), pp. 1345–1352, 2006.

[4] J. Bechtel, A. Erasmi, M. Misfeld and HH. Sievers, *Rekonstruktive Aortenklappenchirurgie: Ross-, David- und Yacoub-verfahren.* Herz 31(5), pp. 413-422, 2006.

[5] G. Marom, R. Haj-Ali, M. Rosenfeld, HJ. Schäfers and E. Raa-nani, *Aortic root numeric model: annulus diameter prediction of effective height and coaptation in post-aortic valve repair.* J Thorac Cardiovasc Surg 145(2),406-411, 2013.

[6] H. Hadjar, R. Friedl, HH. Sievers, P. Hunold, B. Stender, A. Schlaefer, *Patient-specific finite-element simulation of aortic valve-sparing surgery.* Computer Assisted Radiol-ogy and Surgery (CARS 2012), 2012.

[7] P. Hammer, C. Pacak, R. Howe and P. Nido, *Collagen bundle orientation explains aortic valve leaflet coaptation.* Functional Imaging and Modeling of the Heart, pp. 409-415, 2013.

[8] J. Hagenah, M. Scharfschwerdt, C. Metzner, A. Schlaefer, HH. Sievers, and A. Schweikard, *An approach for patient specific modeling of the aortic valve leaflets.* Biomedizinische Technik (BMT 2014), 2014.

[9] J. Hagenah, M. Scharfschwerdt, B. Stender, S. Ott, R. Friedl, HH. Sievers and A. Schlaefer, *A setup for ultrasound based assessment of the aortic root geometry.* Biomedizinische Technik (BMT 2013), 2013.

[10] J. Hagenah, *Erstellung eines patientenindividuellen Modells der Aortenklappe*, Bachelor thesis, Universität zu Lübeck, 2013.

[11] AJ. Smola and B. Schölkopf, *A tutorial on support vector regression*, Statistics and Computing 14(3), pp. 199-222, 2004.

[12] CC. Chang and CJ. Lin, *LIBSVM : A library for support vector machines*, ACM Transactions on Intelligent Systems and Technology 2(27), pp. 1-27, 2011.

Edge-preserving ring artifact correction for CT imaging

S. K. Lüth [1], M. Elter [2], and I. Schasiepen [2]
[1] Medizinische Ingenieurwissenschaft, Universität zu Lübeck, svenja.lueth@miw.uni-luebeck.de
[2] Siemens AG, Erlangen, {matthias.elter, ingo.schasiepen}@siemens.com

Abstract

Defective or miscalibrated detector elements in computed tomography (CT) lead to concentric circular artifacts in the image superimposing the actual object and thus deteriorating the image quality. Existing approaches for image-based ring artifact correction are either difficult to parametrize or make use of coordinate transformations leading to loss of edge quality. This paper proposes a post-processing method for ring artifact reduction with focus on edge-preserving. Each volume slice is subjected to a radial median filter optimized for edge preservation, a difference image is calculated and a circular size-varying smoothing filter is applied to evenly eliminate artifacts in any distance from the rotation center. The resulting image mainly containing ring artifacts is subtracted from the original image yielding an almost artifact-free outcome. The developed algorithm allows a successful suppression of ring artifacts for both clinical and industrial CT data with negligible impact on the object edges.

1 Introduction

Sensitivity changes or malfunction of detector elements lead to line artifacts in the sinogram which are reconstructed to concentric ring-shaped artifacts in the image [1]. Due to the circular image acquisition scheme in CT, this problem mostly occurs with a fixed alignment of X-ray source and detector in combination with the inhomogeneous sensitivity of a flat-panel detector [2], [3].
Ring artifacts severely affect the diagnostic analysis of the images, as well as complicating further processing steps, e.g. image segmentation or registration. Thus, a ring artifact correction (RAC) is necessary. The different approaches for RAC can be divided into two groups [4]: pre-processing methods based on the sinogram and post-processing methods based on the reconstructed image. These approaches set the focus on a minimum number of parameters, the best possible artifact removal in a specified region of interest (ROI) or adaptability to different image and artifact characteristics [4], [5]. As the preservation of edges is often neglected, an edge-preserving post-processing algorithm is presented as a further development of [6].

2 Material and Methods

In this section, a post-processing algorithm for the suppression of ring artifacts in reconstructed CT data is developed. The basis for examination is formed by a database of 40 datasets originating from different CT scanners with different acquisition modalities and containing various kinds of clinical as well as industrial objects to achieve a maximum diversity of image characteristics. Each dataset consists of a reconstructed volume with a stack of z image slices of size $x \times y$, respectively.

2.1 Ring artifact correction algorithm

Starting with the reconstructed image slice **I**, the first step of the basic algorithm in post-processing RAC [6] is to apply a median filter in radial direction on lines running through the center of rotation. The difference image of the original and the median-filtered image **M** yields a correction image **R = I - M** that mainly contains artifacts. As **R** does not only consist of rings but also of noise, it is subjected to a circular smoothing filter removing non-ring structures as well as reducing noise in the ring structures to leave high frequencies unaffected by the RAC. Finally, the smoothed ring image **S** is subtracted from **I** to get the corrected output image **O = I - S**, cf. Fig. 1.

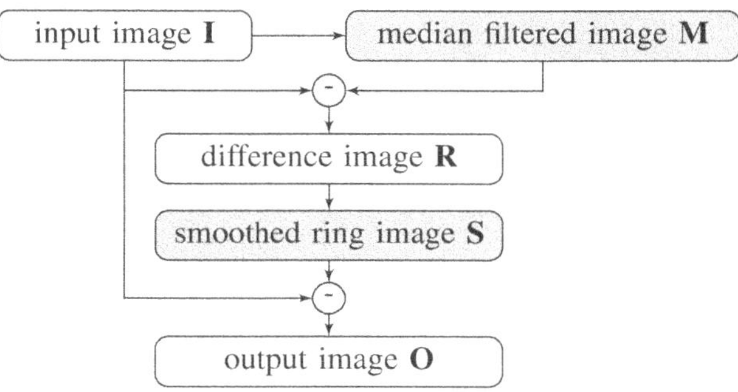

Figure 1: Illustration of the basic algorithm. The presented advancements only affect the highlighted nodes.

Existing approaches mainly preserve object edges by choosing a ROI and only perform the RAC on this section. In fact, the edge sharpness of the transition from the ROI to outlying structures is not impaired, but the image impression is rather unsatisfying as the ring artifacts outside the ROI are not corrected. Further, the ROI segmentation raises a problem and the edges within are blurred due to filtering. The enhancements of the developed method are an edge-preserving modification for median filtering and the elimination of small rings in proximity to the rotation center by a resizable smoothing filter.

2.2 Adaptive radial median filter

We suggest the use of an adaptive median filter whose kernel size automatically adapts if an object edge is detected. According to [7], a good choice for edge detection is a Sobel filtering in x- and y-direction (S_X and S_Y) and calculation of the gradient strength

$$G(x,y) = \sqrt{S_X(x,y)^2 + S_Y(x,y)^2}. \tag{1}$$

For the purpose of determining whether an edge occurs, the gradient strength is converted into a binary mask. To ensure the applicability for varying ranges of attenuation values in different kinds of CT data, the gradient values are normalized to a fixed interval [0;1] allowing the use of a universal threshold to binarize the gradient image. Due to changes in the image contrast along the z-axis of the volume, the gradients of adjacent slices are taken into account while generating the binary mask: the averages of the respective minimum and maximum gradients of neighboring slices are determined to be the gradients used for normalization. This prevents single high- or low-contrast slices from masking too little or too many edges.

Masked structures are excluded from RAC. Thus, severe problems occur if the ring gradients are larger than the object edges. To avoid masking artifacts and leaving them uncorrected, a modified Hough transform is used to remove ring structures from the binary mask (Fig. 2). Given the center of rotation, an iteration over possible ring radii determines whether the inspected radius includes a ring and thus has to be corrected. Therefore, the pixels set to *edge* along a concentric circle are summarized and normalized by dividing by the circumference. If this ratio exceeds a threshold, all pixels along the concentric circle are set to *no edge* in the mask. Unfortunately, this method fails if the image contains too many object edges. An improvement is the additional use of directional information. The direction of ideal concentric circles is computed and compared to the direction angles calculated from the Sobel information

$$\theta(x,y) = \arctan\left(\frac{S_Y(x,y)}{S_X(x,y)}\right). \tag{2}$$

A ring artifact exhibits edges orientated inwards and outwards in radial direction. To avoid different angle information on opposing sides of the ring, the angular range is reduced from $[-\pi;\pi]$ to $[-\frac{\pi}{2};\frac{\pi}{2}]$. Even though the pixel is set to *edge*, if the directions do not coincide, it is not considered as ring artifact and thus does not get corrected.

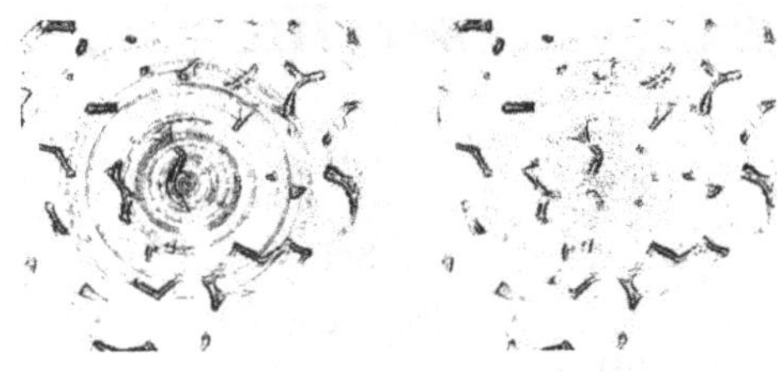

Figure 2: Binary masks from the metal foam dataset. Artifacts with large gradients are set to *edge* and thus excluded from RAC (left). Wrongly masked ring structures are removed from the binary mask via Hough transform (right).

For median filtering at position (x,y), the corresponding pixel in the binary mask is checked. If set to *edge*, the original value is copied and the algorithm continues with the next image pixel. Otherwise, the value at position (x,y) is the first entry in a vector of values to filter. Thence, the preceding and subsequent pixel coordinates in radial direction are determined. The edge map is checked for the occurrence of edges in both directions from (x,y). If *no edge* is traced, the pixel values are appended to the vector. The algorithm continues with further subsequent and precedent positions until either the maximum kernel radius is reached or an edge is detected. In both cases, the median is calculated from the hitherto filled vector, the value is assigned to the current pixel position and the algorithm continues with the next image pixel.

A fast median calculation is not trivial and thus deserves a closer examination. References [8] and [9] present a theoretical overview of the problem and provide solution statements. We compared four approaches on a n-element array, but as all analysed algorithms show negligible memory usage, we only focused on speed.

1. Modified bubble sort
   Quit sorting after half the array is sorted, middle array element is the median. *IsChanged*-flag to avoid redundant comparisons. Complexity: $\mathcal{O}(n^2)$.
2. C++ template function `std::sort`
   Based on divide-and-conquer quicksort, uses heap sort when number of elements exceeds constant `_ISORT_MAX = 32`. Complexity: $\mathcal{O}(n\ log(n))$.
3. C++ template function `std::partial_sort`
   Based on heap sort. Build heap and extract the minimum m times, then stop. Last element in right order is the median. Complexity: $\mathcal{O}(n + m\ log(n))$.
4. C++ template function `std::nth_element`
   Based on quickselsort [10], but applies insert sort for small arrays. Exploits the fact that the quicksort pivot element is arranged at its correctly sorted position. Just continues with the subarray that contains m-th element. Complexity: $\mathcal{O}(n)$, worst case $\mathcal{O}(n^2)$.

Regarding varying ring constitutions due to different artifact origins, it is necessary to find a common way to eliminate rings of different thickness. One approach is to take a small fixed-size median filter (e.g. size 5) and apply it both to the original image and to a downsampled version. Another way is to increase the median kernel size (up to 21 in some datasets) and only apply it to the original image. Both methods are compared with focus on the conservation of object edges.

2.3 Adaptive circular smoothing filter

The difference image **R** contains both noise and ring structures and is thus subjected to a circular smoothing. A severe problem is the choice of the filter size: a constant kernel size appropriate for the major part of the image would repeatedly run around inner ring artifacts with a small circumference.

We suggest a one-dimensional Gaussian kernel whose size is proportional to the distance from the center of rotation and therefore covers a constant angle. The maximum kernel size depends on the opening angle β. To accelerate the calculations, a Gaussian kernel for every needed size is computed and stored in a look-up-table. During filtering, the kernel corresponding to the present distance from the rotation center is applied in circular direction.

Especially in the center region, the kernel size falls below a reasonable size for smoothing. Therefore, an offset is introduced to artificially increase the kernel support. In this way, the image noise in the inner region can be successfully preserved while even small rings are removed.

The last step in RAC is to subtract the smoothed ring image from the original image.

3 Results and Discussion

An objective evaluation of RAC would require a ground-truth image for comparison. Due to the real images in the test cases, such kind of reference does not exist and the use of typical similarity measures is not possible. Although artificially introduced artifacts in images would allow a quantitative judgement on the degree of success, their difference to real applications is too large to provide a reliable statement. Hence, the efficacy of the presented RAC algorithm was confirmed by visual impression throughout the development process.

We compared two methods to remove artifacts of different thickness: downsampling and enlargement of the median support. Both methods have the potential to suppress thicker ring artifacts, but already with small median kernel sizes (e.g. 5 pixels) the downsampling approach shows a noticeable edge deterioration (Fig. 3). Furthermore, interpolation is needed twice for median filtering and for upsampling which causes interpolation errors. Since the calculation effort increases with larger kernel sizes, we compared different median-finding algorithms to minimize the computing time. The average runtime for RAC on the 512×512×4 chicken dataset shown in Fig. 3 without any median computation is 3.34 s. As shown in Table 1, the quickselsort-based C++ template function `nth_element` suits best for any size of array length. We empirically determined a filter size of 9 pixels for median filtering as an appropriate compromise between calculating time and the suppression of various ring thickness in test volumes.

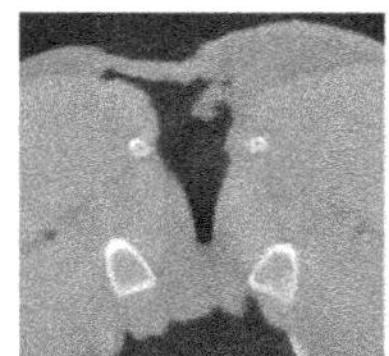
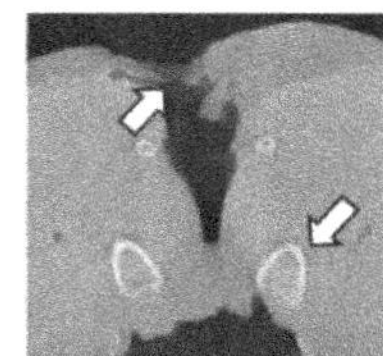
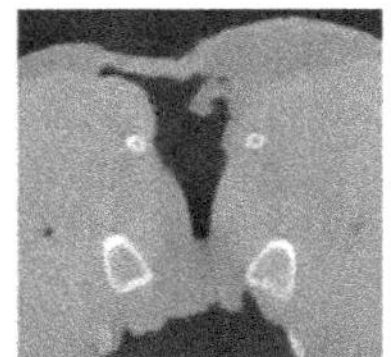

Figure 3: Original image (left) compared to the basic algorithm with factor 4 downsampling (5 pixels median filter, middle) and to edge-preserving RAC with adaptive median filter (21 pixels median filter, right). Images are cropped.

Table 1: Average computing time for RAC on the 512×512×4 chicken volume with different median-finding algorithms. System specification: Microsoft Windows 7 Ultimate 64 bit, Intel Xeon E5440 2.83 GHz, 32GB RAM.

		kernel size / pixels		
	Algorithm	9	21	41
1.	Bubble sort	4.08 s	5.32 s	8.37 s
2.	`std::sort`	4.01 s	4.84 s	5.50 s
3.	`std::partial_sort`	3.99 s	4.59 s	5.56 s
4.	`std::nth_element`	3.95 s	4.47 s	5.30 s

The basis for edge-preserving median filtering is a binary mask of the object edges. Several edge detection algorithms were examined regarding practicability for the problem [11]. The Sobel filter offers edge detection based on the spatial derivative in combination with binomial smoothing perpendicular to the differentiation direction. Additionally, it allows the calculation of edge directions (cf. (2)). The normalization of the gradient to a fixed interval [0;1] permits the application on any kind of CT data. Based on the edge strength and the image contrast, the user may vary the edge threshold (e.g. 0.4) whether there are weak edges (increase threshold, e.g. 0.9) or strong edges (lower threshold, e.g. 0.15) to be masked.

In case the artifact gradients are stronger than the object edges, the ring artifacts get masked and thus not corrected. This problem may be solved by eliminating ring structures from the mask using a Hough transform. A major disadvantage is the failure of this method if there are nearly concentric object edges. Experiments have shown that the edge direction calculated from the Sobel filtered image points towards the exact center of rotation with a tolerance of approximately 10°. This deviation has a strong impact on the accuracy of this method.

In fact, the edge-preserving characteristic of the adaptive median filter is shown by calculation of the difference image. When applying the edge mask, the amount of object details in the ring image is significantly reduced and a closer examination of the edge sharpness in the corrected image hardly shows any losses. Each of the 40 test datasets was processed without any noticeable edge smearing.

Existing approaches often use a coordinate transform because sophisticated radial and circular filtering in Cartesian coordinates equals simple filtering of columns or rows in polar coordinates. Approaches in both coordinate systems were compared in [5]. Even though the polar method was shown to be more effective in the center region, the polar image has to be divided into several domains for median filtering and the coordinate transform leads to interpolation errors. We managed to avoid the poor performance of Cartesian coordinates in the center region by introducing the adaptive Gaussian filter. In the context of this paper, each filtering step is performed in Cartesian coordinates.

The size-varying Gaussian kernel represents a major amendment in RAC, especially in the center region. For every distance to the center, it covers the same angular range and thus corresponds to a filtering of a constant time period during the CT measurement. In contrast to the invariant kernel size in the basic RAC algorithm, the radius of the adaptive Gaussian kernel is comparatively small in the vicinity of the center. Hence, there is no risk for the kernel to surround one ring more than once, whereby even small rings can successfully be eliminated. Due to the strong occurrence of ring artifacts in the center, this constitutes a significant improvement for RAC. Another important fact is the ability of the adaptive Gaussian filter to remove ring artifacts with varying intensity. Varying ring intensities are smoothed over a smaller ring section and can thus be removed more successfully.
The kernel support was artificially enlarged for a better smoothing result in the center region. While this magnification has a big effect on the inner rings, the angular range covered in outer regions nearly stays constant. We empirically determined an offset of 6 pixels to yield good results. By use of a look-up-table containing precalculated Gaussian kernels, the calculation time can be noticeably reduced: Compared to 512^2 calculations for a 512×512 pixel slice, only 0.1% of this effort is needed with precalculated kernels.

4 Conclusion

In this work, a novel method for effective suppression of ring artifacts in CT images is presented. The goal was to preserve the object edges the best possible in both clinical and industrial CT volumes, independently of tissue-specific attenuation coefficients. In contrast to existing approaches, we succeeded in retaining the object edges in the whole image slice at once and not just in a specified region of interest. Since a post-processing method was developed which operates on reconstructed volumes, no geometry information is required. The edge detection works fully automatically as well as the sensitivity to parameter settings is significantly reduced.
The presented algorithm requires knowledge of the rotation center which can usually be determined from the scanner geometry. If the assumed geometry is not correct or simply not known, the center has to be identified manually. Hence, a method for the automatic location of the rotation center constitutes a useful extension to the presented algorithm.

Acknowledgement

The work has been carried out at Siemens AG, Erlangen.

5 References

[1] E. M. Anas, S. Y. Lee and K. Hasan, *Removal of ring artifacts in CT imaging through detection and correction of stripes in the sinogram.* Physics in Medicine and Biology, vol. 55, no. 22, pp. 6911–6930, 2010.

[2] T. M. Buzug, *Computed Tomography.* Springer, Berlin/Heidelberg, 2008.

[3] J. F. Barrett and N. Keat, *Artifacts in CT: recognition and avoidance.* Radiographics, vol. 24, no. 6, pp. 1679–1691, 2004.

[4] E. M. Anas, J. Kim, S. Y. Lee and K. Hasan, *Comparison of ring artifact removal methods using flat panel detector based CT images.* Biomedical Engineering online, vol. 10, no. 1, p. 72, 2011.

[5] D. Prell, Y. Kyriakou and W. Kalender, *Comparison of ring artifact correction methods for flat-detector CT.* Physics in Medicine and Biology, vol. 54, no. 12, p. 3881, 2009.

[6] T. Flohr, *Method for post-processing of a tomogram, and computed tomography apparatus operating in accordance with the method.* US Patent US6047039, April 2000.

[7] M. Sharifi, M. Fathy and M. T. Mahmoudi, *A classified and comparative study of edge detection algorithms.* in: Proc. of the International Conference on Information Technology: Coding and Computing, 2002. IEEE, pp. 117–220, 2002.

[8] A. Schönhage, M. Paterson and N. Pippenger, *Finding the median.* Journal of Computer and System Sciences, vol. 13, no. 2, pp. 184–199, 1976.

[9] D. E. Knuth, *The Art of Computer Programming: Sorting and Searching, volume 3.* Addison-Wesley, 2nd edition, 1998.

[10] C. Martinez, *Partial Quicksort.* in: Proc. of the 6th ACM-SIAM Workshop on Algorithm Engineering and Experiments and 1st ACM-SIAM Workshop on Analytic Algorithmics and Combinatorics, pp. 224–228, 2004.

[11] D. Marr and E. Hildreth, *Theory of edge detection.* in: Proc. of the Royal Society of London. Series B. Biological Sciences, vol. 207, no. 1167, pp. 187–217, 1980.

Fully Automated Camera Calibration for X-ray Inspection and Computed Tomography Systems

M. Meike [1], B. Kratz [2] and F. Herold [2]
[1] Medizinische Ingenieurwissenschaft, Universität zu Lübeck, Meike@miw.uni-luebeck.de
[2] YXLON International GmbH Hamburg, {Baerbel.Kratz,Frank.Herold}@hbg.yxlon.com

Abstract

YXLON International develops X-ray inspection and computed tomography systems for industrial applications including quality assurance or size measurements. A visual camera can be placed inside these inspection systems. We developed an automated camera calibration algorithm to get the intrinsic and extrinsic camera parameters which are further used in combination with X-ray images. By determining the extrinsic camera parameters we get a transformation between the camera and the machine coordinate system. The extrinsic camera calibration is done with a common calibration object and the optimization of the camera projection matrix while the intrinsic camera parameters are determined separately in a previous step with the well known chessboard technique. An algorithm to determine sample points from the calibration object in the camera image with subpixel accuracy and a theoretical approach to get the extrinsic parameters by optimization will be presented. Finally the automatic sample point detection is verified.

1 Introduction

X-ray based computed tomography (CT) provides a three dimensional view into objects. In this work we focus on systems for industrial applications considering up to 600 kV radiation dose to inspect and penetrate even massive, strongly absorbing objects e.g. car wheels or turbine blades. Typical applications are pore diameter and wall thickness analysis, determination of shape and positioning tolerances, actual and target comparison as well as surface detection. We present an automatic camera calibration algorithm for YXLON inspection systems, which is also adaptable for similar set-ups. The resulting images can be used as further information about the object of interest, e.g. by registering the object to the Cartesian coordinate system. Also an adjustment between X-ray coordinate systems and visual camera coordinate systems is possible. The camera is able to detect a larger field of view (FOV) than the X-ray detector, as it can be seen in Fig. 1. In order to determine the camera position to the manipulator exactly, in section 2 we will present an algorithm to calibrate machine coordinates to camera coordinates automatically.

Camera calibration is a fundamental point in three dimensional computer and machine vision [1]. For our application we need detailed information about the camera parameters. Camera parameters can be subdivided into intrinsic and extrinsic parameters: While intrinsic parameters give information about the 'inner' camera properties, e.g. radial (barrel) and tangential distortion as well as image sensor scaling, extrinsic parameters provide position information through translation and rotation of the camera in relation to the world coordinate system origin [2]. In Fig. 2 a transformation from the camera (C) to a world coordinate system (W) is shown. The intrinsic parameters are determined in a previous step with the so-called chessboard technique [3]. Usually the chessboard technique provides both, computation of intrinsic and extrinsic camera parameters. We split this computation and used the method described in this paper to increase accuracy of the extrinsic parameters. Since intrinsic parameters are camera specific, they only depend on the camera and lens setting and so only need to be defined once. To get the extrinsic parameters we created an inexpensive and simple calibration object and used a stan-

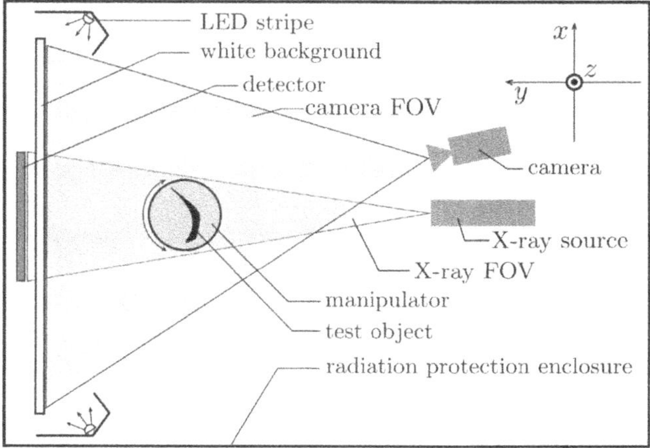

Figure 1: Top view of the geometry of the used system. The test object is moved in the cabin by the manipulator. In addition, a visual camera is provided which needs to be calibrated automatically.

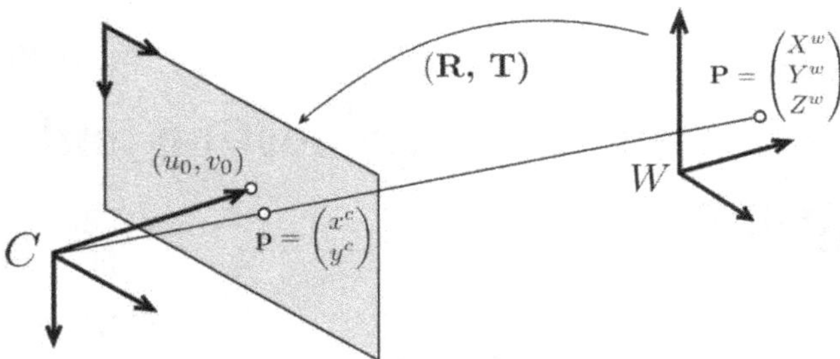

Figure 2: Camera (C) and world coordinate system (W) are shown. The principle point (image center) is given by (u_0, v_0). The coordinate system transformation is given by $\mathbf{R}$ and $\mathbf{T}$. A point in the world coordinates system $\mathbf{P}$ is projected to the image plane and given by $\mathbf{p}$.

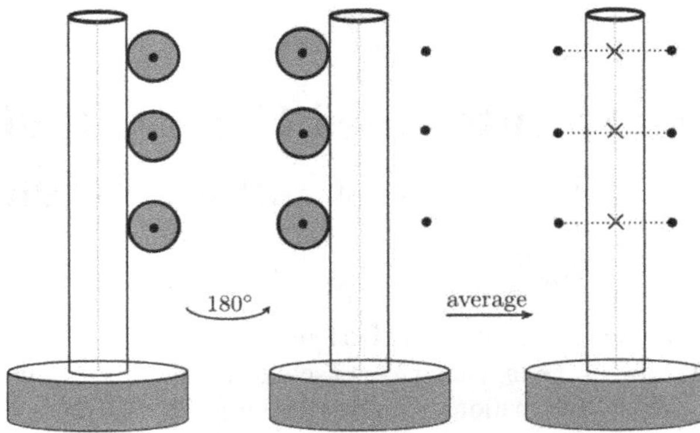

Figure 3: Model of the calibration object fixed on the manipulator and the process of determining the sample points coordinates in the camera image. Each dot represents a center of mass of one sphere. The used sample points are shown as a cross in the middle of the calibration object (rotation axis).

dard algorithm for camera projection matrix recovery with the given intrinsic parameters. This algorithm needs sample points in the three dimensional space, which we receive from the calibration object in relation to the manipulator position. The points are projected to the image plane and then the sample points are extracted by evaluating the center of gravity of spheres, which are attached to the calibration object (see Fig. 3). These sample points are provided to a system of equations which models the projection of a scene to the camera plane (see Fig. 2). By optimizing this system of equations we get an optimal camera projection matrix. The extrinsic parameters also need to be determined only once as long as the camera's position is not manipulated.

2 Material and Methods

For the development of an automatic camera calibration algorithm a test system, where the object is moved and rotated on a manipulator, detector and X-ray source are moveable in all three spatial dimensions while the manipulator is only fixed in height, has been used.

The calibration object is built of a cylindrical shaped rod made of carbon-fiber-reinforced plastic (CFRP) and three excentric ceramic spheres. Shape and material provide the possibility to distinguish spheres and rod in the X-ray image and also to determine the center of gravity of each sphere in the camera image assuming a specific rotation angle of the manipulator (see Fig. 3). Details on the right manipulator rotation are described later on.

The first step before the usage of visual camera-based information is to determine the intrinsic and extrinsic camera parameters to avoid optical aberrations and to get the exact transformation of the camera- to machine coordinates. The used camera has a resolution of 659×494 pixels (monochromatic) and a pixel size of $9.9\,\mu\text{m}^2$. Moreover, the lens has a focal length of 8 mm with manual focus and iris. We assumed a pinhole camera model [4] where general camera parameters can be described by the matrices $\mathbf{K}, \mathbf{R}$, and $\mathbf{T}$, given by

$$\mathbf{K} = \begin{pmatrix} f_x & 0 & u_0 \\ 0 & f_y & v_0 \\ 0 & 0 & 1 \end{pmatrix}, \tag{1}$$

$$\mathbf{R} = \begin{pmatrix} r_{11} & r_{12} & r_{13} \\ r_{21} & r_{22} & r_{23} \\ r_{31} & r_{32} & r_{33} \end{pmatrix}, \tag{2}$$

$$\mathbf{T} = \begin{pmatrix} T_x \\ T_y \\ T_z \end{pmatrix}. \tag{3}$$

$\mathbf{K}$ represents the intrinsic parameters and $\widetilde{\mathbf{T}} = -\mathbf{RT}$ with $\mathbf{R}$ describing the three dimensional rotation and $\mathbf{T}$ the translation of the camera position to the world coordinate system origin (see Fig. 2). The image center is given by u_0 and v_0. The image scale factors in image u_0 and v_0 axes direction are denoted as f_x and f_y. The projection of a three dimensional scene to the image plane can be described by

$$\begin{pmatrix} x^c \\ y^c \\ 1 \end{pmatrix} = \mathbf{K}(\mathbf{R}|\widetilde{\mathbf{T}}) \begin{pmatrix} X^w \\ Y^w \\ Z^w \\ 1 \end{pmatrix} \tag{4}$$

To estimate $\mathbf{R}$, $\mathbf{T}$, and $\mathbf{K}$, we need sample points in the machine coordinate system $\mathbf{P_i} = (X_i^w, Y_i^w, Z_i^w)$ and their projected image coordinates $\mathbf{p_i} = (x_i^c, y_i^c)$. In Fig. 2 this relation is shown. The sample points are points on the rotation axis of the CFRP rod (see Fig. 3).

To get an overdetermined system of equations we need at least six sample points which are not coplanar, because we have 12 variables and each sample point yields to two equations. To achieve a higher accuracy and to avoid errors we used up to six alignments.

To get the three dimensional positions of a sample point, we use the x- and y-machine coordinates of the manipulator which represents the rotation axis (see Fig. 1). To get

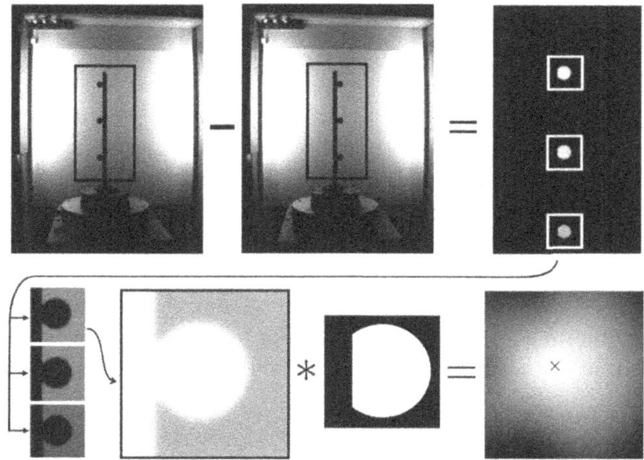

Figure 4: Scheme of the convolution of the sphere detection mask and the ROI image of one image. If the sphere lies on the other side of the rod stick, the mask will be mirrored. The maximum gray value coordinates of the resulting image correspond to the center of gravity of the sphere.

the height of each sphere an alignment of the sphere's center of gravity to the central X-ray beam is made. The height of a sample point can afterwards be deduced from the z-position (height) of detector and X-ray source. This height adjustment is done initially at the beginning of the calibration progress. We can now easily get the three dimensional machine coordinates of all three spheres.

To get the two dimensional image coordinates of the center of gravity of the three spheres $\mathbf{p}_i = (x_i^c, y_i^c)$ the following image processing basics were used. An LED mounting with white LED stripes next to the white background avoids a direct optical path from the LEDs to the camera. The camera is directed to the white illuminated surface in front of the X-ray detector, so the camera image shows a pure black shadow of the test object. To avoid an error through a skewed fixed calibration object or other inaccuracies, two images are acquired. The first image is taken with manipulator rotation angle α and a second with $\alpha + 180°$. The average of the center of gravity of one sphere from both images yields exact coordinates of the sample point which is centered on the rotation axis (see Fig. 3).

To ensure that the spheres are located as uncovered as possible of the rod for all images, for every new position the rod is rotated around the manipulator rotation axis in a specific interval $I := \alpha_1, ..., \alpha_N$. For every angle in I an image is taken. For all images A_i with $i \in [1, 2, ..., N]$ we sum all gray values $A(x, y)$ and search for the index of the darkest image

$$i_{\text{dark}} = \{i | \min_I (\sum_{y=1}^{Y} \sum_{x=1}^{X} A_i(x, y)) \forall i\}. \tag{5}$$

With the index i_{dark} we found the perfect manipulator angle for one alignment of the calibration object. We then take a pair of images (180° rotated) and determine the approximate position and size of each sphere in both images and set an area around every sphere to the region of interest (ROI). This is done by subtracting the corresponding images, using morphological operators and a gray value projection in x- and y-direction. To achieve subpixel accuracy when computing the center of gravity we supersample this ROI with bilinear interpolation and convolve it with an adapted circular shaped mask (see Fig. 4). The maximum gray value of the convolved image represents the center of gravity of a sphere.

We now have all necessary sample points coordinates to solve our system of equations [5]. With $\mathbf{M} = \mathbf{K}(\mathbf{R}|\widetilde{\mathbf{T}})$ we can write $\mathbf{p}_i = \mathbf{M}\mathbf{P}_i$. When reshaping $\mathbf{M}$ to a one-dimensional vector $\mathbf{m} \in \mathbb{R}^{1\times 12}$ the linear system of equations is given by

$$\mathbf{A}\mathbf{m} = \mathbf{0} \text{ with } \mathbf{m} = \begin{pmatrix} m_{11} & m_{12} & \dots & m_{34} \end{pmatrix}^{\mathrm{T}}, \tag{6}$$

$$\mathbf{A} = (\mathbf{A}_1 | \mathbf{A}_2), \tag{7}$$

$$\mathbf{A}_1 = \begin{pmatrix} X_1^w & Y_1^w & Z_1^w & 1 & 0 & 0 & 0 & 0 \\ 0 & 0 & 0 & 0 & X_1^w & Y_1^w & Z_1^w & 1 \\ & & & & \dots & & & \\ X_N^w & Y_N^w & Z_N^w & 1 & 0 & 0 & 0 & 0 \\ 0 & 0 & 0 & 0 & X_N^w & Y_N^w & Z_N^w & 1 \end{pmatrix}, \tag{8}$$

$$\mathbf{A}_2 = \begin{pmatrix} -x_1^c X_1^w & -x_1^c Y_1^w & -x_1^c Z_1^w & -x_1^c \\ -y_1^c X_1^w & -y_1^c Y_1^w & -y_1^c Z_1^w & -y_1^c \\ & \dots & & \\ -x_N^c X_N^w & -x_N^c Y_N^w & -x_N^c Z_N^w & -x_N^c \\ -y_N^c X_N^w & -y_N^c Y_N^w & -y_N^c Z_N^w & -y_N^c \end{pmatrix}. \tag{9}$$

Since we have twelve parameters ($\mathbf{M} \in \mathbb{R}^{3\times 4}$) and one sample point yields to two equations (8, 9) we need at least six sample points, which are not coplanar (two different alignments) to get an overdetermined system of equations. To achieve a higher accuracy and to avoid errors we incorporated up to six alignments. We then get a system of equations which is solved by an optimization algorithm.

All following methods are planed as future work. We intend to use a Powell's Dog-Leg optimization algorithm to estimate the optimal camera projection matrix $\mathbf{M}$. To compute the extrinsic camera parameters we have to obtain $\mathbf{R}$ and $\mathbf{T}$ from $\mathbf{M}$ with given intrinsic parameters from the previous chessboard calibration, which simplifies the extraction of the extrinsic parameters. We split the camera projection matrix $\mathbf{M}$ into the first 3×3 submatrix $\mathbf{B}$ and the last column of $\mathbf{M}$ denoted by $\mathbf{b}$, so that $\mathbf{M} = (\mathbf{B}|\mathbf{b})$. Considering the composition of $\mathbf{M}$ we can write $\mathbf{B} = \mathbf{K}\mathbf{R}$ and $\mathbf{b} = \mathbf{K}\mathbf{T}$ [5]. Thus the extrinsic parameters could be computed by the following equations

$$\mathbf{R} = \mathbf{K}^{-1}\mathbf{B} \text{ and} \tag{10}$$

$$\mathbf{T} = \mathbf{K}^{-1}\mathbf{b}. \tag{11}$$

Table 1: Accuracy of sample point detection. Comparison between automatic and manually detected sample points. All values are given in pixels and in the world coordinate system.

Img.	Manual	Automatic	Error Dist.
	(241.75, 420.75)	(241.95, 420.65)	0.224
1	(312.00, 421.00)	(312.05, 421.05)	0.071
	(382.00, 421.00)	(382.05, 421.00)	0.050
	(211.25, 257.75)	(211.40, 257.60)	0.212
2	(308.75, 257.75)	(308.70, 257.90)	0.158
	(406.25, 258.25)	(406.50, 258.20)	0.255
	(154.75, 418.25)	(154.60, 418.30)	0.158
3	(301.50, 420.00)	(301.65, 420.00)	0.150
	(449.00, 419.50)	(449.00, 419.55)	0.050

Table 2: Comparison between the rotation axis coordinates in all three images. All values are given in pixels.

Image	Manual	Automatic	Error Dist.
1	420.92	420.90	0.02
2	257.92	257.90	0.02
3	419.25	419.28	0.03

3 Results and Discussion

Since the implementation of the optimization algorithm is still in progress, we present a verification of the center of gravity detection accuracy. Therefore the calibration object has been placed at three different positions in a CT test-system and acquire camera images. The respective rotation of the manipulator is done manually. We determine the center of gravity of every sphere manually by drawing a perfect circle around the sphere's shape and deriving the center of the circle by building the average of all coordinate pairs inside this circle. With this method we gain an accuracy of 0.5 pixels. Notice that the height of one sample point is the average of two spheres on the same height (see Fig. 3). The axis coordinate is derived from the average of all three imaginary spheres coordinates. In Table 1 a comparison between manually and automatically determined sample points of the three test image pairs is made. The error distance is the euclidean norm between the two points. In Table 2 the manual and automatic detection of the manipulators rotation axis is shown.

For all test images the error distance between automatic and manual sample point detection is less than 0.255 pixels. Our method's accuracy depends on the supersampling factor of the ROI images of the spheres. The work presented has been done with a factor of ten and resulted in a subpixel accuracy of 0.1 pixel. The manual detection only achieved an accuracy of 0.5 pixels because of the regular shaped mask we determined the circle with. A systematic error of ± 0.25 pixels can be assumed with this method. In Table 2 it can be seen that the axis detection is very accurate. The error for each image is not greater than 0.03 pixels and shows subpixel accuracy.

4 Conclusion

Preparing a test system with the camera, developing a calibration object and the sample point detection software was presented and done so far and can already be used in practice. Our tests showed, that the detection algorithm is accurate and stable, and can be used for further applications. The algorithm is not complete at this time. The next steps are the implementation of the system of equations and the optimization algorithm. After calculating the camera projection matrix the extrinsic camera parameters have to be extracted by an inversion of the camera projection matrix.

Acknowledgement

The work has been carried out at YXLON International GmbH in Hamburg. A big thanks for support, guidance and encouragement, and for the opportunities provided to me during my time at YXLON to all colleagues and especially to Baerbel Kratz and Frank Herold. Thanks for support by the Universität zu Lübeck to Prof. Thorsten M. Buzug from the Institute of Medical Engineering.

5 References

[1] C. S. Fraser, "Automatic camera calibration in close range photogrammetry," *Photogrammetric Engineering & Remote Sensing*, vol. 79, no. 4, pp. 381–388, 2013.

[2] R. Hartley and A. Zisserman, *Multiple view geometry in computer vision.* Cambridge university press, 2003.

[3] A. De la Escalera and J. M. Armingol, "Automatic chessboard detection for intrinsic and extrinsic camera parameter calibration," *Sensors*, vol. 10, no. 3, pp. 2027–2044, 2010.

[4] R. Szeliski, "Computer vision: algorithms and applications," 2010. http://szeliski.org/Book/.

[5] Z. Zhang, *Emerging Topics in Computer Vision*, ch. Chapter 2: Camera Calibration, pp. 4–43. Upper Saddle River, NJ, USA: Prentice Hall PTR, 2004.

[6] Z. Zhang, "A flexible new technique for camera calibration," *Pattern Analysis and Machine Intelligence, IEEE Transactions on*, vol. 22, no. 11, pp. 1330–1334, 2000.

Analysis of an Automatically Computed Abstraction Parameter in Sketch-based Image Retrieval Using Angular-Radial Partitioning

M. Duchrow [1], A. Mertins [2]
[1] Medizinische Ingenieurwissenschaft, Universität zu Lübeck, duchrow@miw.uni-luebeck.de
[2] Institute for Signal Processing, Universität zu Lübeck, mertins@isip.uni-luebeck.de

Abstract

Sketch-based image retrieval has gained importance through rapid technological development like smartphones and tablet computers. In this work, sketch-based image retrieval using angular partitioning is implemented in Matlab. The opportunity of an improvement through an automatically computed abstraction parameter is investigated. Therefore, this work tries to find a relationship between the best value for this abstraction parameter and image properties of the query and the database images. For comparison the average normalization retrieval rank is measured. The results show that there is no relationship between the best value for the abstraction parameter and the pixel intensities nor the size of the different images.

1 Introduction

The rapid development of the computer technology in the recent years provides many new opportunities. Touch-screens simplify man-machine communication by enabling inputs with hand or pencil. So the user is able to pass directly down visual information to the computer. Small, efficient touch-screen devices like smartphones and tablet computers have become our everyday attendant and allow internet researches everywhere and at all time. Moreover, acquiring and storing images in digital form has become much easier and faster, which resulted in the availability of extensive large image databases [1].

However, the development in the image search field has not kept pace with the technological advance. Textual methods are still state of the art for most users like a decade ago, even though they often result in insufficient and inefficient outcomes. Hereby text and alphanumeric symbols are used to describe images. Today's text-based image search systems, like the well-known Google image search, allow to specify the query by adding different parameters like size or dominant color, but it is impossible to define where in the image different search words are arranged. Also different people will use different words to describe the same image based on their cultural and educational background. It is therefore difficult for the user to transform the exact image, which he imagines in his head, into a suitable text-based query [2]. This problem can be solved by applying content-based image retrieval methods, whereby content features are used for image retrieval instead of a textual description. The three main image content features are color, texture and shape [1].

Sketch-based image retrieval (SBIR) has gained much importance due to today's extension of touch-screen devices. It enables an intuitive and simple user interaction and, according to the adage "An image is worth a thousand words", it also allows an easier description of complex, content-rich images like landscapes and drawings. In SBIR, the task is to use a simple black and white hand-drawing sketch to find one or multiple images with similar content in an image database. The difficulty is that the image database contains conventional color or gray-scale images and thus has a fundamentally different modality than the sketch. Therefore, an appropriate method for feature extraction, which produces comparable characteristics of both types of originals, has to be applied to solve this problem. Considering the non-existing color and texture in a simple line-drawing, only shape remains as useful image feature. It is also important to evaluate the robustness of the retrieval system in view of distortions and rotations for the reason that not all people are well-trained artists and will not draw perfect sketches.

In this work the SBIR by angular partitioning approach by Chalechale et al. [1] is examined. It tries to link the abstraction parameter with image properties like pixel density or image size.

2 Material and Methods

To perform SBIR, the original image data has to be transformed into a new abstract structure, which enables a similarity measurement between the color images of the database and the hand-drawn, black and white sketch [1].

If a user sketches an image, he will most likely start by drawing the edges. In consequence, information of edges has to be a feature of high value while searching in a color image database by using a sketch query. Accordingly, the implemented algorithm uses edge detection for feature extraction.

2.1 SBIR Using Angular Partitioning

SBIR using angular partitioning was introduced by Chalechale et al. in 2004 in [5]. The beginning of the abstraction of the query and of the database images are obtained in two different ways. The database image abstraction starts by only maintaining the luminance while excluding the hue and saturation. As a consequence, the color images are transformed into gray intensity images. Afterwards, the Canny edge operator is used for obtaining edge maps. Hereby, the standard deviation of the Gaussian filter is chosen as $\sigma = 1$ and the size of the Gaussian mask as nine pixels. For only retaining strong edges, the values of high and low thresholds for the magnitude of potential edge points are chosen automatically by firstly computing the 1-D discrete convolution of the Gaussian 1-D filter G and the derivative of the Gaussian used in the Canny edge operator g:

$$H(k) = \sum_i G(i)g(k+1-i). \tag{1}$$

In the next step the vertical and horizontal edge maps X and Y are estimated:

$$X(u,v) = \left[\sum_{j=1}^{V} I'(u,j)H(v-j)\right]' \tag{2}$$

and

$$Y(u,v) = \sum_{i=1}^{U} I'(i,v)H(u-i), \tag{3}$$

with $u = 1,2,...,U$ and $v = 1,2,...,V$. U and V are defined as the number of rows or columns in the gray intensity image I. Afterwards, the magnitude of the edge points is obtained by:

$$\Gamma(u,v) = \sqrt{X(u,v)^2 + Y(u,v)^2}. \tag{4}$$

Then the minimum index ι in the 64-bin cumulative histogram of $\Gamma(u,v)$, which is greater than $\alpha \cdot U \cdot V$, where $\alpha = 0.7$ equals the percentage of non-edge points in the image, is used for calculating the threshold values:

$$thresh\_high = \beta \cdot \iota \tag{5}$$

and

$$thresh\_low = 0.4 \cdot \beta \cdot \iota. \tag{6}$$

The abstraction parameter β controls the degree of the strength of the edge points, whereby the higher β, the lower the number of edge points [1].

The query image is abstracted by simply applying black and white morphological thinning. Afterwards the thinned sketch contains only the main structure of the users demand. Its spatial distribution of pixels is now comparable to the edge maps of the abstract database images. In the next step, the bounding boxes of both kind of images are calculated. Thereafter, the area of each bounding box is normalized to $J \times J$ pixels, using the nearest neighbour interpolation. Converting different size images to an equal, predefined size leads to scale invariance. Working in the bounding box of images ensures robustness against translations [1].

Afterwards, the surrounding circle of the resulting so-called abstract image Ω is divided into K angular partitions (slices). The number of angular partitions in the abstract image K determines the angle between adjacent slices $\varphi = 2\pi/K$. The scale invariant image feature $\{f(i)\}$ is now represented by the number of edge points in each slice of Ω and calculated as follows:

$$f(i) = \sum_{\theta=\frac{i2\pi}{K}}^{\frac{(i+1)2\pi}{K}} \sum_{\rho=\frac{mR}{M}}^{\frac{(m+1)R}{M}} \Omega(\rho,\theta), \tag{7}$$

for $i = 0,1,...,K-1$ and $m = 0,1,...,M-1$. R is defined as the radius of the surrounding circle and M is the number of radial partitions accordingly. To obtain robustness against rotation, the 1-D discrete Fourier transform of $f(i)$ is used:

$$F(u) = \frac{1}{K}\sum_{i=0}^{K-1} f(i)e^{-j2\pi ui/K}. \tag{8}$$

As shown in [1] the magnitude of $F(u)$ equals to the magnitude of the 1-D discrete Fourier transform of a rotated image. Therefore $\Upsilon = \{F(u)\}$ for $u = 0,1,..,K-1$ is chosen as final image feature. Fig. 1 shows a rough example of the whole abstraction process.

For similarity measurement between images the Manhattan distance is used. Let Υ_I be the feature vector of a database image and Υ_Q represents the query feature vector, then the similarity is calculated as:

$$d(I,Q) = \sum_u |\Upsilon_I(u) - \Upsilon_Q(u)|. \tag{9}$$

The lower $d(I,Q)$, the higher is the retrieval rank.

2.2 Retrieval Performance Criteria

In image retrieval research, the average normalized modified retrieval rank (ANMRR) is a widely used performance evaluation measurement, because it uses not only the recall and precision information, but also takes advantage of the rank information among the retrieved images [1],[4]. The ANMRR is calculated as follows, whereby Q equals the absolute number of queries, $NG(q)$ represents the number of ground truth images for a query q and T is defined as $T = min\{4 \cdot NG(q), 2 \cdot GTM\}$ with $GTM = max\{NG(1), NG(2), ..., NG(Q)\}$:

$$ANMRR = \frac{1}{Q}\sum_{q=1}^{Q} NMRR(q). \tag{10}$$

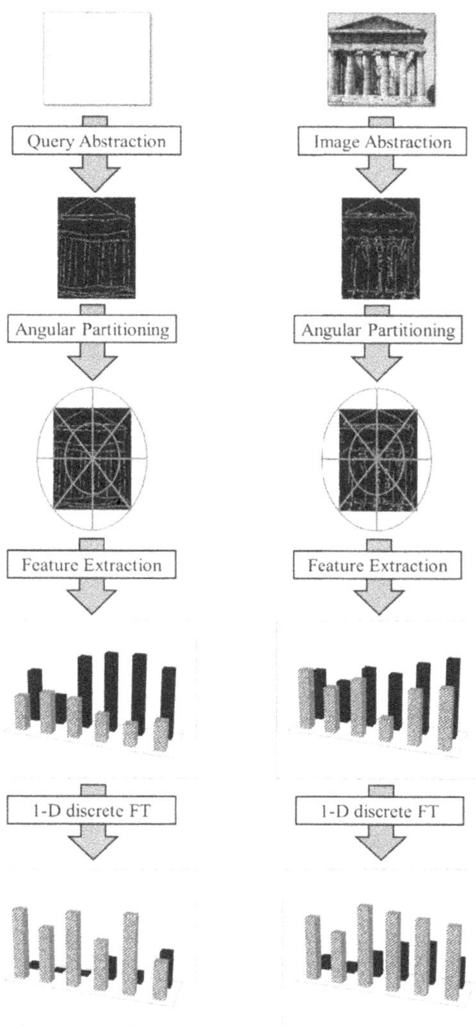

Figure 1: A rough example of the abstraction process. In the first step query and database image are abstracted in different ways. Black and white morphological thinning is applied on the query before resizing the bounding box area to a predefined pixel size. The database image is converted into gray-scale and then the Canny edge operator is applied before also resizing the bounding box area. Afterwards both images are radial and angular partitioned. Then, the feature vector is extracted by summing up the edge points of each slice. After the 1-D discrete Fourier transform is applied on both, the feature vectors are in a comparable, abstract structure.

$$NMRR(q) = \frac{MRR(q)}{T(q) + 0.5 - 0.5 \cdot NG(q)} \tag{11}$$

$$MRR(q) = AVR(q) - 0.5 - \frac{NG(q)}{2} \tag{12}$$

$$AVR(q) = \sum_{i=1}^{NG(q)} \frac{Rank(i,q)}{NG(q)} \tag{13}$$

$$Rank(i,q) = \begin{cases} i & \text{if } i \leq T(q) \\ T(q)+1 & \text{if } i > T(q) \\ 0 & \text{otherwise} \end{cases} \tag{14}$$

The values of the ANMRR will always range between zero and one, whereby according to the definition of the ANMRR, the lower value means a better retrieval performance [4].

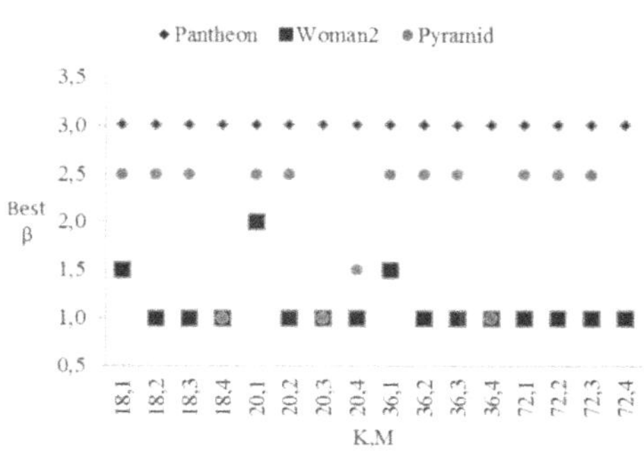

Figure 2: Best NMRR β value in dependence on different angular and radial partition adjustments K,M

2.3 Test Setup

The software MATLAB©was used for implementing the algorithms and methods, described before, and also for computing the results.

A database of $1,179$ JPEG images was created with a wide range of different motives like animals, landscapes, paintings or textures. Most images got a size of 120×80 or 384×256 pixel, but for evaluating scale invariance, each sketched image was additionally stored in up to nine further images, which sizes diversify from 60×40 Pixel to 600×400 Pixel. 25 black and white queries were simulated by using a computer drawing software.

For the angular partitioning parameter four different values were chosen with $K \in \{18, 20, 36, 72\}$ and for each value of K, four radial partitioning parameter and five abstraction parameters were used with $M \in \{1, 2, 3, 4\}$ and $\beta \in \{1, 1.5, 2, 2.5, 3\}$. The resizing value $J = 257$ was chosen as proposed in [1]. The NMRR of each sketch was measured for all possible adjustments and pixel densities and image sizes of the query and database images were computed and compared.

3 Results and Discussion

The best retrieval performance was obtained for $K = 72$, $M = 2$ and $\beta = 2.5$ with an ANMRR value of 0.593. With an automatically computed β, which chooses the β with the best NMRR value, this ANMRR could possibly be improved to 0.439.

3.1 Dependence on query image

According to the results, which are partially displayed in Fig. 2, each query image seems to prefer one β for the best NMRR results.

In Table 1 it can be seen that there is no notable relationship between this best β and query image characteristics like pixel density before and after the abstraction process or

Table 1: Comparison between query image properties (pixel density before and after abstraction, image size) and the best possible or the most frequently used β value

Sketch	ø best β	Most frequently used best β	Pixel density before abstraction	Pixel density after abstraction	Size before resizing
Karate	1.1	1.0	0.928	0.138	152 × 131
Goat and Sun	1.3	1.0	0.938	0.078	193 × 156
Grande Arche	1.3	1.0	0.894	0.228	62 × 72
Flag Brazil	1.3	1.5	0.889	0.145	134 × 220
Woman2	1.5	1.5	0.893	0.117	273 × 146
Flag FRD	1.6	1.0	0.931	0.087	68 × 110
Hawk3	1.7	1.0	0.976	0.057	60 × 65
Ace of Hearts	1.9	2.0	0.958	0.060	316 × 223
Pyramid	2.1	2.5	0.960	0.068	111 × 200
Rose	2.2	1.5	0.971	0.054	237 × 219
Jolly Roger	2.2	2.5	0.887	0.151	135 × 211
Bird	2.3	3.0	0.941	0.120	161 × 117
Goat	2.4	2.5	0.934	0.092	112 × 239
Hawk2	2.4	2.0	0.969	0.150	59 × 131
Ski-Jump	2.7	3.0	0.941	0.096	195 × 120
Cocktail	2.9	3.0	0.934	0.112	116 × 48
Palms	2.9	3.0	0.892	0.112	376 × 255
Building	2.9	3.0	0.892	0.037	279 × 255
Woman1	2.9	3.0	0.890	0.143	239 × 122
Pantheon	3.0	3.0	0.951	0.049	253 × 376
Hawk1	3.0	3.0	0.942	0.212	65 × 161
Flag Cuba	3.0	3.0	0.861	0.174	139 × 221
Plate	3.0	3.0	0.950	0.091	224 × 239
Child	3.0	3.0	0.961	0.133	214 × 133

the query size before resizing. The three query image properties vary independent of the best β value. For example the pixel density after abstraction of 93.8% of the sketch "Goat and Sun" uses most frequently a best β value of 1.0, but $\beta = 3.0$ is the most suitable choice for "Hawk1" with a pixel density of 94.2%. "Karate" has a pixel density before abstraction of 13.8% and a best β value of 1.0, what is contrary to "Child" with a most frequently used $\beta = 3.0$ and a pixel density of 13.3%. Also the image size can not be linked mathematically to a high or low value of β. "Flag Cuba" has an image size of 139 × 221 pixel with best $\beta = 3.0$, but "Flag Brazil", which is resized to 134 × 239 pixel chooses $\beta = 1.0$ most frequently. So it is not possible to automatically compute a value for β based on this three query image properties.

3.2 Dependence on database image

Table 2 shows an extract of the results of the comparison between the database images and the chosen β value for the lowest retrieval distance d for an adjustment of $K = 72$ and $M = 2$. Here it can be seen that there is also no notable relationship between the image properties and the best chosen β. Neither database image size nor pixel density seem to have a measurable impact on the choosing of the best suitable value of β. There is not one image size in Table 2, where the best β value is equal for all three displayed queries. Also, it is not possible to link the pixel density of the abstracted database images with the best possible choice of β. For example the sketch "Hawk2" has a pixel density of 6.7% for an image size of 384 × 256 pixel and a best β of 1.0, but "Rose" uses $\beta = 2.5$ for a pixel density of 6.9% and an image size of 120 × 80 pixel. So this image properties can also not be used for an automatic computation of the abstraction parameter β.

Table 2: Comparison between database image properties, like pixel density and image size, and the best possible used value of β for an adjustment of $K = 72$ and $M = 2$

Image Size	Hawk2 Pixel Density	Best β	Pillar Pixel Density	Best β	Rose Pixel Density	Best β
384 × 256	0.067	1.0	0.090	2.5	0.072	1.5
120 × 80	0.073	1.0	0.103	2.5	0.069	2.5
257 × 257	0.059	1.5	0.091	2.5	0.055	2.5
450 × 300	0.054	1.0	0.087	2.5	0.113	1.5
600 × 400	0.050	1.0	0.083	2.5	0.116	1.0
60 × 40	0.075	1.0	0.126	2.5	0.078	2.0
256 × 384	0.057	1.0	0.084	2.5	0.101	2.0
128 × 128	0.067	1.5	0.104	1.5	0.069	3.0
333 × 500	0.048	1.0	0.093	2.5	0.100	1.5
256 × 171	0.049	1.5	0.097	2.5	0.096	3.0

4 Conclusion

This work shows that the query image properties, pixel density before and after abstraction or image size before resizing cannot be used for automatically computing an abstraction parameter value β to improve SBIR using angular partitioning. Furthermore it can be concluded that there is no relationship between this best value of β and the database image properties, image size and pixel intensity, even though it was proposed in [3].

Further work has to be done, to find the link between a suitable image feature and an automatically computed value of β. This could include a comparison between edge histograms and best computed β values to investigate the possibility of a shape based relationship.

Acknowledgement

The work has been carried out at the Institute for Signal Processing, Universität zu Luebeck. Special thanks to Lars Hertel for his valuable linguistic and visual hints.

5 References

[1] A. Chalechale, G. Naghdy and A. Mertins, *Sketch-Based Image Matching Using Angular Partitioning*. IEEE Transactions on Systems, Man, Cybernetics - Part A: Systems and Humans, vol. 35, no. 1, pp. 28–41, 2005.

[2] C. Wang, Z. Li, L. Zhang, *MindFinder: image search by interactive sketching and tagging*. In: WWW'10: 19th International World Wide Web Conference, pp. 1309–1312, 2005

[3] A. Chalechale, *Content-based retrieval from image databases using sketched queries*. PhD thesis, School of Electrical, Computer and Telecommunications Engineering, Wollongong, Australia: University of Wollongong, 2005.

[4] C. Gao, N. Sang and Q. Tang, *Evaluating the measurement scales of semantic features for remote sensing images retrieval*. Available: http://www.isprs.org/proceedings/XXXVIII/part1/ [last accessed on 15.01.2015].

[5] A. Chalechale, F. Naghdy, P. Premaratne and A. Mertins, *Angular-Radial Decomposition Algorithm for Sketch-Based Image Retrieval*. Proc. Eighth World Multi-Conference on Systemics, Cybernetics and Informatics (SCI), 2004.

11
Image Processing II

Performance of Förstner- and Rohr operators based on structure tensors versus Hessians

F. Sannmann [1], T. Polzin [2], and J. Modersitzki [2]
[1] Medizinische Ingenieurwissenschaft, Universität zu Lübeck, sannmann@miw.uni-luebeck.de
[2] Institute of Mathematics and Image Computing, Universität zu Lübeck, {polzin, modersitzki}@mic.uni-luebeck.de

Abstract

In this work the performance of Förstner and Rohr operators for detecting landmarks in 3D thoracic CT images is evaluated regarding usage of first order and second order derivatives. Förstner and Rohr operators detect landmarks based on principal curvatures of the intensity function. Usually, these operators are based on the structure tensor which approximates the Hessian matrix using gradient information. The structure tensor approach is compared to explicitly computed Hessians. The evaluation will be based on the performance of thin-plate-spline registration using the automatically detected point landmarks. Additionally, the computation time of the structure tensor versus the Hessian is given.

1 Introduction

Detecting landmarks in lung CT data has been the subject of research for some years [10]. Landmarks can be used to support image registration by adding more information to establish a good initalization or tune parameters. Furthermore, landmarks are used for evaluation of registration accuracy [3, 7]. In [9] three operators to detect landmarks based on the principal curvatures of the grey-value intensity function are given. Landmarks are defined as distinctive points in the image where the intensity difference to the neighboring points is very high. This is characterized by a large slope in the intensities of the image. To detect extreme values Förstner and Rohr defined three operators. These operators are all based on an approximated Hessian matrix, aiming at calculating the principal curvatures of the grey value intensity function. This paper will compare the performance of the operators based on structure tensors to the performance of the same operators based on an explicitly computed Hessian-Matrix. The work will be carried out on 3D-Computed Tomography (CT)- Images. The five thoracic image pairs are taken as extreme phases of 4D-CT data sets provided by the DIR-Lab [3]. For each image the expiration as well as inspiration phase along with a set of 300 landmark pairs placed by experts are given.

2 Material and Methods

For the task of image registration, at least two images are given. They are often denoted as template (T) and reference (R) image, respectively. We are handling d-dimensional grey value images with compactly supported domain Ω: $T,\ R\colon \mathbb{R}^d \supset \Omega \rightarrow \mathbb{R}$. Image registration is used to find a transformation $\varphi\colon \mathbb{R}^d \rightarrow \mathbb{R}^d$ such that $T \circ \varphi$ becomes similar to R. In particular corresponding points and regions of R and T should be properly aligned. The similarity of R and $T \circ \varphi$ is modeled based on a suitable distance measure D. The goal is to minimize the distance while keeping the transformation φ plausible. As image registration is an ill-posed problem, usually, a regularizer S is employed [6]. The registration problem is solved by minization of the joint functional:

$$\varphi^* = \arg\min_{\varphi} D\left[T \circ \varphi, R\right] + \alpha S[\varphi] \qquad (1)$$

Corresponding point landmarks, which could be anatomical points like vessel bifurcations in the context of medical imaging, can be used as additional information to guide the registration. When $L \in \mathbb{N}$ corresponding points r_i and t_i, $i \in \{1, 2, ..., L\}$ in reference and template image are found, the transformation φ can be computed resulting in $\varphi(r_i) \approx t_i$, $i \in \{1, 2, ..., L\}$. The concrete mapping depends on the type of modelled transformations. Affine and rigid transformations are frequently used and their parameters can be determined by solving a least square problem, cf. [6]. The transformation used in this work is based on thin plate splines taken from, e.g., [9, 6].

2.1 Thin-Plate-Spline-Registration

Thin-Plate-Spline (TPS) registration is a technique, which is thouroughly explained in [9], [8] and [6]. TPS-registration creates a smooth φ based on radial basis functions. It is based on landmarks and the transformation is computed by solving a system of linear equations that contains information on every landmark. From this information the coefficients for the basis functions and hence the transformation are deduced. For further explanations see [8] and for information on the FAIR-based implementation in MATLAB see [6].

2.2 Structure Tensor and Hessian

In the following sections, we restrict to the case $d = 3$ and consider images $g\colon \mathbb{R}^3 \to \mathbb{R}$. In [9] three operators based on principal curvatures of images are defined with the goal of detecting landmarks. The operators depend on the structure tensor which approximates the Hessian matrix by averaging the tensor product of the gradient vector,

$$\nabla g = \begin{pmatrix} g_x \\ g_y \\ g_z \end{pmatrix} \tag{2}$$

where g_x, g_y and g_z denote the partial derivatives of g along the x-,y- and z-axis, respectively. The structure tensor $\mathbf{C}_g$ is defined as

$$\mathbf{C}_g = \overline{\nabla g\,(\nabla g)^T} = \begin{pmatrix} \overline{g_x^2} & \overline{g_x g_y} & \overline{g_x g_z} \\ \overline{g_x g_y} & \overline{g_y^2} & \overline{g_y g_z} \\ \overline{g_x g_z} & \overline{g_y g_z} & \overline{g_z^2} \end{pmatrix}. \tag{3}$$

The averaging (denoted by the overlining) can be performed by convolution with a Gaussian Kernel and distributes information across the neighbourhood. It enables a full rank $\mathbf{C}_g$ whereas $\operatorname{rank}(\nabla g\,(\nabla g)^T) = 1$ and hence $\det(\nabla g\,(\nabla g)^T) = 0$. The Hessian matrix $\mathbf{H}$ consists of the second partial derivatives in all three dimensions and is symmetric:

$$\mathbf{H} = \begin{pmatrix} g_{xx} & g_{xy} & g_{xz} \\ g_{yx} & g_{yy} & g_{yz} \\ g_{zx} & g_{zy} & g_{zz} \end{pmatrix}. \tag{4}$$

For the analysis of the principal curvaturves and thus detecting landmarks the eigenvalues of the two matrices are used. To avoid computing the eigenvalues, the determinant and the trace of the matrices are computed. The determinant is equal to the product of the eigenvalues while the trace identifies as the sum of the eigenvalues. For numerical computation of the derivatives the method of central finite differences was used as defined in [1].

2.3 Förstner and Rohr Operators

The three operators defined by Förstner and Rohr depend on the determinant and trace of $\mathbf{C}_g$. The Förstner3D-Operator is defined as $\operatorname{tr}(\mathbf{C}_g^{-1})$, which is to be minimized to find possible landmarks. This problem is equivalent to maximizing the inverse of $\operatorname{tr}(\mathbf{C}_g^{-1})$. Instead of the inverted matrix the adjoint matrix $\operatorname{adj}(\mathbf{C}_g)$ is used [1]. This leads to

$$\text{Förstner3D} = \frac{1}{\operatorname{tr}(\mathbf{C}_g^{-1})} = \frac{\det \mathbf{C}_g}{\operatorname{tr}(\operatorname{adj}(\mathbf{C}_g))} \to \max. \tag{5}$$

For $d = 3$ generally $\operatorname{tr}(\operatorname{adj}(\mathbf{C}_g)) \neq \operatorname{tr}(\mathbf{C}_g)$, due to this another operator is defined

$$\text{Op3} = \frac{\det \mathbf{C}_g}{\operatorname{tr} \mathbf{C}_g} \to \max. \tag{6}$$

The third operator, to be evaluated throughout this work, is the Rohr3D-Operator which omits computations of traces:

$$\text{Rohr3D} = \det \mathbf{C}_g \to \max. \tag{7}$$

While the definitions shown here, taken from [9], use the structure tensor $\mathbf{C}_g$ we also computed these operators using the Hessian matrix $\mathbf{H}$ instead. The operator responses have to be computed for the whole image. From the resulting image only the voxels featuring local maxima are used as landmarks. However, as we are interested in the breathing motion of the lungvolumes, lung segementations were used to detect landmarks only inside the lungs. The segmentations were generated with the method published in [5].

2.4 Increasing Robustness

Landmarks, that we are interested in, are located at corners like vessel bifurcations. These points are interesting, because they can be matched more reliably to the corresponding points in the second image than, e.g., points lying on a plain edge of a vessel. The Förstner and Rohr operators have been designed to feature high values at corners. Due to this we filter our landmark candidates by applying a threshold on the operator responses. Nevertheless, because of numerical approximations, partial volume effects and deteriorated images there might be similar values in a neighborhood around the feature we would like to extract. This may affect the landmark matching and does not improve the final registration result as directly neighboring points are moving almost equal. To cope with the described situation a non-maximum-suppression was performed on a $5 \times 5 \times 2$ voxel neighborhood. Only the remaining points were used for the blockmatching and the following registration.

2.5 Matching Landmarks

The images used for this work [3] show normal, i.e. not forced, breathing movement. Therefore only a limited amount of movement between inspiration and expiration scans can be seen. Furthermore, the CT scanner and its parameters like acquisition dose were the same and patients did not suffer from lung diseases (some had esophageal cancer treatments [3]). For this setting blockmatching is a suitable technique to transfer landmarks from the reference image to the template image. For a neighborhood (also called block) with the centre r_i in the reference image blockmatching means that a corresponding block in the template image has to be found. The center of the located block becomes the corresponding landmark t_i in the template image. In this work a block has a size of $15 \times 15 \times 7$ voxel and approx. $1.5 \times 1.5 \times 1.75\ \text{mm}^3$ respectively. To limit the search range and time only a certain search window of the template is used. It was $11 \times 11 \times 7$ voxels. The normalized cross correlation (NCC) [6] is used here to determine similarity of two blocks.

$$D^{\mathrm{NCC}}(\hat{\mathbf{R}}, \hat{\mathbf{T}}) = 1 - \frac{\left\langle \hat{\mathbf{T}}, \hat{\mathbf{R}} \right\rangle_2^2}{\|\hat{\mathbf{T}}\|_2^2 \|\hat{\mathbf{R}}\|_2^2}, \tag{8}$$

where $\hat{\mathbf{R}}$, $\hat{\mathbf{T}} \in \mathbb{R}^{15 \cdot 15 \cdot 7} = \mathbb{R}^{1575}$ denote a block of the reference and template image respectively that has been rearranged into a vector. It holds that $0 \leq D^{\mathrm{NCC}}(\hat{\mathbf{R}}, \hat{\mathbf{T}}) \leq 1$. A landmark in the template image is accepted if D^{NCC} is minimal in comparison to all other blocks in the search range.

3 Experiments and Results

The data that was used for the experiments were five publicly available thoracic 4D data sets from the DIR-Lab [3]. We chose the scans during maximal inspiration and expiration because breathing movement is shown and for each of this scans 300 expert annotated landmarks are provided. The inspiration scan was used as reference whereas the expiration scan was used as template image. Each of the data sets had an axial resolution of 256×256 voxels (ranging from 0.97×0.97 to 1.16×1.16 mm^2) and a number of slices varying between 94 and 112 (slice thickness 2.5 mm). Segmentation masks generated according to [5] were applied to focus the next steps on the lungs. We performed landmark detection on each reference image with all three explained operators first based on the structure tensor and afterwards all three operators were used again based on the Hessian matrix. Landmark candidates were then reduced as described in Sec. 2.4 and transferred to the Förstner/Rohr filtered template images. In the following section the quality of the detected landmarks will be discussed as well as the computation time for the matrices on which the operators were based.

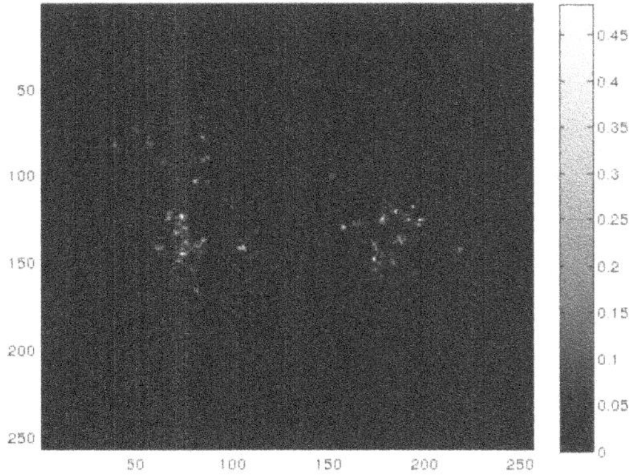

Figure 1: Axial slice of Förstner3D image based on $\mathbf{C}_g$.

3.1 Landmark Detection

Using the Förstner and Rohr Operators to detect landmarks based on the structure tensor as well as the Hessian matrix

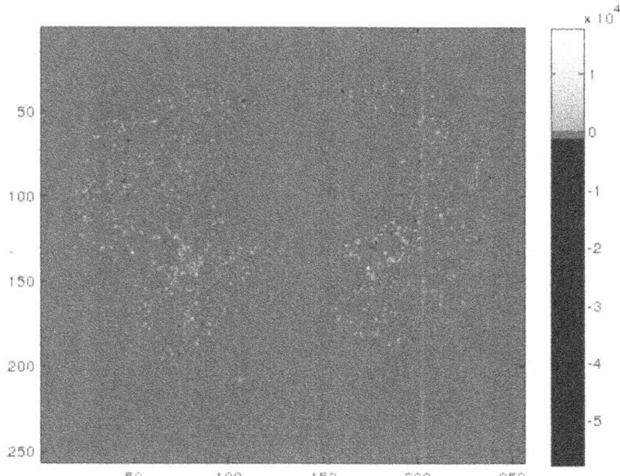

Figure 2: Axial slice of Förstner3D image based on $\mathbf{H}$.

led to six landmark images per data set. In Fig. 1 the response of the Förstner3D operator based on the structure tensor is shown as an axial slice. The maximum grey value is 0.5. The minimum is 0 the bright points correspond to distinctive points in the original image. In Fig. 2 the operator response based on the Hessian matrix is shown for the same slice. Here, the minimal value in the image is $-6 \cdot 10^{-4}$ while the maximum is $2 \cdot 10^{-4}$. The fundamental difference between operator responses based on the structure tensor versus the Hessian matrix is the range of the response values. Using $\mathbf{C}_g$ the values are always nonnegative while using the Hessian matrix negative values occur. Although these negative responses happen, the range of most contrast is between 0 and $1 \cdot 10^-4$. The responses of the other operators showed similar properties as the Förstner3D operator.

Landmarks should be distinctive points which are used in this case to support the registration function. To improve the registration of the lungs, landmarks should be widely spread across the image, because in the TPS-registration each landmark has most influence in a small neighborhood. In Fig. 3 a 3D-Plot of accepted landmarks is shown. The gross shape is similar to human lungs and many landmarks have been detected.

3.2 Time Evaluation

All calculations were performed on a computer with four cores and a frequency of 3.4 GHz (Intel i7-2600), 16 GB RAM and Ubuntu 12.04 OS. Evaluating the computation time for the structure tensor and the Hessian matrix revealed that it takes about 3 seconds to compute all structure tensors for an image of the size $256 \times 256 \times 94$ while it takes 7 to 9 seconds to calculate the Hessian matrices for the same image. DIR-Lab [2] also provides images with a resolution of up to $512 \times 512 \times 130$, however, when trying to perform the computation on these images either MATLAB crashed or the calculation of the Hessian matrix took longer than 12 minutes. Although we used sparse matrices to compute finite differences as matrix-vector-multiplication the computer was running out of memory. To handle this problem

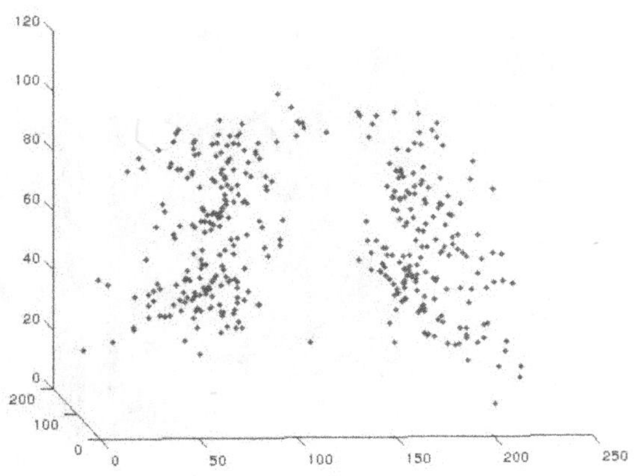

Figure 3: Detected landmarks plotted in 3D.

matrix-free implementations should be used. This would need many for-loops that are computed very slowly in MATLAB. Therefore a C++ implementation with a link to MATLAB via MEX interface could be a solution to this problem.

4 Conclusion

The evaluation of computation time showed that computing the hessian explicitly took approximately three times as long as computing the structure tensor. However, when the memory of the computer was not exceeded a calculation time of 10 seconds at maximum is ok.
Using the structure takes less time to compute. This approach is currently used for landmark detection and we were also able to perform it on the high resolution images. Further evaluation will involve using the detected landmarks for a TPS-Registration and evaluate the results on the given expert landmarks. An alternative computation of the Hessian matrix is used in [4] to detect blood vessels. They convolve the image with the second derivatives of a Gaussian-kernel.

Acknowledgement

The work for this paper has been carried out at the Institute of Mathematics and Image Computing, University of Lübeck.

5 References

[1] T. Arens, C. Karpfinger, U. Kockelkorn, K. Lichtenegger, H. Stachel, F. Hettlich: *Mathematik*. Spektrum Akademischer Verlag, 2011.

[2] E. Castillo, R. Castillo, J. Martinez, M. Shenoy, T. Guerrero: *Fourdimensional deformable image registration using trajectory modeling*. Physics in Medicine and Biology 55, 305-327, 2009.

[3] R. Castillo, E. Castillo, R. Guerra, V. E. Johnson, T. McPhail, A. K. Garg, T. Guerrero: *A framework for evaluation of deformable image registration spatial accuracy using large landmark point sets*. Physics in Medicine and Biology 54, 1849-1870, 2009.

[4] A. F. Frangi, W. J. Niessen, K. L. Vincken, M. A. Viergever: *Multiscale vessel enhancement filtering*. In Medical Image Computing and Computer-Assisted Intervention, 130-137, 1998.

[5] B. Lassen, J.-M. Kuhnigk, M. Schmidt, S. Krass, H.-O. Peitgen: *Lung and Lung Lobe Segmentation Methods at Fraunhofer MEVIS*. In 4th International Workshop on Pulmonary Image Analysis, 185-199, 2011

[6] J. Modersitzki: *FAIR Flexible Algorithms for Image Registration*. SIAM, 2009.

[7] K. Murphy, B. van Ginneken, J. M. Reinhardt, et al.: *Evaluation of Registration Methods on Thoracic CT: the EMPIRE10 Challenge*. IEEE Transactions on Medical Imaging 11, 1901-1920, 2011.

[8] T. Polzin: *Lungenregistrierung mittels automatisch detektierter Landmarken*. Master's Thesis, Lübeck 2012.

[9] K. Rohr: *Landmark-based Image Analysis*. Kluwer Academic Publishers, 2001.

[10] C. Duscha, R. Werner, H. Handels:*Optimization of the Detection Performance of Förstner-Rohr-Type Operators in Abdominal and Thoracic Tomographic Image Data*.In: T. M. Buzug et al (eds.), Student Conference 2013, Medical Engineering Science, Lübeck, Grin Verlag, 35-38, 2013.

Dimensionality reduction of multidimensional image descriptors for medical image registration

J. Degen [1], J. Modersitzki [2,3], and M. P. Heinrich [4]

[1] Medizinische Ingenieurwissenschaft, Universität zu Lübeck, degen@miw.uni-luebeck.de
[2] Institute of Mathematics and Image Computing, Universität zu Lübeck, jan.modersitzki@mic.uni-luebeck.de
[3] Frauenhofer MEVIS, Project Group Image Registration, jan.modersitzki@mevis.frauenhofer.de
[4] Institute of Medical Informatics, Universität zu Lübeck, heinrich@imi.uni-luebeck.de

Abstract

Similarity measurements are among challenging and relevant research topics in multimodal image registration. The frequently used mutual information disregards spatial information, which is shared across modalities. A recent popular approach, called modality independent neighbourhood descriptor, is based on local self similarities of image patches and thus allows for spatial information. Since this image descriptor generates vectorial representations, it is multidimensional, which results in a disadvantage in terms of computation time. In this work, we present a problem-adapted solution to this, by using principal component analysis and Horn's parallel analysis for dimensionality reduction. Furthermore, the influence of dimensionality reduction in global rigid image registration is investigated. It is shown that the registration results obtained from the reduced descriptor have same high quality in comparison to those found for the original descriptor.

1 Introduction

In medicine, an ever increasing number of medical devices and imaging methods can be observed, which all have their respective merits. Physicians take great interest in combining these different techniques to improve the diagnosis or image guided interventions. Therefore multimodal image registration is needed, whose aim is to find the best possible correspondence of anatomical and functional structures between images obtained from different modalities. An important part of image registration is a distance measure, which evaluates the similarity between the registered images. The definition of a suitable distance measure is a difficult task in multimodal image registration because there are amongst others intensity variations caused by several physical phenomena, which were measured by the different imaging devices. In order to overcome these problems, a new image descriptor for defining the similarity between two images has been introduced – the modality independent neighbourhood descriptor (MIND) [1] . The idea is to reduce a multimodal registration problem to a monomodal one by mapping both images to a common comparable space [2] . To capture as many features the image descriptor is multidimensional. This increases the computation time that is necessary for distance calculations.
The purpose of this paper is to clarify whether the dimensionality of the descriptor can be reduced without causing significant loss of quality in the registration results. The benefits due to the dimensionality reduction are noise removal and reduced computing time and memory requirement. The principal component analysis (PCA) is used as a dimensionality reduction method [4]. With a subsequent Horn's parallel Analysis (PA), the problem specific number of principal components is selected [5]. Finally, the registration results based on the reduced and the complete descriptor are compared.

2 Material and Methods

This section presents an overview of the background to this work with a focus on the introduction of the image descriptor MIND. Furthermore, the PCA and Horn's PA are briefly explained. For a detailed description see [4] and [5].

2.1 Modality independent neighbourhood descriptor

The basic idea of MIND is the concept of local self-similarity, which has been previously used in image denoising [3]. Multimodal images gave a non corresponding intensity distribution, but they still represent the same anatomical structures. We take advantage of the assumption that the particular structure within a local neighbourhood can be described by the similarities of small image patches and is preserved across modalities. This principle is illustrated in Fig. 1 where it is exemplarily shown that an edge can be extracted from both images by using self-similarities. The formulation of an image descriptor based on this concept has several benefits. MIND is independent of the modality and the related contrast, while allowing a simple intensity-based registration. Due to the usage of

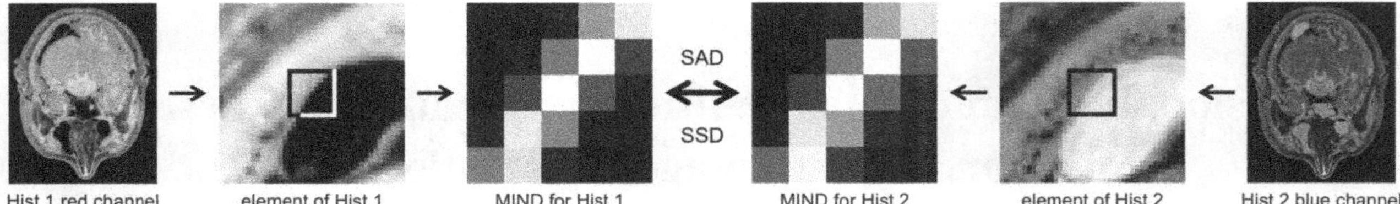

Figure 1: On the right and on the left histological images of the head, obtained from different color channels are shown. The MIND descriptors of the elements at the center of the marked rectangles are presented in the middle. This example illustrates that the concept of local self-similarities is suitable for extracting image features and the descriptors are comparable using monomodal distance measurements, e.g. sum of absolute/ squared differences.

patches, it is sensitive to a variety of features, such as corners, edges and textures.
The real-valued measurements are stored in an array I with corresponding spatial dimensionality d. The positions of the elements of I are denoted by $x_j = [x_j^1, \dots, x_j^d] \in \mathbb{N}^d$. MIND is defined in form of a Gaussian-function with a patch-based distance D_P and a variance estimate V as the essential components.

2.1.1 Patch-based distance

The patch-based distance is defined as the sum of squared differences (SSD) of all elements $I(x_j)$ within the two patches centred at two different positions x_j. As this calculation has to be performed for each element of I, a convolution can be used instead of an element-wise calculation of the SSD. A convolution with a d-dimensional kernel C_P of the same size as the size of the patch P is a very efficient method to generate the patch-based distances, yielding:

$$D_P(I, x_j, C_P, r) = C_P * (I - I_r)^2 \quad \forall r \in R \quad (1)$$

$$\text{with} \quad I_r(x_j) = I(x_j + r) \quad \forall x_j, \quad (2)$$

were r is an element of the set of search positions R within the search region (see Section 2.1.3). I_r is the array I translated by r in terms of (2). The patch-based distances are calculated for each search position according to (1) and stored in an $(d+1)$-dimensional array D_P. We have chosen a Gaussian filter kernel for C_P.

2.1.2 Variance measure

The local variance measure V is calculated directly from the patch distances. V is defined as the average of the directly neighbouring patch distances for each element x_j. The formula can be written as:

$$V(I(x_j), C_P) = \frac{1}{|N|} \sum_{n \in N} D_P(I, x_j, C_P, n). \quad (3)$$

N defines the four-neighbourhood in two dimensions or the six-neighbourhood in three dimensions.

2.1.3 Spatial search region

It is important to define the search region since it has a large influence on the descriptor. Not only the size of the search region has to be chosen. In addition, three different spatial configurations are at our disposal (for more details see [1]). We have used a dense sampling. In this case, the search positions r are elements of the set

$$R = \{-k, \dots, 0, \dots, k\}^d \setminus \{0\}^d \quad k \in \mathbb{N}. \quad (4)$$

All neighbours of the current element $I(x_j)$ within a fixed neighbourhood, defined by k, are included for the calculation of MIND. When selecting the size and the configuration of the search region, note that the computing time is directly proportional to the number of search positions. In general, the search region as well as the patches are symmetrical, but they do not have to be square.
Using the previously described components, the general formula for MIND can be specified in following manner:

$$\text{MIND}(I(x_j), C_P, r) = \frac{1}{z} \exp\left(-\frac{D_P(I, x_j, C_P, r)}{V(I(x_j), C_P)}\right) \quad (5)$$

with z as an normalization constant, so that all entries of MIND are in a range of 0 to 1. This formulation of a Gaussian-function results in high entries for MIND, if two patches are similar, which leads to small distances. Otherwise there occur low entries, if the patches are dissimilar and therefore having large patch-based distances. The registration process using MIND is divided into two main parts: Initially the descriptors are determined for each modality independently. In the subsequent registration procedure the optimal transformation parameters are searched by comparing the descriptors using monomodal similarity metrics.

2.2 Principal component analysis

PCA as introduced by Pearson and Hotelling is a widely used method for dimensionality reduction of large data sets, whereat the contained variance should be preserved as much as possible [4]. Thus, relevant information from the data is extracted and noise could be removed. A linear combination with so-called principal components (PCs), which describes a variety of data, is being searched. These PCs describe an orthogonal linear transformation of the data into a linear subspace. The calculation of the PCs is based on the principal axis theorem. Initially the covariance matrix Σ of the given data set is determined. In the next step Σ is diagonalized so that $\Sigma = U^T \Lambda U$ by eigendecomposition. The matrix U contains the eigenvectors of Σ and Λ is a diagonal matrix with the corresponding eigenvalues. These matrices are arranged so that the eigenvector corresponding to the largest eigenvalue is in the first column of U, etc. U is a new orthonormal basis, which decorrelates the data and retains as much of the variance as possible. A crucial issue while performing a PCA is the number of significant principal components, which provides a sufficiently good approximation of the data. An optical method for determining the number of relevant components is the scree plot, which demonstrates the curve shape of the eigenvalues that resembles the letter L or an elbow [4]. One can determine the vertex of this L-curve from which all components to the right should be discarded. Because this approach requires a subjective decision, the automatic method described in the following section is preferred.

2.3 Horn's parallel analysis

John L. Horn introduced the parallel analysis as a novel method to determine the number of factors to retain from the factor analysis [5]. He suggested to compare the empirically obtained eigenvalues with those of uncorrelated, normally distributed random variables. For this purpose, one has to generate a data set of uncorrelated, normally distributed random variables with the same number of observations and variables as the original data set. Then the eigenvalues of this data set can be calculated. This process is repeated many times using a Monte Carlo simulation. Finally, the eigenvalues of the original data set can be considered in parallel with the 95 percent quantile of the eigenvalues obtained from the random data set [5]. With increasing sample size, the distribution of the eigenvalues of random variables approximates a straight line parallel to the x-axis. Only factors with eigenvalues above this line are considered significant. Similarly, the PA can be used to determine the relevant components of a PCA. In this contribution the MATLAB® file *pa_test* was used to generate the random eigenvalues. Thereby, the random data sets are generated by permutation of the original data set and the eigenvalues are determined by means of a PCA.

3 Results and Discussion

The following experiments were carried out on data sets of the Visible Human Project® [6]. Transverse histological images of the head, which were recovered with different color channels and T1- as well as T2-weighted coronal MRI-images of the thorax were used.

3.1 Dimensionality reduction of MIND

In the following, we explain our proposed approach to reduce the dimensionality of MIND. First, the descriptors of the given data sets were determined by using a dense sampling search region with $k = 2$ and a Gaussian filter kernel with the size of five elements in each dimension. Subsequently, a PCA with both descriptors at the same time is performed, because otherwise, the order of the components would be different. For this purpose, the descriptors have been concatenated in such a way that the number of observations equals double the number of elements in the data set and the number of variables corresponds to the cardinality of R. The resulting coefficient matrix is used to reduce the descriptors in its dimension. The reduced MIND arises from the multiplication of the entire MIND and a certain part of the coefficient matrix. In order to decide which part of the coefficient matrix is to be used, it has to be decided which principal components are regarded as significant. To answer this question, a PA is performed and the result is displayed in a scree plot together with the eigenvalues obtained from the PCA. Fig. 2 illustrates the scree plots for both data sets. As seen from the left scree plot, the com-

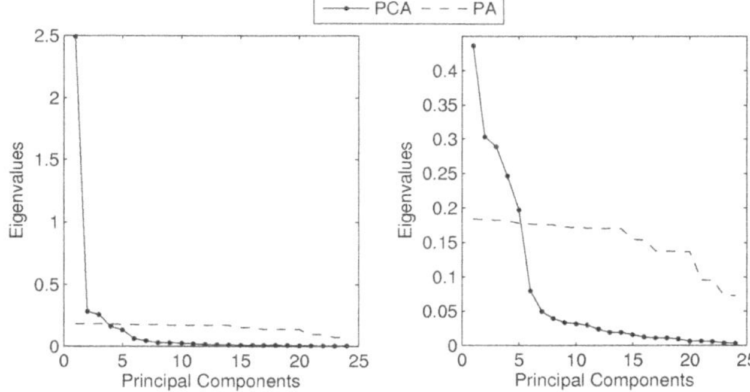

Figure 2: On the left side the eigenvalues of the histological data set are shown together with the eigenvalues obtained from the PA. On the right side there is the scree plot of the MRI data set.

parison with the eigenvalues obtained from the PA suggests that the first three principal components approximate the histological data set satisfactorily. For the MRI data set, however, five PCs have to be taken into account, since the corresponding eigenvalues are bigger than those of the random variables. The magnitudes of the eigenvalues are very different for the considered data sets. While in the histological data set, the high eigenvalue of the first PC is followed by very small eigenvalues of the other PCs. In contrast, the eigenvalues of the MRI data set are more evenly distributed. This can be also observed in Table 1, where the percentages of total variance explained by each of the first five PCs are listed. As seen from Table 1, 83.04 % of the total variance

Table 1: Percentages of the explained variance

	PC 1	PC 2	PC 3	PC 4	PC 5
Hist	68.25	7.74	7.05	4.47	3.62
MRI	23.19	16.11	15.36	13.08	10.48

are explained by the selected three PC. In the MRI data set, the first five PCs explain 78.22 % of the total variance. For a visual example of our proposed dimensionality reduced MIND the three components for the histological data set are depicted in Fig. 3. It can be seen that at some places the representations of the reduced MIND appears to be similar to the results of an edge detection. Besides edges other image details are also included in the reduced MIND. Further-

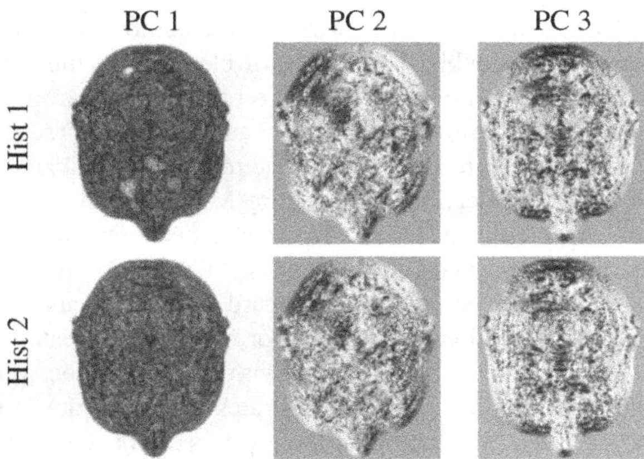

Figure 3: Representation of the reduced MIND for the histological data set. The rows represents the two different color channels from which the histological images were taken. Column by column, the three slices of the reduced descriptors are shown.

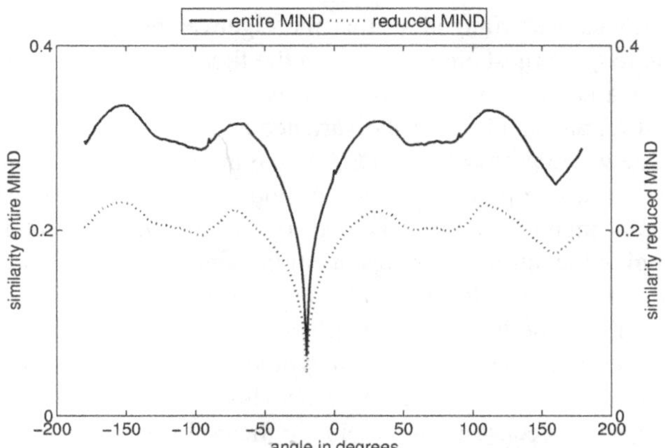

Figure 4: The registration results of the global rigid registration with the entire as well as the reduced MIND. The correct alignment of both images is found equally with the reduced MIND and the registration results are of the same quality as those of the original MIND.

more, it becomes clear that the descriptors are comparable with each other.

3.2 Global rigid registration using MIND

After the reduced descriptors have been determined, a comparison of the registration results corresponding to the entire and reduced MIND is made. By way of example, a global rigid registration is used. One of the histological measurements is set as reference while the other one is defined as template. The reference is rotated clockwise by 20 degrees compared to the template. Successively the template is rotated by angles ranging from -180 to 180 degrees (with a step size of 1°). For each angle, the PCA and the resulting descriptors are recalculated. Then, the sum of absolute differences (SAD) of the descriptors corresponding to the particular elements of I are determined. To calculate the similarity of both modalities under the given angle, the results for the SAD of all descriptor elements are summed up. These results are shown in Fig. 4. As can be seen, the optima of both registration functions are located by -20 degrees, where it was to be expected since a counterclockwise rotation-direction was used. Due to the difference of a rotation about 20 degrees and the fact the the brain looks similar up-side down there is an other local minimum at 160 degrees. However, the optimum can be uniquely determined in a range of 60 degrees, which is acceptable for medical image registration, since rotations of smaller angles are common.

4 Conclusion

In summary it can be said that the dimensionality reduction of MIND preserves the quality in the registration result. However, the presented method should be applied to more complex registration problems. In particular, variational deformable image registration is an interesting application area due to the numerous existing regularization parameters. Furthermore, it could be sought of an efficient possibility for not having to recalculate MIND in every step of the registration process.

Acknowledgement

The work has been carried out at the Institute of Medical Informatics and the Institute of Mathematics and Image Computing, Universität zu Lübeck.

5 References

[1] M. P. Heinrich, M. Jenkinson, M. Bhushan, T. Matin, F. V. Gleeson, S. M. Brady, and J. A. Schnabel, "Mind: Modality independent neighbourhood descriptor for multi-modal deformable registration," *Medical Image Analysis*, vol. 16, no. 7, pp. 1423–1435, 2012.

[2] A. Sotiras, C. Davatzikos, and N. Paragios, "Deformable medical image registration: A survey," *IEEE Transactions on Medical Imaging*, vol. 32, no. 7, pp. 1153–1190, 2013.

[3] A. Buades, B. Coll, and J.-M. Morel, "A non-local algorithm for image denoising," in *IEEE Computer Society Conference on Computer Vision and Pattern Recognition, CVPR 2005.*, vol. 2, pp. 60–65, 2005.

[4] I. Jolliffe, *Principal Component Analysis*. New York: Springer, 2002.

[5] J. Horn, "A rationale and test for the number of factors in factor analysis," *Psychometrika*, vol. 30, no. 2, pp. 179–185, 1965.

[6] M. J. Ackerman, "The visible human project," *Proceedings of the IEEE*, vol. 86, no. 3, pp. 504–511, 1998.

An Efficient Implementation of an Affine Point-based Registration using the Expectation Maximization-ICP in C++

D. Puls [1], J. Krüger [2] and H. Handels [2]

[1] Medizinische Ingenieurwissenschaft, Universität zu Lübeck, dennis.puls@miw.uni-luebeck.de
[2] Institute of Medical Informatics, Universität zu Lübeck, {krueger,handels}@imi.uni-luebeck.de

Abstract

Point-based registration plays an important role in medical image analysis. The Expectation Maximization Iterative Closest Point algorithm (EM-ICP) extends the Iterative Closest Point algorithm (ICP), which is a standard method for landmark-based registration of medical images. Based on an existing implementation of the EM-ICP we have implemented the affine transformation for the EM-ICP in the programming language C++. Furthermore, we have optimized the implementation of the rigid transformation. In the paper we show that the registration with the affine transformation in the current implementation outperforms the implementation of the rigid transformation in cases of scaling and shearing. Additionally we combine the rigid and the affine transformation. The experiments demonstrate the performance improvement of the registration with the affine transformation w.r.t. the registration with the rigid transformation. Furthermore, we clarify that the registration with the affine transformation is faster than the rigid transformation in comparable registration cases.

1 Introduction

For the human interior visualization, image acquisition methods are used, which generate medical image data. As part of a diagnosis these image data should be reliable compared to each other. For this purpose, an image data registration is performed. This provides a transformation to minimize the difference between two medical images. A way to determine the transformation is the point-based registration. Therefore, we need landmarks on distinct positions in the image data. The medical images are represented as point-clouds. A standard method for the landmark-based registration is the Iterative Closest Point algorithm (ICP) by Besl [1]. This method is fast and robust, but the ICP presupposes the existence of one-to-one correspondences between point-clouds. This encounters a problem if these correspondences do not exist. Furthermore, the ICP assumes that the number of the points of the point-clouds is the same. To avoid this problems, the Expectation Maximization Iterative Closest Point algorithm (EM-ICP) has been created by Granger et al. [2]. The method is presented in section 2. In [3] Tamaki et al. suggest a fast and parallel implementation of the EM-ICP in C++. Their implementation uses the rigid transformation. Thus, based on the code by Tamaki we have implemented the affine transformation, with more degrees of freedom. This transformation is considered in section 2. After testing the implementation, we show that the usage of the affine transformation improves the EM-ICP, which is described in section 3.

2 Material and Methods

Images are represented as point-clouds $S = (s_i | i = 1, \dots, N_s)$ with $s_i = (x, y, z)^T$ and $M = (m_j | j = 1, \dots, N_m)$ with $m_j = (x, y, z)^T$. x, y and z are three coordinates. The EM-ICP registrates two point-clouds with the transformation T. The transformed point-cloud is determined with $S' = T \star S$. The symbol "$\star$" respresents in this context the application of T to S. In comparison with the ICP algorithm, the main idea of the EM-ICP is to regard no one-to-one correspondences, but probabilistic correspondences between two point-clouds. This problem is given as a minimization problem.

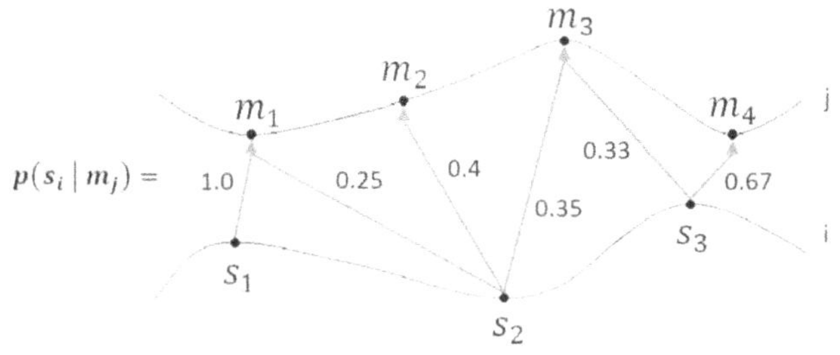

Figure 1: Correspondences scheme of the EM-ICP. One point of the point-cloud M corresponds to each point of the point-cloud S with a probability $p(s_i | m_j, T)$. Correspondences with the value 0 are not shown.

2.1 EM-ICP (expectation maximization-iterative closest point)

The idea of the EM-ICP is to maximize the probability that m_j is correspondent to the transformed $s_i \in S$ by adapting transformation T:

$$p(s_i|m_j, T) = p(T \star s_i|m_j). \tag{1}$$

Each of the N_s points has a probability of correspondence to all N_m points. The lower the distance between two points, the greater is the probability that points correspond to each other (cf. fig. 1).

As described in [4], no closed formula solution exists. Therefore, it is proposed to see the unknown correspondences $H \in \mathbb{R}^{(N_s \times N_m)}$ as randomly distributed variables with $H_{ij} \in \{1, 0\}$ and to maximize the log-likelihood of the whole data allocation $p(M, H|S, T)$. Thus, T is determined by the expectation maximization-method (EM-method) with the minimization criterion

$$\begin{aligned} C_{EM}(T, E) = \sum_i^{N_s} \sum_j^{N_m} E(H_{ij})(m_j - T \star s_i)^T \\ \cdot \Sigma_j^{-1}(m_j - T \star s_i) \end{aligned} \tag{2}$$

with Σ_j as the covariance matrix of the point distances. $E(H_{ij})$ describes the expectation that one point m_j matches each of the s_i points (see fig.1) and is given by

$$E\left(H_{ij}\right) = \frac{\exp\left(-\mu\left(m_j, T \star s_i\right)\right)}{\Sigma_k \exp\left(-\mu\left(m_j, T \star s_i\right)\right)} \tag{3}$$

with

$$\begin{aligned} \mu\left(m_j, T \star s_i\right) = \frac{1}{2}\mu\left(m_j - T \star s_i\right)^T \\ \cdot \Sigma_j^{-1} \mu\left(m_j - T \star s_i\right) \end{aligned} \tag{4}$$

In this context the Mahalanobis distance is used to compute $p(s_i|m_j, T)$. The probabilities are normalized to 1, with the assumption that every point s_i in S has corresponding points in M.

Subsequently the expectation maximization steps are considered. Based on the expectation of the log-likelihood, in the expectation-step (E-step) the correspondence probability is calculated with (3). In the subsequent maximization-step (M-step) the correspondence probability $E(H_{ij})$ is fix and C_{EM} is minimized with respect to T. Thus, we get the equation for the E-step:

$$\begin{aligned} (T_M, t) = \underset{T_M, t}{argmin} \sum_i^{N_s} \sum_j^{N_m} E(H_{ij}) \\ \cdot \|(m_j - ((T_M \cdot s_i) + t)\|^2. \end{aligned} \tag{5}$$

In context of this equation, a transformation consisting of a matrix T_M and a translation vector t. To determine T_M and t, an iterative procedure with alternating E- and M-steps is used.

2.2 Transformations

For the EM-ICP, two transformations are used here. These are the rigid and the affine transformations. The affine transformation extends the rigid transformation degrees of freedom.

As a basis of our implementation we have used the existing implementation of Tamaki et al. [3].

2.2.1 Rigid Transformation

In the implementation of [3], the rigid transformation is used. This transformation consists of a rotation matrix $R \in \mathbb{R}^{3\times3}$ and a translation vector $t_R \in \mathbb{R}^3$. Here, three rotation angles α_1, α_2 and α_3 are integrated in the rotation matrix $R = R^{(\alpha_1)}R^{(\alpha_2)}R^{(\alpha_3)}$. By setting these angles, the coordinate vector $(x, y, z)^T$ can be rotated in three spatial directions with respect to the coordinate origin.

To realize this transformation, Tamaki et al. have implemented the horn's quaternion method. For further information about this method and its implementation see [5] and [3]. The number of iterations (iterative procedure; cf. section 2.1) can be chosen individually and depends on the complexity of the transformation. Also the time for calculating the final transformation parameters depends on the number of iterations. The resulting point-cloud $S' = (s'_i|i = 1, \ldots, N_s)$ is given by

$$s'_i = R \cdot s_i + t_R. \tag{6}$$

This transformation can rotate and translate one point-cloud relatively to another.

For medical image data the affine transformation provides a higher degree of freedom with additional shearing and scaling.

2.2.2 Affine Transformation

Similar to the rigid transformation, the affine transformation consists of a translation vector $t_A \in \mathbb{R}^3$ and an affine matrix $A \in \mathbb{R}^{3\times3}$. But in the affine transformation more degrees of freedom are available. Thus, a 3D object can be rotated, sheared, translated and scaled by twelve parameters. First, to find the translation vector, (5) is derived with respect to t_A, resulting in:

$$t_A = \frac{\sum_{j=1}^{N_m}(m_j \sum_{i=1}^{N_s} E(H_{ij}))}{N_s} - \frac{A\sum_{i=1}^{N_s} s_i}{N_s}. \tag{7}$$

With this vector the two point-clouds are translated to their barycenter, leading to the resulting point-clouds $M_c = (m_{j_c}|j = 1, \ldots, N_m)$ and $S_c = (s_{i_c}|i = 1, \ldots, N_s)$ with

$$m_{j_c} = m_j - \left(\frac{\sum_j^{N_m} \left(m_j \sum_i^{N_s} E(H_{ij}) \right)}{N_s} \right) \tag{8}$$

and

$$s_{i_c} = s_i - \left(\frac{A \sum_i^{N_s} s_i}{N_s} \right). \tag{9}$$

The barycenter is the joint coordinates center of both point-clouds. With the new coordinates the translation vector is specified a few times. Subsequently the minimization criterion is derived with respect to A. We get:

$$A = \sum_i^{N_s} \sum_j^{N_m} (E(H_{ij})(s_{i_c} m_{j_c}^T)) \cdot \left(\sum_i^{N_s} \sum_j^{N_m} (E(H_{ij})(s_{i_c} s_{i_c}^T)) \right)^{-1} \tag{10}$$

The procedure of computing t_A, recomputing barycenters and computing A (one *iteration block*) is repeated (iterative algorithm), in which the number of iteration blocks could be chosen freely. On the basis of this calculation the transformation parameters will be recalculated until the maximum number of iteration blocks is reached. The algorithm is clarified in the following pseudo code:

Pseudo Code Affine Transformation

1: $A \leftarrow I$, $t_A \leftarrow 0$, $E(H_{ij}) \leftarrow 0$.
max. number of iteration blocks ← it_blocks.
2: **while** (current iteration) < (max. number of iteration blocks)
3: calculate Σ
4: **for** t = 1:10 (max. iteration number freely defined)
5: calculate t_A
6: calculate m_{j_c} and s_{i_c}
7: recalculate and normalize $E(H_{ij})$
8: **end for**
9: calculate A
10: **end while**
11: output t_A and A

The resulting point-cloud $S' = (s'_i|i = 1, \ldots, N_s)$ is given by

$$s'_i = A \cdot s_i + t_A. \tag{11}$$

3 Results and Discussion

By testing the implementation we have made some optimization decisions. First, Tamaki et al. had not implemented a directly calculation of the variance Σ in (2), but one freely chosen value is used. Here Σ is reduced iteratively. But the variance is a very important and sensitive parameter in the algorithm, because this parameter determines which points correspond to each other. To stabilize this part of the implementation we have calculated the variance at each step. Furthermore, tests have shown that this method requires fewer iterations, because Σ is not approximated in each iteration, but calculated directly. Accordingly less time for both registration methods is needed. This is especially advantageous for point-clouds with many points. In this context the affine matrix performs the registration faster.

An important purpose of this work was it to extend the existing implementation of the EM-ICP algorithm. The problem was that this implementation had used only the rigid transformation for the registration. In real medical images the rigid transformation of the image data is insufficient to registrate images correctly to each other. The affine transformation extends the registration with more degrees of freedom, which leads to a higher registration result.

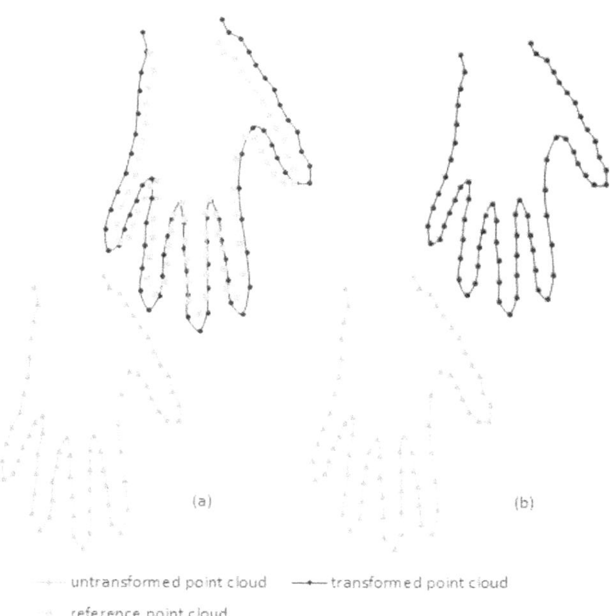

Figure 2: Illustration of the rigid transformation (a) and the affine transformation (b). The lower grey point-clouds in (a) and (b) are the point-clouds, which shall be transformed relatively to the upper grey reference point-clouds in (a) and (b). The results are the black point-clouds. In (a) it is not possible to registrate the point-clouds exactly to each other. In (b) the registration is successful because of the possibility to scale the one point-cloud relatively to the reference point-cloud. The black transformed point-cloud in (b) lies exactly under the upper grey reference point-cloud.

Fig. 2a shows the registration with the rigid transformation and 2b the registration with the affine transformation.

As we had performed the registration for different images we have observed that the registration with the affine matrix has failed in some cases. The cause refers to the correspondence probability of the EM-ICP. After the translation to the barycenter, corresponded points are not close enough to assign these points correctly to each other. This is especially the case if the transformations have big transformation parameters. Because of the larger number of degrees of freedom, the registration in above-mentioned situations fails. To fix this failure, the rigid transformation as a more robust transformation is preceded. Fig. 3a shows the failure and 3b the correction. Because it cannot be assumed that there is no large and complex transformation, the whole registration should be performed by a combination of the rigid and affine registration.

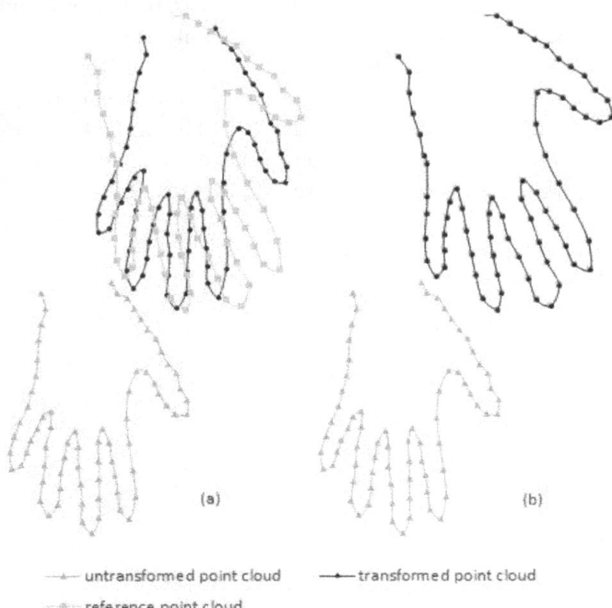

Figure 3: Illustration of the affine registration without (a) and with (b) the preceded rigid transformation. The lower grey point-clouds in (a) and (b) are the point-clouds, which shall be transformed relatively to the upper grey reference point-clouds in (a) and (b). The results are the black point-clouds. In (a) the registration stops, because of a local minima. Thus, the transformed and the reference points are not aligned correctly. In (b) the transformed und reference points are aligned perfectly. The transformed point-cloud in (b) lies exactly under the upper grey reference point-cloud.

4 Conclusion

In the medical imaging analysis the registration is significant to compare medical images for the diagnosis. The EM-ICP outperforms the ICP with respect to the quality of the registration results in many cases (cf.[2], [3]). In this paper we have shown, that our implementation can perform a registration for two 2D image data by affine transformation. Furthermore, one-to-one correspondences are not needed and the registration is more robust. In contrast to the ICP, it is not necessary that the number of points of the point-clouds is the same. A preceded rigid transformation is useful in many image registration cases for higher robustness.

Acknowledgement

The work has been carried out at the Institute of Medical Informatics of the Universität zu Lübeck.

5 References

[1] P.J. Besl, N.D. McKay, *A Method of Registration of 3D Shapes*. 1992.

[2] S. Granger, X. Pennec, *Multi-scale EM-ICP: A fast and robust approach for surface registration*. in: Computer Vision ECCV 2002, vol. 2353 of Lecture Notes in Computer Science, pp. 418–432, 2002.

[3] T. Tamaki, M. Abe, B. Raytchev, K. Kaneda, *Softassign and EM-ICP on GPU*. First International Conference on Net-working and Computing (ICNC), 2010.

[4] H. Hufnagel, *A Probabilistic Framework for Point-Based Shape Modeling in Medical Image Analysis*. Vieweg +Teubner, pp. 29–32, 2011.

[5] Berthold K. P. Horn, *Closed-form solution of absolute orientation using unit quaternions*. in: Journal of the Optical Society of America, vol. 4, pp. 629–642, 1987.

Enabling on-Demand Features for Decision Forests – An Approach to Lesion Segmentation in MR-Volumes –

A. Rüsch [1], O. Maier [2], and H. Handels [2]
[1] Medizinische Ingenieurwissenschaft, Universität zu Lübeck, ruesch@miw.uni-luebeck.de
[2] Institute of Medical Informatics, Universität zu Lübeck, {maier, handels}@imi.uni-luebeck.de

Abstract

Many segmentation algorithms are only marginally successful in extracting lesions, tumors or other structures from medical images due to similar gray values, shape variations from patient to patient and the soft-edged tissues. A promising alternative is to use Random Decision Forest (RDF) with a special feature kind. The on-demand feature is given as a function and not prepared as a pre-calculated set of feature values. The function is called during the node optimization process. Based on randomized function parameters, the on-demand features have an infinite possibility space. Recent articles have shown possible functions for on-demand features and their applications to improve medical image processing. This work describes the main functionality of on-demand features and how to use them in combination with each other or pre-calculated features. We do not present results on medical image processing yet because of the high complexity, but a proof of concept is given.

1 Introduction

This article presents a special machine learning algorithm based on Random Decision Forests (RDFs) [1]. Working with this statistical classification algorithm, we focus on so called "on-demand features". They are used to generate a possibly infinite number of features during the training phase. Recently, a few articles were released, that propose possible applications for on-demand features.

Criminisi *et al.* [1] applied them to detect and localize anatomical structures in CT-volumes. They called them "visual features". The RDF was trained by comparing randomly generated sub boxes of a given CT-volume over a long range within the image. By saving the position and size of those boxes and re-utilize them during prediction, it is possible to generate features with long range spatial context. Thus, the relative position of organs to other structures can be used to improve the segmentation.
Mitra *et al.* [2] used on-demand features to segment chronic ischemic infarcts from multi-modal MRI. They designed a data processing concept including Markov Random Fields as a pre-processing application for a RDFs. Besides pre-calculated features such as the intensities of every modality, they used three different on-demand features which they call "contextual features". The first feature is the comparison of the intensity of one point in different modalities through subtraction. The second feature is the difference between the cuboid means of two volumes in different modalities. The third calculates the difference of intensity along a 3D line in the same modality. It assumes that gray matter and white matter appear as partial volumes and cerebrospinal fluid borders them.
Zikic *et al.* [3] employed on-demand features under the name "context-sensitive features" and used them for brain tumour tissue segmentation. However they changed the pre-processing application for the RDF to Gaussian Mixture models, the same on-demand features that Mitra *et al.* [2] used are described.
Geremia *et al.* [4] invented new features to segment Multiple Sclerosis lesions in multi-channel MR images. Their Decision Forest was trained with three features: The first is represented by the intensity of a prior channel and the last two are on-demand features which they named "context-rich features". One of them is calculated by comparing the mean value of two randomly generated boxes in one channel to the intensity of a spatial point in another channel. The other on-demand feature is the difference of a point of interest and its symmetric counterpart in the same channel with respect to the mid-sagittal plane.

Because of the good results published in difficult areas such as abdominal CTs [1] and brain MR images [2], [3], [4], we are highly motivated to use on-demand calculated features in RDFs for other medical image computation processes. Furthermore, mixing on-demand and pre-calculated features to improve the classification result and possibly decrease the calculation effort should be possible.

2 Material and Methods

The RDF is a learning tool used for classification, regression, density estimation and more [5]. We base our method on the implementation in the scikit-learn package [6]. The RDF is extended to handle on-demand features, given by a function and variables, as well as pre-calculated features at the same time.

2.1 The Random Decision Forest

A Random Decision Forest is an ensemble of Random Decision Trees (RDTs). RDTs are mostly like normal Decision Trees. However, to inject randomness into the algorithm, the training is different to the original in two regards. First, only a subset of all possible samples is selected to train a tree by sampling from the pool of all possible samples uniformly and with replacement [7]. This process is named bootstrap aggregating, in the literature briefly termed bagging. The second randomness input is called randomized node optimization [8]. From the reduced search space given by bagging, every node has only a small randomly chosen sub space of features available [9]. These are very important steps to ensure, that every tree within a forest is different. The outcome of a RDF is a probability distribution generated by averaging the probability results of every tree. The class with the highest probability is then chosen as the classification result. For more information on the general functionality of RDFs see [5], [8] and [7].

2.2 The pre-computed features

The features used in general RDFs are pre-computed and organized in vectors. Once they are set, they will not change during the forest training or application. During node optimization, the values of the given samples from a specific feature are called and used to find a threshold that splits the samples with the highest information gain possible. Note that this feature type always has a fixed position. They are not context sensitive.

2.3 The on-demand features

The goal is now to instantiate features on demand within a node. To do so, a function is passed, that represents the on-demand feature. This function is used to generate a set of samples, in stead of taking them from a given vector, to optimize the node split and find a threshold. The input parameters to the function can be pre-defined or random. Its internal algorithm can use pre-defined parameters to include meta data and knowledge of the user, the random parameters can find unknown relations of the samples. Consequently, context information can be included in the feature instantiations. The higher the applied degree of randomness is, the more different features can be generated from a single function. We have to distinct between the terms "on-demand feature", which is the passed function, and the "on-demand feature instantiations". The on-demand feature has the possibility to generate an infinite number of feature instantiations by changing the input parameters to the function. The instantiations are the complement to the pre-computed features.

If the on-demand feature instantiation can split the samples well, a unique identifier of the chosen feature instantiation must be stored within the node in addition to the threshold, to reproduce it during application. This identifier is represented by the on-demand functions input parameters.

The great benefit of on-demand features is the possibly infinite variation. Randomly generated parameters represent a nearly unlimited possibility space. During the RDF training different trees can be build from the same on-demand feature constellation because of randomized parameters. To minimize the computational burden, only a small subset of all possible features can be realized explicitly.
To get a better understanding, imagine we try to segment MS lesions in a MR image. The on-demand feature created by Geremia *et. al.* [4] should be used for this purpose. A sample of a randomly generated feature instantiation is calculated by subtraction of the mean of two subregions R_1 and R_2 in one channel from the intensity of a spatial point in another channel. An example constellation of these boxes can be seen in Fig. 1. The channels are for example a T1 and a T2 weighted MR image. In Fig. 1 the sample index s is used as an offset for the boxes. The offset vectors and the size of the boxes need to be stored if this feature instantiation splits the samples best.

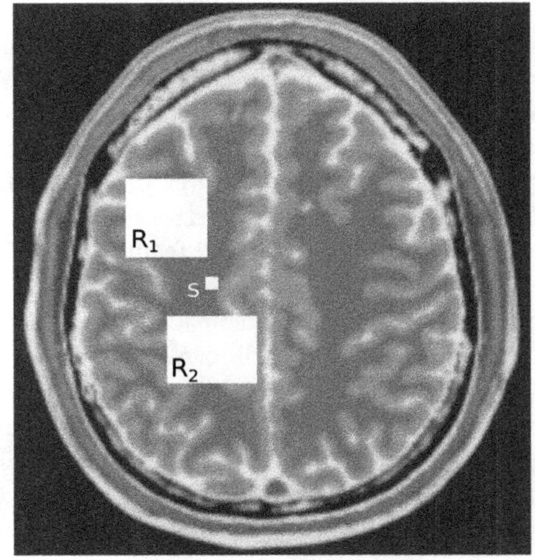

Figure 1: This T2 weighted MR image with MS lesions shows parts of the on-demand feature used in [4]. The boxes R_1 and R_2 have different randomly generated sizes and offset verctors. The offset vector relates to the sample s, which is a pixel position in this case. The MR image used in this example is taken from [10].

2.4 Combining different feature types

Combining pre-calculated and on-demand features can cause benefits especially in image processing. Sample features such as gray-values are cheap in respect of storage and calculation effort. If the cheap information is not able to split the samples well, an on-demand feature possibly is. To make sure that both have potential to become the basis for a node split, we must be aware of the ratio of different feature types.

2.4.1 Mixing pre-computed and on-demand features

Since we still use RDFs, the feature of choice is randomly picked from a pool of features. We need to ensure that the given on-demand feature is not seen as a single feature but as an additional infinite feature pool, filled with possible on-demand feature instantiations. To control the ratio of on-demand instantiations and pre-calculated features, it is possible to increase the maximum number of both feature types separately. During training, the randomly chosen feature is then called either from the pre-computed or the on-demand pool, as long as the specific maximum of calls is not reached.
To find the right ratio between both feature types is not an easy task. A massive use of on-demand instantiations can cause trees without any pre-calculated features. The use of a high number of pre-calculated features contrary to the on-demand instantiations reduces the usability of on-demand features, as they are designed to be used in a large number.

2.4.2 Multiple on-demand features

Besides mixing pre-computed and on-demand features, it is possible to use different on-demand features. Doing so, the ratio of these features must be defined as well. If there are two on-demand features for instance, they can be called with a equal distribution. But in some cases it can be useful to call one feature more often since it relates more to randomness than the other. We can think of these two on-demand features as two different imaginary feature pools filled with their own possible instantiations. We can now give every pool a maximum number of feature calls. Increasing one number will automatically increases the number of triggers to this feature, because of the random selection algorithm.

2.5 Implementation details

To realize the new feature type we implemented the on-demand algorithm by extending the "scikit-learn" library [6], which performs well with normal decision trees and highly randomized decision trees for classification purposes. It comes with implemented optimization functions to find the best node split threshold. The library is based on Cython which combines usability and efficiency. Cython compiles a code written in Python into C code. The compiled C code is faster than the Python version. However, we still can call the methods from a Python script, which increases the usability.
The on-demand called function is given as a class. Therfore, we can easily save data as member variables and define member functions to calculate more complex features. The input variables which need to be stored in the node are ordered in a struct. This allows the user to use as many and complex features as he wants.
It is essential that the class used in the training is the same as in the test phase. Otherwise the calculated features can not guarantee the expected node split.

3 Results and Discussion

The proposed method is examined through a proof of concept to evaluate feasibility and usability.

3.1 Results

To show that the on-demand functionality is given and that it can improve the classification outcome, a proof of concept is given here. We use a forest of 10 trees and trees with a depth of 2 nodes. At each point, only 1 feature is chosen. A sample vector x_p of 4 samples with a single pre-calculated feature is used to train the forest as it can be seen in (1).

$$\begin{aligned} x_p &= [0,1,0,1] \\ y &= [0,0,1,1] \\ x_o &= [1,1,0,0] \end{aligned} \tag{1}$$

The samples are classified into 2 classes, based on the ground truth given by a vector y. The on-demand feature is generated by a function $f(s)$ dependent on the sample index s. Its output is given as vector x_o. Note that this vector does not really exist, the feature instantiation is calculated on demand within the node, depending on s.

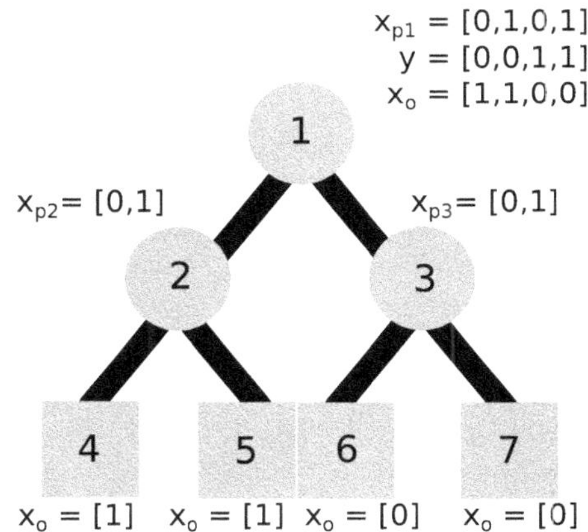

Figure 2: The given example tree selects the normal feature first. It can be seen that a split right in the middle of the sample vector x_{p1} is done. According to the feature value, this is a random split. There is no linear split that can classify the input vector based on its values correctly to the ground truth y in the first place. If there were just this one feature, the classification process would stop and fail at this point. Now we can use the on-demand calculated features to add a split node level and generate a new feature as we need it. Thus, the separated sample vectors are given to the next split node level. Here the on-demand feature function $f(s)$ takes the sample index s to produce a feature that can be used to classify the input sample vector.

It can easily be seen in Fig. 2, that the feature given in x_p will not lead to useful classification. However, if we add the on-demand feature, the number of available features increases and a perfect split is possible, in worst case when the second node is reached.

3.2 Discussion

The functionality of on-demand features is reached as shown. In this example, we used a single pre-computed and a single on-demand feature. The probability to be chosen first is equal for both features. Since we wanted to keep many possibilities in using different features, we had to take care about ratios.

In the near future, we plan to employ the on-demand features for lesion detection in MR-volumes. Then, tests on run-time and accuracy can be made. It is necessary to keep the run-time in training and testing phase in mind. Depending on the given function, training times of up to a few days, using a normal PC, are to be expected in medical image processing. To improve the usability for medical purposes, a selection of most common on-demand feature functions should be pre-implemented.

4 Conclusion

In this paper we described on-demand features for Random Decision Forests. They promise good classification results in difficult areas of medical image processing. These classifications can be used for voxel-wise segmentation processes as well.
The shown alterations of RDFs have much potential in classification areas where normal features can not improve the segmentation outcome. We can use meta data or random parameters to generate new features. If pre-computed features do not lead to a satisfying segmentation, a high number of on-demand feature instantiations should be used. Doing so, relations between structures, that can not be seen readily are revealed in a probabilistic way.
Further reseach is needed to test the run-time in training and test phase and to improve the calculation and memory management. The implementation of a set of the most common on-demand features, including an on-demand feature for lesion detection in MR-volumes, improving the run time and the reduce of memory space are our aspirations for the near future.

Acknowledgement

The work has been carried out at the Institute of Medical Informatics, Universität zu Lübeck.

5 References

[1] A. Criminisi, J. Shotton, and S. Bucciarelli, "Decision forests with long-range spatial context for organ localization in CT volumes," in *MICCAI workshop on Probabilistic Models for Medical Image Analysis (MICCAI-PMMIA)*, 2009.

[2] J. Mitra, P. Bourgeat, J. Fripp, S. Ghose, S. Rose, O. Salvado, A. Connelly, B. Campbell, S. Palmer, G. Sharma, S. Christensen, and L. Carey, "Classification forests and markov random field to segment chronic ischemic infarcts from multimodal MRI," in *Multimodal Brain Image Analysis* (L. Shen, T. Liu, P.-T. Yap, H. Huang, D. Shen, and C.-F. Westin, eds.), vol. 8159 of *Lecture Notes in Computer Science*, pp. 107–118, Springer International Publishing, 2013.

[3] D. Zikic, B. Glocker, E. Konukoglu, J. Shotton, A. Criminisi, D. Ye, C. Demiralp, O. M. Thomas, T. Das, R. Jena, and S. J. Price, "Context-sensitive classification forests for segmentation of brain tumor tissues," in *MICCAI 2012 Challenge on Multimodal Brain Tumor Segmentation*, October 2012.

[4] E. Geremia, B. Menze, O. Clatz, E. Konukoglu, A. Criminisi, and N. Ayache, "Spatial decision forests for MS lesion segmentation in multi-channel MR images," in *Medical Image Computing and Computer-Assisted Intervention – MICCAI 2010* (T. Jiang, N. Navab, J. Pluim, and M. Viergever, eds.), vol. 6361 of *Lecture Notes in Computer Science*, pp. 111–118, Springer Berlin Heidelberg, 2010.

[5] A. Criminisi, J. Shotton, and E. Konukoglu, "Decision forests for classification, regression, density estimation, manifold learning and semi-supervised learning.," Tech. Rep. MSR-TR-2011-114, Microsoft Research, Oct 2011.

[6] F. Pedregosa, G. Varoquaux, A. Gramfort, V. Michel, B. Thirion, O. Grisel, *et al.*, "Scikit-learn: Machine learning in Python," *Journal of Machine Learning Research*, vol. 12, pp. 2825–2830, 2011. and Blondel, M. and Prettenhofer, P. and Weiss, R. and Dubourg, V. and Vanderplas, J. and Passos, A. and Cournapeau, D. and Brucher, M. and Perrot, M. and Duchesnay, E.

[7] L. Breiman, "Random forests," *Machine Learning*, vol. 45, no. 1, pp. 5–32, 2001.

[8] A. Criminisi and J. Shotton, *Decision Forests for Computer Vision and Medical Image Analysis*. Springer, February 2013. http://research.microsoft.com/en-us/projects/decisionforests/.

[9] F. Schroff, A. Criminisi, and A. Zisserman, "Object class segmentation using random forests," in *Proc. British Machine Vision Conference (BMVC)*, 2008.

[10] C. A. Cocosco, V. Kollokian, R. K.-S. Kwan, G. B. Pike, and A. C. Evans, "Brainweb: Online interface to a 3D MRI simulated brain database," *NeuroImage*, vol. 5, p. 425, 1997.

Ischemic Stroke Lesion Segmentation
– Setup of a Challenge –

L. Friedmann [1], O. Maier [2], and H. Handels[3]
[1] Medizinische Ingenieurwissenschaft, Universität zu Lübeck, friedman@miw.uni-luebeck.de
[2] Institute of Medical Informatics, Universität zu Lübeck {maier, handels}@imi.uni-luebeck.de

Abstract

This paper describes the setup of a medical image segmentation challenge for automatic extraction of ischemic stroke lesions in multi-spectral MRI images. The results of this competition will be presented in October 2015 in the form of a workshop at the Medical Image Computing and Computer Assisted Intervention (MICCAI) conference. The general reason for organizing a challenge is reviewed and the medical background explained. The provided datasets and their preprocessing are described and the evaluation and ranking system presented. In the results the established online platform of the challenge is explained.

1 Introduction

In medical image processing a large number of methods for different tasks exist. But a general problem seems to be, that the fitness of those methods are not always comparable [1]. The reason for that is, that the methods are evaluated on private datasets. To overcome this problem, in [1] challenges are mentioned as a solution for benchmarking and ranking computer vision techniques.
The challenge setup described in this paper is established for a challenge of Ischemic Stroke Lesion Segmentation (ISLES), which will be presented at the Medical Image Computing and Computer Assisted Intervention (MICCAI) in Munich, in October 2015. The challenge is organized with cooperation partners of the Brain Tumor Segmentation (BRATS) challenge. The task is backed by a well established clinical and research motivation and a large number of already existing methods.

1.1 Anatomy of a Challenge

A challenge strives to provide a public dataset that represents the diversity of the given task and a platform, which is fair and offers a direct comparison of the methods fitness with suitable evaluation measures. According to [2], the general anatomy of a challenge can be explained by following notes:

- The output/task is defined
- A public dataset is provided
- The evaluation system is defined
- Participants apply their algorithm to the whole dataset
- The dataset should be representative for the type of data in research and clinical practice
- The reference standard is described
- The evaluation is carried out

To present the results of a successfully organized challenge, the MICCAI conference provides a stage for the participating researchers.

1.2 Medical Background

A stroke is a sudden occurrence of brain disease, which often involves the loss of functions of the central nervous system. It is caused by disturbance in the blood supply of the brain. Strokes can be classified into the groups: Ischemic, caused by undersupply of blood in a brain area, and hemorrhagic, caused by leaking blood in a brain area due to a broken vessel. In Fig. 1 an FLAIR MRI image with a lesion after an ischemic stroke is shown.

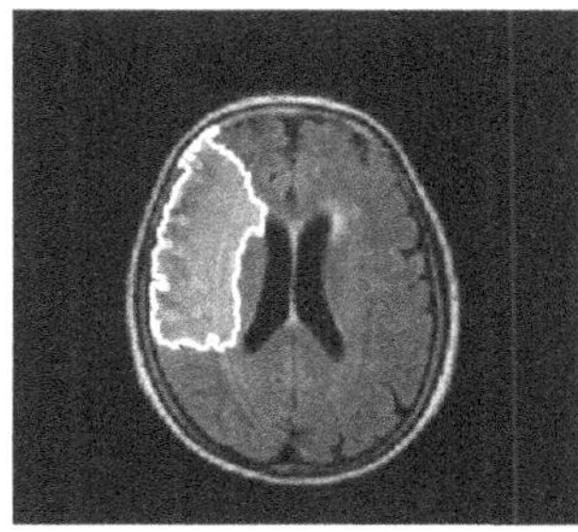

Figure 1: Shown is an axial FLAIR MRI image of a patient after an ischemic stroke. The lesion area is hyperintense and highlighted with a white border.

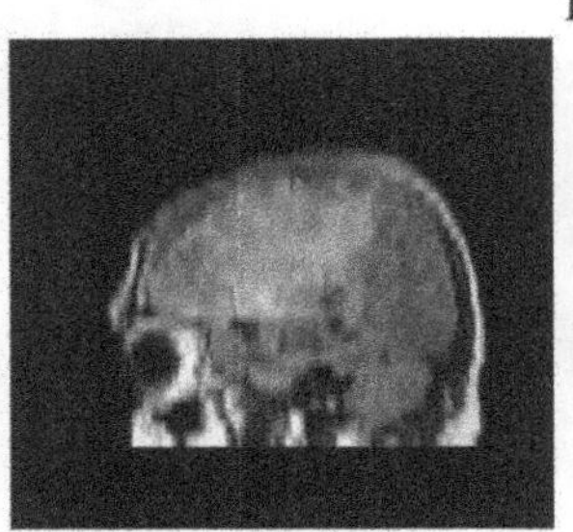
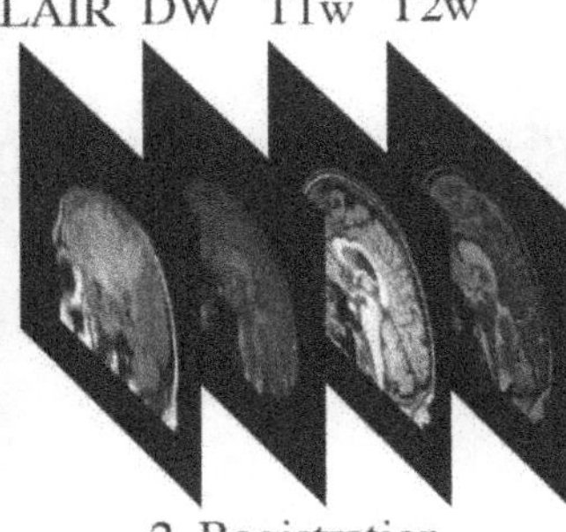

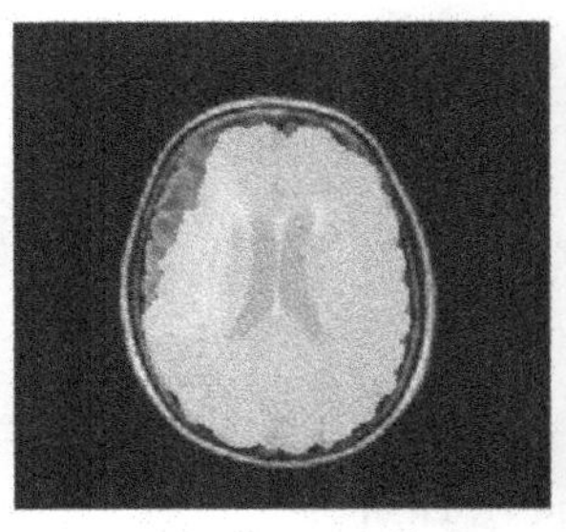
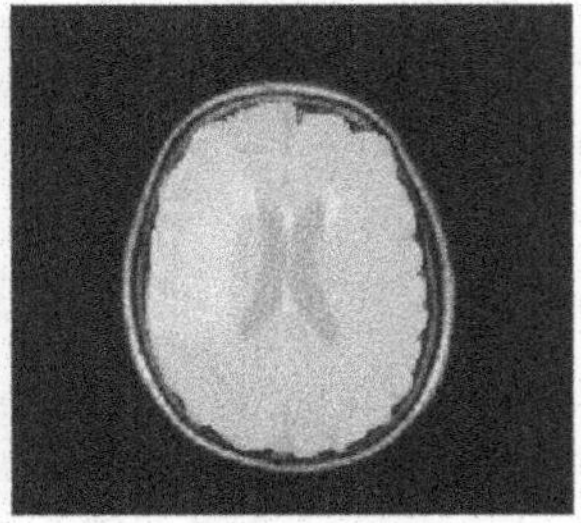

1. FLAIR Resampled 2. Registration 3. Skull stripping 4. Manual skull stripping

Figure 2: The pre-processing is performed in four main steps: Firstly, the original FLAIR image is resampled to the isotropic 1 mm^3 resolution. Secondly, all other MRI sequence images are rigidly registered on the resampled FLAIR image. Thirdly, a brain mask is automatically acquired on the T1w image and finally the brain mask is manually optimized.

These lesions can be identified in multi-spectral MRI data. With this challenge, we aim to take a step forward to computer-aided methods for automatic segmentation of brain lesions. One clinical application could be the better understanding of specific brain area functions by connecting the caused dysfunction with the affected brain area. The required processes would strongly benefit by automatic segmentation algorithms.

2 Material and Methods

To provide a challenge which is fair, easy to participate in and offers a possibility to compare new and existing methods of the field, a pre-processing of the data, an automatic evaluation and a ranking system on a public platform are needed.

2.1 Data and Pre-processing

The provided data scans were carefully selected from appropriate discharge reports of patients, among which an ischemic stroke was diagnosed. The general representativity of the dataset for all type of data in research and clinical practice was regarded by including different case characteristics like embolic strokes, single strokes, secondary lesions, movement artifacts and imaging artifacts.

For all cases, the dataset contains scans with the MRI sequences fluid-attenuation inversion recovery (FLAIR), T2-weighted (T2w) with Turbo Spin Echo (TSE), T1-weighted with Turbo Field Echo (TFE) and diffusion-weighted images (DWI) with an Apparent Diffusion Coefficient (ADC) map. Table 1 gives an overview of the data details.

Table 1: Data details

Cases	50-100
Training cases	ca. 50
Centers	2
Expert segmentation sets	2
MRI sequences	FLAIR, T2w TSE, T1w TFE, DWI with ADC map

The dataformat Compressed Neuroimaging Informatics Technology Initiative format (*.nii.gz.) was chosen.

As reference datasets, the ground-truths were manually prepared by expert segmentation.

The pre-processing is performed in the following four steps and visualized in Fig. 2:

1. The FLAIR images were resampled to the isotropic 1 mm^3 resolution with cubic b-spline interpolation.
2. The DW, T1w and T2w images were semi-automatically, rigidly co-registered onto the proper resampled FLAIR image by b-spline based mutual information registration.
3. An automatic skull stripping was performed on all co-registered T1w images and the brain masks were saved.
4. The brain masks were manually optimized and applied on all images.

The resampling was performed, because most images had an in-plane resolution of 1 mm^2. In many cases, a slice thickness higher than 1 mm was given, which led to up-interpolation to a higher resolution than the original one.

To perform an algorithm on multi-modal MRI images, a registered dataset of one patient as a basis is essential. After the rigid registration onto the resampled FLAIR image, all images are registered and resampled to the isotropic resolution.

The skull stripping is needed to preserve the patients anonymity. By cutting out the brain, the face of the patient can not be reconstructed.

After the automatic skull stripping, in most cases, a manual optimization of the brain mask was performed to receive a satisfying result. The automatic skull stripping algorithm tends to find edges inside or at the border of a brain lesion, when it actually should find the edges between the brain and the cerebrospinal fluid (Fig. 2).

2.2 Evaluation System

The quality of a segmentation is evaluated by five different measures, of which the three following are used to compute

the rank in the ranking system by comparing to the reference ground-truth: The Dice's coefficient (DC) measures the overlap of two volumes, the average symmetric surface distance (ASSD) the fitting of surfaces and the Hausdorff distance (HD) the maximum distance between surfaces.
In addition to those the precision and recall measures are provided to reveal over- or under-segmentation, but will not be considered in the computation of the team ranks, because they are represented in the DC value.

2.2.1 Dice's Coefficient

According to [3] the DC value of two sets of voxels A and B is defined as

$$DC = \frac{2|A \cap B|}{|A| + |B|}. \tag{1}$$

A value of 0 specifies no overlap, a value of 1 perfect similarity. The DC value tends to return higher values for larger volumes: About 0.9 for an acceptable lung segmentation and 0.6 for MS lesions, which are comparable to the ischemic stroke lesions.
Worthy of special mention is that the DC value is the harmonic mean of precision and recall.

2.2.2 Average Symmetric Surface Distance

The ASSD represents the average distance over all volume surface points, averaged over both directions. According to [4], when bearing in mind two sets of surface points A and B, the average surface distance (ASD) is given as

$$ASD(A, B) = \frac{\sum_{a \in A} \min_{b \in B} d(a, b)}{|A|} \tag{2}$$

where $d(a, b)$ is the Euclidean distance between the points a of the surface A and b of the other surface B. Because $ASD(A, B) \neq ASD(B, A)$, the $ASSD$ is then given as

$$ASSD(A, B) = \frac{ASD(A, B) + ASD(B, A)}{2}. \tag{3}$$

The ASSD value is measured in mm. A lower value represents a better segmentation. In contrast to the DC value, the ASSD value works equally well over all sizes of considered volumes.

2.2.3 Hausdorff Distance

The HD value is defined as the maximum distance between two sets of points. According to [5] we first define

$$h(A, B) = \max_{a \in A} \min_{b \in B} d(a, b) \tag{4}$$

where $d(a, b)$ is again the Euclidean distance. A more general definition of the Hausdorff distance is

$$HD(A, B) = \max\{h(A, B), h(B, A)\} \tag{5}$$

which defines the maximum distance between A and B, while (4) measures the maximum distance from A to B, which is the reason why h is called the directed Hausdorff distance.

2.2.4 Precision and Recall

According to [6] precision (also called positive predictive value) and recall (also known as sensitivity) of two sets of points can be defined as

$$precision = \frac{TP}{TP + FP} \tag{6}$$

and

$$recall = \frac{TP}{TP + FN}, \tag{7}$$

where TP (true positive) are the overlapping points, FP (false positive) are the wrong segmented points in the segmentation and FN (false negative) are the non-segmented points in the reference.
Both measure take values between 0 and 1. A higher precision value in comparison to a lower recall value reveals under-segmentation and vice-versa, which is exemplified in Fig. 3.

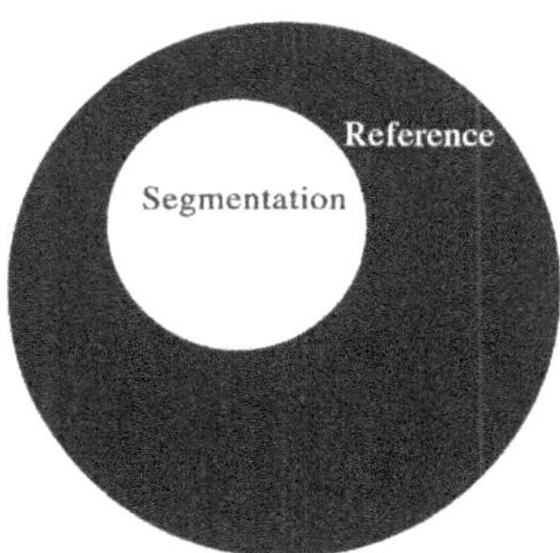

Figure 3: In this example under-segmentation is shown: All points of the segmentation are correct, but the majority of points were missed. This results in a high $precision = 1$ and a low $recall \sim 0.2$.

2.3 Ranking System

Due to the fact, that the different evaluation measures cannot be compared to each other, a ranking system was established. The basic idea is to obtain a ranking of each evaluation measure first. Thereby comparisons of respective ranks are possible.
To obtain the overall ranking, the following steps are performed:

1. Compute the DC, ASSD and HD values for each dataset and for all teams.

2. Determine each teams rank for DC, ASSD and HD value separately for each dataset.

3. Compute the mean rank over all three evaluation measures per dataset to acquire the teams rank for each dataset.
4. Compute the mean rank over all dataset-specific ranks to obtain the teams final rank.

This procedure is visualized in detail in Fig. 4.

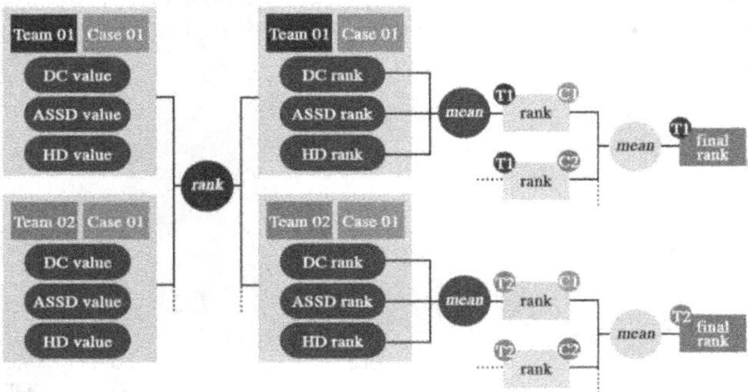

Figure 4: At first, all evaluation measures for all datasets of each team are computed and separately compared to each other to obtain the evaluation measure ranks for each dataset. Secondly, the average ranks for each team of all datasets are determined. Out of those the final rank is generated by computing the mean value.

By not averaging the actual evaluation measures, but rather the ranks in each, the ranking system is not affected by special cases, which are either very easy or difficult.
In the following special cases of the ranking system are described:

- If a label for a case has not been uploaded or could not be processed, the associated team will be assigned the last rank for all evaluation measures.
- A complete mismatch of the ground-truth and the submitted segmentation label (e.g.: $DC = 0$) leads to the last rank for all evaluation measures for the associated team.
- If multiple teams share a single rank, the lower ranks will be left empty.

2.4 Implementation of an Online Platform

To provide the information about the ISLES challenge, the rules for participation, the dataset and the evaluation and ranking system, an online platform was implemented. It can be visited at www.isles-challenge.org. The download and evaluation results for the participants are outsourced to the Virtual Skeleton Database Project in corporation with the organizers of the BRATS challenge.

3 Results and Discussion

The platform was successfully implemented and it provides an overview of information about the challenge and it notifies the participants about important changes or deadline changes. Furthermore, the rules for the participation are noted, the datasets are described in detail and the medical background of the challenge is presented. In addition, the evaluation and ranking system is precisely explained.
Links to the Virtual Skeleton Database are provided. Through that database, the participants can receive the dataset and submit their results in form of their segmentation labels of the lesions. The submitted data will be evaluated automatically and the results will be shown in a table. The table provides the participants with the exact values of each evaluation measure and the overall rank.

4 Conclusion

The next months will show, if the ISLES challenge will find resonance with the researchers of the field and if automatic methods for ischemic lesion segmentation will be presented at the MICCAI 2015. But due to the successful setup of the ISLES platform and prosperous challenges in the past years of our cooperation partners, it is very likely that this challenge will be well received. Through this platform, it will be possible to test and compare different methods of segmentation on a public dataset. This will promote and motivate researchers in the field of medical image processing. It will help benchmark and to rank new and existing methods.

Acknowledgement

The work has been carried out at the Institute of Medical Informatics, Universität zu Lübeck.

5 References

[1] A. L. Yuille, *Computer vision needs a core and foundations*. in: Image and Vision Computing 30, pp. 469–471, 2012.

[2] B. v. Ginneken, *Why challenges?*. Available: http://grand-challenge.org/Why_Challenges/ [last accessed on 27.01.2015], 2014

[3] C. D. Manning and H. Schütze, *Foundations of Statistical Natural Language Processing*. Mit Pr, Massachusetts, 1999.

[4] A. S. El-Baz, L. Saba and J. S. Suri, *Abdomen and Thoracic Imaging*. Springer, New York/Heidelberg/Dordrecht/London, 2014.

[5] D. P. Huttenlocher, G. A. Klanderman and W. J. Rucklidge, *Comparing Images Using Hausdorff Distance*. in: IEEE Transactions on Pattern Analysis and Machine Intelligence, Vol. 15, No. 9, pp. 850–863, 1993.

[6] F. Guillet and H. J. Hamilton, *Quality Measures in Data Mining*. Springer, Berlin/Heidelberg, 2007.

www.ingramcontent.com/pod-product-compliance
Lightning Source LLC
Chambersburg PA
CBHW082308210326
41598CB00029B/4477

* 9 7 8 3 9 4 5 9 5 4 0 0 3 *